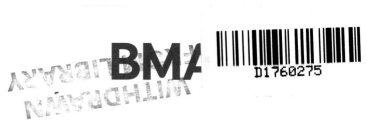

Female Genital Plastic and Cosmetic Surgery

Female Genital Plastic and Cosmetic Surgery

EDITED BY

Michael P. Goodman MD, FACOG, AAACS, IF, NCMP, CCD

Caring for Women Wellness Center
Davis, CA, USA

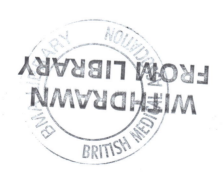
WILEY

This edition first published 2016 © 2016 by John Wiley & Sons, Ltd

Registered Office
John Wiley & Sons, Ltd, The Atrium, Southern Gate, Chichester, West Sussex, PO19 8SQ, UK

Editorial Offices
9600 Garsington Road, Oxford, OX4 2DQ, UK
The Atrium, Southern Gate, Chichester, West Sussex, PO19 8SQ, UK
111 River Street, Hoboken, NJ 07030-5774, USA

For details of our global editorial offices, for customer services and for information about how to apply for permission to reuse the copyright material in this book please see our website at www.wiley.com/wiley-blackwell.

Library of Congress Cataloging-in-Publication Data

ISBN HB 9781118848517

A catalogue record for this book is available from the British Library.

Wiley also publishes its books in a variety of electronic formats. Some content that appears in print may not be available in electronic books.

Cover image: ©lowball-jack/istockphoto

Set in 8.5/12pt Meridien by SPi Global, Pondicherry, India
Printed and bound in Singapore by Markono Print Media Pte Ltd

Contents

List of contributors

Marci Bowers
Director, Division of Transgender Surgery
Mills-Peninsula Hospital
Burlingame, CA, USA

Linda Cardozo OBE, MD, FRCOG
Professor of Urogynaecology
King's College Hospital
London, UK

Orawee Chinthakanan MD, MPH
International Urogynecology Associates of
Atlanta and Beverly Hills
Vaginal Rejuvenation Center of Atlanta
Atlanta Medical Research, Inc.
Alpharetta (Atlanta), GA, USA

Andrew T. Goldstein MD, FACOG, IF
Director, the Centers for Vulvovaginal Disorders
Washington, DC; New York, NY;
Clinical Professor, Department of Obstetrics and Gynecology
The George Washington University School of Medicine
Washington, DC, USA

Pablo Gonzalez Isaza MD
Division of Urogynecology and Pelvic
Reconstructive Surgery
Department of Obstetrics and Gynecology
Hospital, Universitario San Jorge
Pereira, Colombia

Sarah L. Jutrzonka PhD
Pacific Graduate School of Psychology
Palo Alto University, Palo Alto, CA, USA

Gustavo Leibaschoff MD
General Secretary, World Society of Cosmetic Gynecology
President, International Union of Lipoplasty
Dallas, TX, USA

David Matlock MD, MBA, FACOG
Medical Director
Laser Vaginal Rejuvenation Institute of America
Co-Medical Director
Laser Vaginal Rejuvenation Institute of Los Angeles
Los Angeles, CA, USA

John R. Miklos MD, FACOG, FACS, FPMRS
Director, Urogynecology
International Urogynecology Associates of Atlanta
and Beverly Hills
Adjunct Professor of Obstetrics and Gynecology
Emory University
Atlanta, GA, USA
Vaginal Rejuvenation Center of Atlanta
Atlanta Medical Research, Inc.
Alpharetta (Atlanta), GA, USA

Robert D. Moore DO, FACOG, FACS, FPMRS
Director, Advanced Pelvic Surgery
International Urogynecological Associates of
Atlanta and Beverly Hills
Adjunct Professor of Obstetrics and Gynecology,
Emory University
Atlanta, GA, USA
Vaginal Rejuvenation Center of Atlanta
Atlanta Medical Research, Inc.
Alpharetta (Atlanta), GA, USA

Otto J. Placik MD, FACS
Assistant Professor of Clinical Surgery (Plastic)
Northwestern University Feinberg School of
Medicine, Chicago, IL, USA
Principal Investigator, DeNova Research
Chicago, IL, USA

Dudley Robinson MD, FRCOG
Consultant Urogynaecologist and Honorary Senior Lecturer
Department of Urogynaecology
King's College Hospital
London, UK

Alex Simopoulos
MD, FACOG
FPA Women's Health
Los Angeles, CA, USA

Bernard H. Stern
MD, FACOG
Aesthetic Plastic Surgery International
Alexandria, VA, USA
Aventura Center for Cosmetic Surgery
Elite Plastic Surgery
Aventura FL, USA
Baftis Plastic Surgery
Jupiter, FL, USA

Preface

A women has the opportunity to request alteration of her vulva and/or vagina for a variety of reasons. Clinicians in the office hear of cosmetic and self-esteem rationale, as well as functional complaints. Regarding the vulva, distress with the appearance of "flaps" or "elephant ears" or other protrusions beyond the labia majora; self-consciousness; and distress over potential prominence or slippage of hypertrophic labia from beyond the confines of thong-type undergarments or swimwear predominate on websites, blogs, and office commentary. Discomfort ("chafing") with sports, sexual, and other activities; discomfort with tight clothing; necessity to "re-arrange" the labia for sexual intimacy; and hygienic difficulties predominate functional complaints heard in the office. Redundant labia majora are described as "droopy," or the patient dismays over the appearance of "camel toe."

Sexual issues dominate pelvic floor complaints in women inquiring about a vaginal tightening procedure. They describe a "sensation of wide/smooth vagina" (a term popularized by Jack Pardo S. from Chile and Adam Ostrzenski from the United States) with secondary diminishment of friction, less sensation, and greater difficulty achieving orgasm, at times concomitant with displeasure regarding the visual appearance of the introitus.

Size-reducing labia minoraplasty and/or majoraplasty (LP-m; LP-M), size reduction of redundant clitoral hood folds (RCH), posterior colporrhaphy/perineoplasty (PP), and anterior colporrhaphy/vaginoplasty (VP), the latter two colloquially termed "vaginal rejuvenation" (VRJ), are increasingly common women's cosmetic genital surgical procedures and have been subject to scrutiny both in the press and by investigators and editorialists. Another genital plastic procedure, hymenoplasty (HP), is usually performed for religious and cultural reasons, although occasionally requested as a "gift" for one's sexual partner.

In this text, the first to concentrate on plastic and cosmetic procedures specifically designed for elective comfort, self-esteem, and sexuality reasons, the procedures themselves, their rationale and risks, what is presently known regarding outcome, ethical considerations, and psychosexual considerations are discussed. The importance of proper and adequate surgical and sexual medicine training for surgeons is emphasized, along with the specific anatomic adjustments and psychosexual outcomes produced by these procedures.

The specific surgical procedures are defined and described. The importance of proper patient selection and preparation and adequate patient protection are reviewed, along with reminders of the intensely sexual nature of this work and the importance of counseling patients regarding their personal normality, while at the same time acknowledging their right to seek reconstruction.

Above all, this text hopes to familiarize the gynecologic, the plastic and reconstructive, and the cosmetic surgeon with a crucially important area of a woman's body, the intensity of her concentration and concern about the appearance and function of the area, and the availability and potential pitfalls of methods, predominantly surgical at this time, designed to meet her stated goals. We, your editor, associate editors, and contributors, intend to help raise your awareness of the issue and begin to explore the territories entered with an understanding of women's body image, feelings about their genitalia, and surgical and non-surgical options to safely and effectively achieve personal goals.

Michael P. Goodman
Davis, CA, USA

Acknowledgments

First and foremost, I wish to acknowledge Drs. Marco Pelosi II and III and Dr. Red Alinsod. The vision, perseverance, and educational efforts of these friends have resulted in the education and training of hundreds of genital plastic and cosmetic surgeons who are far more likely to accomplish success rather than failure for their patients. They are fine surgeons and educators.

Of course I am indebted to each and every one of the authors and associate editors (especially my friend Dr. Otto Placik) who have worked their behinds off on this project, and without whose efforts this unique book would not be before you. I am personally indebted to Dr. Gary Alter, from whose 1998 publication I initially learned the labiaplasty technique of modified V-wedge, and Dr. David Matlock, from whom a few years later I learned proper technique for curvilinear resection, and who has carefully trained hundreds of genital plastic/ cosmetic surgeons. They are pioneers in the field.

Martin Sugden, publisher of the Scientific Textbook Division at Wiley, is my mentor in this book, Pri Gibbons and Jasmine Chang is my editor and Radjan Lourde Selvanadin is the project manager. They both have worked "above and beyond." An author could not ask for a more knowledgeable, flexible, and easy to work with pair of professionals.

I offer my thanks to my family, my friends, especially my son, Sam, from whom I was aloof during the full-term gestation of this project. They all hope this is the termination of my writing—at least for a while!

I thank my professional, empathetic, kind, and flexible office staff. Nicole Sanders is our patient care coordinator, office manager, and first assistant. Raechel Davis is our receptionist and first assistant. Elise Eisele and Heather Kochner were our surgical nurses during this text's gestation. There is absolutely no way I could practice genital plastic surgery without this crew!

And last, but certainly not least, I wish to thank my patients. These intrepid and trusting (!!) souls, women on a mission, wonderfully weave through this text, which would not exist without them.

CHAPTER 1

Introduction

Michael P. Goodman

Caring for Women Wellness Center, Davis, CA, USA

> The time is the time. After the time is sometimes the time. Before the time is never the time.
>
> *Francois Sagan*

Female genital plastic/cosmetic surgery (FGPS), aka female cosmetic genital surgery (FCGS), vulvovaginal aesthetic surgery (VVAS), aesthetic (vulvo)vaginal surgery (AVS), or cosmeto-plastic gynecology (CPG), has mounted the stage of twentieth-century cosmesis. Adding in the promise of improvement in sexual function makes for an intriguing debut.

As this elective plastic/cosmetic surgical discipline, like many novel surgical and medical disciplines, traces its genesis to a community rather than academic setting, the succession of different but related names have mirrored the semantic directions of individuals and subspecialty organizations. Although any of the terms noted above will do, for the purposes of this textbook the quite descriptive term FGPS will be utilized.

As women become more comfortable with the idea of elective procedures on their faces, breasts, skin, and so forth designed to enhance their appearance and self-confidence, it is not surprising that they may wish to alter, change, "rejuvenate," or reconstruct even more intimate areas of their bodies [1].

Although surgeons for years have unofficially performed surgical procedures resulting in alterations in genital size, appearance, and function (labial size alteration, perineorrhaphy, anterior/posterior colporrhaphy, intersex and transsexual surgical procedures, and alterations on children and adolescents for benign enlargements of the labia minora), Honore and O'Hara in 1978 [2], Hodgekinson and Hait in 1984 [3], and Chavis, LaFeria, and Niccolini in 1989 [4] were the first to discuss genital surgical alterations performed on adults for purely aesthetic reasons. While there are at present no accurate and ongoing published statistics from either the American Society of Plastic Surgeons, American Academy of Cosmetic Surgeons, or American College of Obstetricians and Gynecologists, it has become apparent in the lay press that aesthetic surgery of the vulva and vagina is gaining significantly in popularity. As far back as 2004, Dr. V. Leroy Young, chair of the emerging trends task force of the Arlington Heights, Illinois, American Society of Plastic Surgeons, commented in a personal communication that he felt that "labiaplasty and vaginal cosmetic surgery are the fastest growing emerging growth trend in cosmetic plastic surgery."

Aesthetic surgery of the vulva and vagina has heretofore not been officially described as such, nor "sanctioned" by specialty organizations, as they are community rather than university or academically driven. The operations themselves, however, are really not new; the only new thing is the concept that women may individually wish to alter their external genitalia for appearance or functional reasons, or tighten the vaginal barrel to enhance their sexual pleasure. However, since any surgery has potential for causing morbidity including pain and distress (both physical and psychological) if not performed properly, and especially since FGPS involves concepts and procedures that are not yet fully researched

Female Genital Plastic and Cosmetic Surgery, First Edition. Edited by Michael P. Goodman.
© 2016 John Wiley & Sons, Ltd. Published 2016 by John Wiley & Sons, Ltd.

nor understood, guidelines for training, surgical technique, and patient selection should be discussed.

This textbook will give an overview of the most commonly performed procedures: labiaplasty of the minora and majora (LP-m; LP-M), size reduction of redundant clitoral hood epithelium (RCH), clitoral hood exposure for symptomatic phimosis (RCH-p), perineoplasty (PP), vaginoplasty (VP), colpoperineoplasty (CP; a combination of VP and PP), and hymenoplasty (HP), and will discuss rationale for surgery, ethical issues, patient expectations, patient selection and patient protection, complications, training issues, psychosexual issues, the procedures themselves, and all presently available outcome data. "Vaginal rejuvenation" (VRJ), a slippery and colloquial—although frequently used—term used to mean elective VP, PP, and/or CP (and for some, even LP) will be discussed.

First performed by community gynecologists or plastic surgeons in response to occasional patient requests in the mid-/late 1990s and early 2000s, by the mid-2000s the alternative of surgical alteration or reconstruction for "enlarged" labia/clitoral hood, and vaginal operations geared primarily to a goal of tightening for reasons of enhancement of sexual satisfaction, became more widely available and a subject of comment, blog, search, and consultation.

Although certainly the vulva and vagina are areas under the purview of gynecology and gynecologic training, *virtually no training* is offered in OB/GYN residencies in plastic technique, cosmetic labiaplasty, or pelvic floor surgery designed specifically for enhancement of female sexual pleasure (see Chapter 21). With the subject adequately addressed by only a portion of plastic surgery residencies (and in these, usually LP/RCH only), an individual patient finds herself on her own when endeavoring to navigate a path to successful reconstruction. With little guidance from specialty or regulatory agencies, "caveat emptor" became the rule, and un- or undertrained surgeons began performing these plastic procedures, frequently with less-than-optimal, and occasionally disastrous, results.

A textbook cannot substitute for a teaching program, observation of proper technique, and actual performance of procedures with expert proctoring. However, this text will point the way and provide guidance toward those

ends. It is designed to be a complete teaching guide to be used concomitantly with a hands-on teaching program, designed to develop competency leading to proficiency for female patients putting their trust in the hands of their gynecologic, plastic, or cosmetic surgeon. It is intended to educate the uninitiated and point the way toward the goal of comfort working with—psychologically, sexually, physiologically, and surgically—women who desire a guide to help them achieve their cosmetic, functional, sexual, and psychological goals.

After an introduction to the relatively brief "history" of the surgical specialty and discussion of pertinent anatomy, and after a thorough discussion of patient rationale for surgery, elements of patient protection, and the relevant ethical issues involved, the specifics of the most commonly utilized surgical techniques for both vulvar and vaginal procedures will be dissected and discussed in detail. Following this, patient selection technique and the biomechanics and physiology of tightening operations as they relate to the female orgasmic cascade will be discussed in depth. After a review of surgical risks, individual chapters will be devoted to important topics such as choice of anesthesia, surgical venue, complication avoidance, transgender surgery, and the important topic of revisions and re-operations. The book continues with in-depth discussions of psychosexual issues, up-to-date outcome data, and a chapter devoted entirely to brief "pearls" involving physician and patient protection. The editor's suggestions for implementing training programs and minimal "standards of care" will conclude the book.

References

1. Goodman MP. Female cosmetic genital surgery. *Obstet Gynecol* 2009;**113**:154–96.
2. Honore LH, O'Hara KE. Benign enlargement of the labia minora: Report of two cases. *Eur J Obstet Gynecol Reprod Biol* 1978;**8**:61–4.
3. Hodgekinson DJ, Hait G. Aesthetic vaginal labiaplasty. *Plast Reconstr Surg*, 1984;**74**:414–6.
4. Chavis WM, LaFeria JJ, Niccolini R. Plastic repair of elongated hypertrophic labia minora: A case report. *J Reprod Med* 1989;**34**:3737–45.

CHAPTER 2

Genital plastics: the history of development

Michael P. Goodman

Caring for Women Wellness Center, Davis, CA, USA

With a contribution from David Matlock

The only reason some people get lost in thought is because it's unfamiliar territory.

Paul Fix

Documented since the time of the pharaohs in ancient Egypt, women throughout history have modified their genitalia via adornments, devices, colorations, bleaches, and reductive and expansive techniques.

Although gynecologic surgeons have for years performed surgical procedures resulting in alterations in genital size, appearance, and function (repairs after obstetrical delivery, perineorrhaphy, anterior/posterior colporrhaphy, intersex and transsexual surgical procedures), in addition to reductions for pediatric labial hypertrophy, Honore and O'Hara in 1978, Hodgekinson and Hait in 1984, and Chavis, LaFeria, and Niccolini in 1989 were the first to discuss genital surgical alterations performed for aesthetic and/or sexual reasons (see references 2–4 in Chapter 1).

Traditionally taught in OB/GYN residencies as surgical procedures designed for symptomatic pelvic floor herniations of bladder, urethra, rectum, or peritoneal cavity, but never proposed as a sexual-enhancing surgical procedure, traditional anterior and posterior "repairs" (colporrhaphies) are being adapted to improve sexual function by strengthening the pelvic floor and tightening the vaginal barrel to produce greater friction and vaginal wall pressure. This "shifting" of indications and modification of traditional gynecologic surgery primarily for reasons of enhancement of sexual function has not been without controversy, as gynecologic academic organizations such as the American Congress of Obstetricians and Gynecologists (ACOG) have officially decried this representation [1].

In step with ACOG, the Society of Obstetricians and Gynaecologists of Canada (SOGC) published its Policy Statement No. 300, December 2013 [2], in which they opine that the literature "does not support non-medically indicated female cosmetic surgery procedures considering the available evidence of efficacy and safety." This document appears to be a modification of the ACOG Opinion No. 378, September 2007, referenced above and, as was the ACOG opinion, was written by non-community academics, few if any of whom have any experience in the field of genital plastics or the benefit of consultation with or study of women seeking genital cosmetic care.

The same SOGC document advises practitioners in Canada that "Physicians who choose to undertake cosmetic procedures to the vagina and vulva should be appropriately trained in the gynaecologic and/or plastic surgery aspects of cosmetic surgery of the lower genital tract."

Although multiple articles describing vulvar labiaplasty technique, along with small retrospective case series, are available in the literature from the late 1980s onward (3–15), it was not until the early twenty-first century that procedures designed specifically for reduction of labial and clitoral hood size, narrowing of the hymenal aperture, and increasing vaginal wall pressure by surgical narrowing of the vagina were widely publicized in the lay press and online. As an extension of "women's liberation" and the owning of her own sexuality, and with the advent of social sharing

Female Genital Plastic and Cosmetic Surgery, First Edition. Edited by Michael P. Goodman.

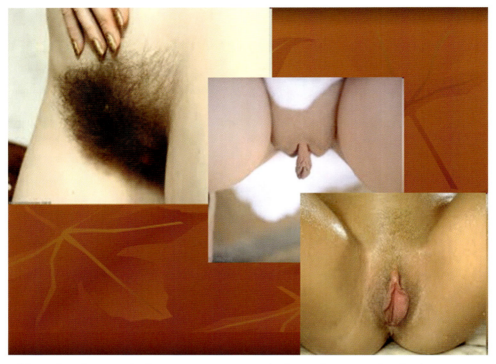

Figure 2.1 Visibility and "cushioning" of vulvar structures. Source: Michael P. Goodman. Reproduced with permission.

sites, more vulvar visibility secondary to various depilation techniques (Figure 2.1), and wishing to improve one's self-image to "feel more comfortable in her own skin," women in increasing numbers are seeking vulvar and vaginal aesthetic and plastic modifications.

While no "official" statistics on the varied FGPS procedures are kept by either the American Academy of Cosmetic Surgeons, the British Association of Aesthetic Plastic Surgeons, or the American Society of Plastic Surgeons (ASPS), the ASPS did note a 30% increase in "VRJ" procedures between 2005 and 2006 (793 to 1,030) but did not keep statistics beyond 2006 (16). The American Society for Aesthetic Plastic Surgery (ASAPS) kept demographic data for "VRJ" procedures in 2007 and found that of 4,505 procedures noted, 38.1% were in the 19–34 age group, 54.4% age 35–50, 2.4% 18 and under, and 5.1% 51 and older (17). According to the ASAPS 2012 statistics presented at their 2013 annual meeting, over 3,500 vaginal rejuvenation (CP, VRJ, PP) procedures were performed, representing a 64% increase from 2011. Informal polls of high-volume genital plastic/cosmetic surgeons by the editors of the journal of the ASAPS, along with the increase in volume of liability actions referable

to genital cosmetic surgery, suggest a continued rise in the public's interest in these procedures. Although, in this author's estimation, obstetrician-gynecologists perform a volume equal to that of plastic surgeons, gynecology specialty organizations have taken no interest in promoting these procedures in any way, including keeping statistics involving numbers performed annually by their members. I suspect both plastic surgery and OB/GYN societies would be surprised at the actual volume.

Mirzabeigi *et al.* in 2009 surveyed members of the ASPS via electronic mail (18); 750 surgeons responded (a 19.7% response rate.) Although selection bias very likely increased the rate, 51% of the sample currently offered labiaplasty, and responding members performed a total of 2,255 procedures in the previous 2 years (2007, 2008).

A major milestone in the development of surgical technique was reported in the 1998 article by Gary Alter, MD (8), describing the "modified V-wedge" procedure for reducing labial volume. Developed in response to the often poor cosmetic appearance and edge sensitivity noted by many patients receiving a linear resection-based labiaplasty performed with large-caliber suture and often a continuous running suture technique, Alter's procedure, although requiring a longer learning curve and representing an increased risk of wound disruption, offered the promise of better cosmetic appearance and little risk of neurological alteration, a potential benefit not proven by prospective research.

Instruction in plastic tissue handling and suturing technique and the specific procedures of cosmetic labiaplasty and aesthetic hood reduction, as well as sexual pleasure-enhancing perineoplasty, is absent from virtually all OB/GYN residency programs. Cosmetic labiaplasty technique is taught in only a percentage of plastic surgery residencies (and pelvic floor surgery rarely taught). Due to the lack of training in academic centers, it was inevitable that community surgeons would respond to the emerging and burgeoning demand for cosmetic female genital procedures. Unfortunately, many gynecologists, by virtue of being vaginal surgeons and having observed or performed a limited number of extirpative labial techniques (for in situ or invasive malignancies) in residency, feel that they are equipped to perform both labial reductive and vaginal floor-tightening procedures for reasons of enhancing sexual pleasure. Although gynecologists are trained in pelvic floor restoration, they are undereducated in the use of these surgical techniques specifically for sexual indications. The reality is that, in the absence of any meaningful instruction in careful plastic technique, or instruction in aesthetic labiaplasty or sexuality-oriented vaginoplasty/perineoplasty, general gynecologists, as well as a large percentage of plastic surgeons, are ill equipped to perform these procedures. Academic physicians, most recently Cheryl Iglesia, MD [19], who write editorials, "regulations," and "practice advisories," are also not specifically trained and/or experienced in these procedures and appear to shun what they do not understand.

In his own words, Dr. David Matlock, one of FGPS's early pioneers, describes his seminal experience.

The history of the development of female genital plastic and cosmetic surgery

David Matlock

My path in FGPS started in 1996. In general, my interest in cosmetic surgery started in 1987 with the implementation of liposuction into my gynecology practice. The tumescent liposuction technique revolutionized liposuction and eventually was employed in other procedures including breast reductions performed via tumescent liposuction. During this time, I was also interested in the

emerging trend of laser technologies for surgery. I took as many hands-on laser courses as available and read the latest textbooks. It wasn't long before I had a desire to apply this cosmetic and laser knowledge to vaginal surgery. My goal at the time was to restore form, function, and appearance.

To formulate my knowledge base and surgical technique I reviewed research papers and pertinent chapters of *Gray's Anatomy*, *Te Linde's Operative Gynecology*, and *Grabb and Smith's Plastic Surgery*. The objective was to extrapolate from scientific knowledge and formulate a procedure consistent with the goals of enhancing form, function, and aesthetic appearance. The vulvovaginal structures of young nulliparous patients in my practice served as a model to emulate in surgery. A big part of cosmetic surgery is restoring youth or creating a more youthful appearance. I took a common gynecologic procedure, anterior, posterior colporrhaphy and perineorrhaphy, with well-documented outcomes, efficacy, risk, and complications and modified it to accomplish cosmetic and sexual objectives. The modifications included a tumescent solution infiltration of the vaginal mucosa, a 980 nm diode laser to perform all the cutting and dissecting, plastic surgery suturing techniques, attention to detail and alignment of structures (hymenal ring, ends of the labia minora and outer border of the labia majora). The patients were also given a pudendal block with 0.5% Marcaine with epinephrine, which provided prolonged post-op pain-control anesthesia. I felt the purpose of the procedure would be better served if I thought more like a plastic surgeon than a gynecologist.

My first case was a 42-year-old G4 P4 with mild stress urinary incontinence and a POP 2 cystourethrocele and rectocele. She was consented for an anterior, posterior colporrhaphy and perineorrhaphy. Her surgery and post-operative course were uneventful. Shortly after resuming normal sexual activity the patient and her husband called me and she said, "Sex is great now." The patient's husband went on to say, "It is like having the same wife, but a new woman." I didn't make much of it at the time. Instead, I kind of filed it away in the back of my mind.

Shortly after this, the patient's friend came in requesting the same procedure because her friend had reported improved sex. This patient was 38 years old with three children. She noted that her sexual gratification had diminished with the birth of each subsequent child. She stated that she didn't have a functional problem such as stress urinary incontinence, rather wanted the procedure to enhance sexual gratification. After careful thought and consideration, I ultimately performed the procedure and achieved similar results as with the first patient. This second patient reported enhancement of sexual gratification for her and her partner. Shortly thereafter, I coined the term Laser Vaginal Rejuvenation (LVR).

Over time, more and more patients came in requesting LVR for enhancement of sexual gratification. It eventually became clear to me that a true need existed for this type of procedure. Prior to launching a program, I wanted to establish parameters to avoid going against the grain of the "medical establishment." These were as follows:

- The procedures were viewed as strictly cosmetic, fee for service, not covered by insurance.
- As with any cosmetic surgery (breast augmentation, breast reduction, liposuction, rhinoplasty, blepharoplasty, etc.), LVR is more about lifestyle, personal preference, and choice.
- Patients had to request the surgery under their own volition. If they were coerced, influenced, or forced, the surgery would be denied.
- If patients had body dysmorphia syndrome, psychological disorders, sexual dysfunction, pelvic pain, unrealistic expectations, and so forth, the procedure would be denied.
- If the patient wanted the procedure to produce vaginal orgasms due to the fact that she only experienced clitoral orgasms, the procedure would be denied. It would also be explained to the patient that perhaps this was normal for her. I wanted to convey that the procedure was for the enhancement of sexual gratification, which among other things is directly related to the amount of frictional forces generated. This was a clinical observation.
- The environment had to be one where patients felt comfortable in opening up to discuss their medical, physical, sexual, and social self.
- Patients' participation in their healthcare and surgical design was strongly encouraged. In the final portion of the consultation, patients were given a mirror and were shown what the procedure entailed.
- The husband/partner was encouraged to be present during the consultation, if the woman so desired.
- A mission statement was developed: Our mission is to empower women with knowledge, choice and alternatives.
- Medical legal concerns: I collaborated with a healthcare attorney to devise a comprehensive informed consent document.

My launch strategy initially involved marketing and media, feeling additionally that research on a new procedure/technique/concept, and so forth is to be done as soon as feasible. Like most new procedures (e.g., laparoscopic hysterectomy) time is required to build caseloads and surgical experience before embarking on research. I felt that it was more prudent to help create awareness among physicians and patients and in so doing caseloads could be developed and ultimately research would be done. I also felt that I was on solid ground since LVR was based upon a standard existing surgical procedure.

I went on and placed an ad in a weekly newspaper. Over time, the practice was inundated with calls, consultations, and surgeries. I had to pull the ad because I couldn't keep up with the demand.

Local, national, and international media began requesting interviews on the subject matter. Additionally, patients started requesting reduction of their labia minora and the excess prepuce. I approached each request with literature searches, extensive review of the anatomy, and lab work on animal models (pig ears). I continued until I successfully

developed a laser reduction labioplasty with the reduction of the excess prepuce and named this technique Designer Laser Vaginoplasty (DLV). Each of the procedures was developed based upon the request of women. All of the procedures were developed with systems and methods in mind, so that they could easily be reproduced and taught to other surgeons. The procedures are as follows:

- [laser reduction] labioplasty of the labia minora;
- reduction of the excess prepuce;
- [laser reduction] labioplasty of the labia majora via a vertical elliptical incision;
- [laser] perineoplasty as a modification of posterior colporrhaphy;
- liposuction of the fatty mons pubis and superior aspect of the labia majora;
- augmentation of the labia majora via autologous fat transfer;
- supra-pubic lift of the vulvar structures;
- [laser] hymenoplasty.

Around 1998, I started getting calls from gynecologists from around the country inquiring about a training program. This was something I had not thought about. While pursuing a healthcare executive MBA program at the University of California at Irvine, I developed a training program with the assistance of my professors and fellow graduate students. By the time I matriculated in 2000, I had a comprehensive business plan to launch a training program called the Laser Vaginal Rejuvenation Institute of America. The course would be three days in length and include eight hours of didactics, a full day of intraoperative observation of the procedures, and a day in the inanimate lab. The lab was where the surgeons would perform all of the procedures on animal models. As of 2013, 411 surgeons including gynecologists, plastic surgeons, and urologists from over 46 countries have been trained.

I have had the privilege of treating patients from all 50 states and over 65 countries. As predicted, FGPS has been brought into the mainstream. Surgeons are performing the procedures throughout the world and the research is flowing!

Politically, the waters remain muddy. Although a robust literature regarding the rationale, safety, and effectiveness of genital plastic/cosmetic procedures exists, and is quoted extensively throughout this text, this literature apparently "disappears" for the authors of "official positions" for the hierarchy of some specialty organizations. ACOG, the organization purporting to represent OB/GYNs, made clear their opinion, discussed above, in 2007. Their position was further discussed in 2012 as a "College Statement of Policy" ("The Role of the Obstetrician-Gynecologist in Cosmetic Procedures") [20], where they opined that "Obstetrician-gynecologists who offer procedure typically provided by other specialists should possess an equivalent level of competence," and that "the obstetrician-gynecologist must be knowledgeable of the ethics of patient counselling and informed consent." This opinion finds no argument from your editor. However, they also advise that "Special care must be taken when patients are considering procedures in a effort to enhance sexual appearance and function, as female sexual response has been shown to be an intricate process determined predominantly by brain function and psychosocial factors, not by genital appearance." As discussed and referenced especially in Chapter 17 in this text, the authors of this statement have not been diligent in their research, as there is a robust literature (21–26) showing exactly the opposite: that female sexual response, while admittedly complex, *is* certainly influenced by genital appearance.

Further "guidance" has been forthcoming from ACOG, following up on their 2007 statement of "caution." In regards to vaginal tightening procedures [1], a new Committee Opinion, replacing a 2008 statement on non-traditional surgical procedures, was issued in October of 2013 [27]. The statement was written by the ACOG's Committee on Ethics and published in the November 2013 issue of *Obstetrics and Gynecology* [27], ACOG's official publication. In it, ACOG acknowledges that "the importance of patient autonomy and increased access to information, especially information on the Internet, has prompted more requests for surgical interventions not traditionally recommended." In drafting the statement, the committee aimed "to provide an ethical framework to guide physicians' responses to patient requests for surgical treatment that is not traditionally recommended." While written more for the eventualities of elective Cesarean section before onset of labor, and prophylactic removal of ovaries in a woman at very significant risk for breast or ovarian cancer, the committee notes that, "depending on the context, acceding to a request for a surgical option that is not traditionally recommended can be ethical," and that "decisions about acceding to patient requests for surgical interventions…should be based on strong support for patients' informed preferences and values."

While the politics remain interesting, the handwriting is on the wall: patient autonomy (see Chapter 6) is paramount, and physicians can and will perform these procedures, provided that the patient is well informed,

not pressured, and the physician adequately trained for the specific procedure he or she plans to perform.

References

1. American College of Obstetrics and Gynecology. Committee Opinion #378. Vaginal "rejuvenation" and cosmetic vaginal procedures. *Obstet Gynecol* 2007;**110**:737–8.
2. Society of Obstetricians and Gynaecologists of Canada. Policy Statement. Female genital cosmetic surgery. *J Obstet Gynaecol Can* 2013;**35**(12):e1–e5.
3. Girling VR, Salisbury M, Ersek RA. Vaginal labiaplasty. *Plast Reconstr Surg* 2005;**115**:1792–3.
4. Rubayi S. Aesthetic vaginal labiaplasty. *Plast Reconstr Surg* 1985;**75**:608.
5. Miklos JR, Moore RD. Labiaplasty of the labia minora: Patient's indications for pursuing surgery. *J Sex Med* 2008;**5**: 1492–5.
6. Pardo J, Sola P, Guiloff E. Laser labiaplasty of the labia minora. *Int J Gynecol Obstet* 2005;**93**:38–43.
7. Heusse JL, Cousin-Verhoest S, Aillet S, Wattier E. Refinements in labia minora reduction procedures. *Ann Chir Plast Esthet* 2009;**54**:126–34.
8. Alter GJ. A new technique for aesthetic labia minora reduction. *Ann Plast Surg* 1998;**40**:287–90.
9. Krizko M, Krizko M, Janek L. Plastic adjustment of the labia minora. *Ceska Gynekol* 2005;**70**:446–9.
10. DiGiorgi V, Salvini C, Mannone F, Carelli G, Carli P. Reconstruction of the vulvar labia minora with a wedge resection. *Dermatol Surg* 2004;**30**:1583–6.
11. Munhoz AM, Filassi JR, Ricci MD, Aldrighi C, Correira LD, Aldrighi JM, Ferreira MC. Aesthetic labia minora reduction with inferior wedge resection and superior pedicle flap reconstruction. *Plast Reconstr Surg* 2006;**118**:1237–47.
12. Choi HY, Kim CT. A new method for aesthetic reduction of labia minora (the deepithelialized reduction labiaplasty). *Plast Reconstr Surg* 2000;**105**:419–22.
13. Goldstein AT, Romanzi LJ. Z-plasty reduction labiaplasty. *J Sex Med* 2007;**4**:550–3.
14. Maas SM, Hage JJ. Functional and aesthetic labia minora reduction. *Plast Reconstr Surg* 2007;**106**:1453–6.
15. Rouzier R, Louis-Sylvestre C, Paniel BJ, Hadded B. Hypertrophy of the labia minora; experience with 163 reductions. *Am J Obstet Gynecol* 2000;**182**:35–40.
16. American Society of Plastic Surgeons. 2005, 2006 Statistics. Available at: http://www.plasticsurgery.org/media/statistics/loader.cfm?url=/commonspot/security/getfile.cfm&PageID=23766 (accessed August 30, 2009).
17. The American Society for Aesthetic Plastic Surgery. Cosmetic Surgery National Data Bank. Available at: http://www.surgery.org/download/2007stats.pdf (accessed August 30, 2009).

18. Mirzabeigi MN, Moore JH, Mericli AF, Buciarelli P, Jandali S, Valerio IL Stofman GM. Current trends in vaginal labioplasty: A survey of plastic surgeons. *Ann Plast Surg* 2012;**68**:125–34.

19. Iglesia CB. Cosmetic gynecology and the elusive quest for the "perfect" vagina. *Obstet Gynecol* 2012;**119**:1083–4.

20. The role of the obstetrician-gynecologist in cosmetic procedures. Approved by the Executive Board, the American College of Obstetricians and Gynecologists, approved November 2008; reaffirmed July 2012.

21. Pujols Y, Meston C, Seal BN. The association between sexual satisfaction and body image in women. *J Sex Med* 2010;**7**:905–16.

22. Ackard DM, Kearney-Cooke A, Peterson CB. Effect of body self-image on women's sexual behaviors. *Int J Eat Disord* 2000;**28**:422–9.

23. Lowenstein L, Gamble T, Samses TV, Van Raalte H, Carberry C, Jakus S, Kambiss S, McAchran S, Pham T, Aschkenazi S, Hoskey K; Fellows Pelvic Research Network. Sexual function is related to body image perception in women with pelvic organ prolapse. *J Sex Med* 2009;**6**:2286–91.

24. Shick VR, Calabrese SK, Rima BN, Zucker AN. Genital appearance dissatisfaction: Implications for women's genital image self-consciousness, sexual esteem, sexual satisfaction, and sexual risk. *Psychol Women Q* 2010;**34**:384–404.

25. Goodman MP, Fashler S, Miklos JR, Moore RD, Brotto LA. The sexual, psychological, and body image health of women undergoing elective vulvovaginal plastic/cosmetic procedures: A pilot study. *Am J Cosmetic Surg* 2011;**28**:1–8.

26. Herbenick D, Reece M. Development and validation of the female genital self-image scale. *J Sex Med* 2010;**7**: 1822–30.

27. American College of Obstetricians and Gynecologists. Committee Opinion #578. Elective surgery and patient choice. *Obstet Gynecol* 2013;**122**:1134–8.

CHAPTER 3
Anatomic considerations

Orawee Chinthakanan, Robert D. Moore, and John R. Miklos

International Urogynecology Associates, Atlanta, GA, and Beverly Hills, CA, USA

Introduction

Pelvic floor dysfunction is a common health issue in women [1], with an 11.1% lifetime risk of undergoing pelvic floor reconstructive surgery [2]. Researchers have predicted that surgery for stress urinary incontinence (SUI) and pelvic organ prolapse (POP) will have increased by 47.2% over the next four decades [1]. In addition, female genital cosmetic surgery has became more available in the general population [3]. Integrity of the pelvic floor is a basis for the physiology of this complex anatomical region, as it is involved in functions such as defecation, urination, and sexual activity. The prevention of POP and maintenance of continence also depend on the pelvic floor supportive system.

This chapter focuses on the functional anatomy of the pelvic floor and relations to female genital cosmetic surgery. The chapter is divided into three sections: general pelvic floor anatomy, external genital anatomy and inter-relationships, and internal anatomy/inter-relationships.

General pelvic floor anatomy

The bony pelvis

The bony pelvis is composed of sacrum, ileum, ischium, and pubis. The pelvis is divided into the major (false) and minor (true) pelvis. The major pelvis is a part of the abdominal cavity that is superior to the pelvic brim. The minor pelvis is an inferior and narrower continuation of the major pelvis (Figure 3.1). The anatomical landmark of major and minor pelvis consists of the pelvic symphysis, coccyx, and sacrum at the back. A wider transverse inlet and narrower obstetrical conjugate predispose the female to subsequent pelvic floor disorders [4]. For pelvic reconstructive surgeons, various parts of the bony pelvis can be used clinically as surgical landmarks. The ischial spine is an anatomical landmark that can be used to identify the sacrospinous ligament. The sacrospinous ligament is attached from the ischial spine to the lateral margins of the sacrum and coccyx, which are located anterior to the sacrotuberous ligament. The sacrotuberous ligament extends from the ischial tuberosity to the coccyx. The greater and lesser sciatic foramena are above and below the sacrospinous ligament. The anterior superior iliac spine (ASIS) is a bony landmark that helps the surgeon's orientation for placing endoscopic ports. The inguinal ligament is attached from the ASIS to the pubic tubercle. The ileopectineal ligament (Cooper's ligament) is attached from the posterior aspect of the inguinal ligament anteriorly to the iliopectineal eminence posteriorly. Cooper's ligament is an important anatomical landmark for Burch colposuspension [5] (Figure 3.1). The arcus tendineus fascia pelvis (ATFP) or white line is an anatomical landmark for paravaginal defect repair (Figure 3.1). The ATFP is a thickening of the endopelvic fascia over the obturator internus muscle, which is attached from the pubic symphysis anteriorly to the ischial spine posteriorly on each side of the pelvis. The vagina and its surrounding connective tissue attach to this dense fibrous structure to form a slinglike structure that runs under the urethra and bladder neck in a position to support the urethra. The average distance of the ATFP is 9 cm and is correlated

Female Genital Plastic and Cosmetic Surgery, First Edition. Edited by Michael P. Goodman.
© 2016 John Wiley & Sons, Ltd. Published 2016 by John Wiley & Sons, Ltd.

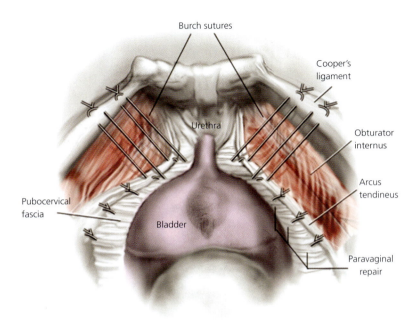

Burch sutures

Cooper's
ligament

Urethra

Obturator
internus

Arcus
tendineus

Pubocervical
fascia

Bladder

Paravaginal
repair

Figure 3.1 Cooper's ligament and the arcus tendineus fascia pelvis (ATFP). Source: Robert D. Moore and John R. Miklos. Reproduced with permission.

with the height [6]. The ATFP and Cooper's ligament can be palpated during dissection into the Retzius (para-vesical) space. These ligaments play an important role in urethral support [7, 8]. Paravaginal defects, commonly seen in patients with anterior vaginal wall prolapse, are due to the detachment of pubocervical fascia from the ATFP, at or near its lateral attachment. The symphysis pubis is also an anatomical landmark for anti-incontinence procedures, that is, retropubic sling, Marshall-Marchetti-Krantz (MMK) procedure, and so forth. The sacral promontory is an important landmark for sacral colpopexy procedures.

Pelvic floor musculature

The skeletal muscles that provide pelvic floor support are the levator ani muscles, the coccygeus, the external anal sphincter, the striated urethral sphincter, and the deep and superficial perineal muscles.

Pelvic floor muscle (pelvic diaphragm)

The pelvic diaphragm, composed of the levator ani and coccygeus muscles, is responsible for supporting pelvic and abdominal visceral organs and maintaining the sta-bility of intra-abdominal pressure. These muscles form

the muscular floor of the pelvis. The levator ani is composed of the pubovisceral and iliococcygeus [9] (Figure 3.2). From many magnetic resonance imaging (MRI) studies, levator ani abnormalities can be identi-fied in women with stress urinary incontinence [10], POP [11], and even after vaginal delivery [12].

The pelvic diaphragm is formed by two muscle groups, the small coccygeus muscle posteriorly, and the much larger and more important levator ani musculature anteriorly. The coccygeus (ischiococcygeus) muscle is originated from the tip and the posterior border of the ischial spine and inserted at the coccyx. The coccygeus muscle is located at the superior aspect of the sacrospi-nous ligament to form the posterior portion of the pelvic diaphragm. The levator ani muscles are composed of two major components, the pubovisceral and the ilio-coccygeal [9]. The pubovisceral portion includes those muscles arising from the pubic bones: the pubococ-cygeus, puborectalis, and puboperineus. The arcus ten-dineus levator ani (ATLA) represents the upper margin of the aponeurosis of the ileococcygeus muscle. The ATLA is a thickened line of the fascia over the obturator internus muscle running in an arching line from the pubis to the ischial spine. The iliococcygeus muscle is

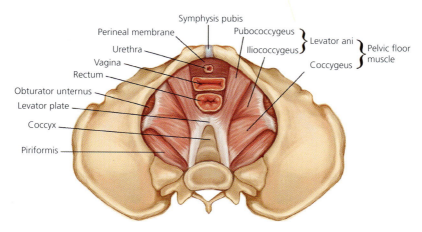

Symphysis pubis
Perineal membrane
Urethra
Vagina
Rectum
Obturator unternus
Levator plate
Coccyx
Piriformis
Pubococcygeus
Iliococcygeus
Coccygeus
Levator ani
Pelvic floor muscle

Figure 3.2 Superior view of the pelvic floor muscle. Source: Orawee Chinthakanan. Reproduced with permission.

a thin lateral portion of the levator ani, which originates from the posterior portion of the ATLA and ischial spine and inserts to the lateral margin of the coccyx and lower sacrum. The pubococcygeus muscle is the thick medial part of the levator ani, originating from the back of the body of the pubis and the anterior portion of the ATLA on each side. The pubococcygeus runs posteriorly almost horizontally to behind the rectum. The medial edge forms the margin of the urogenital (levator) hiatus, which allows passage of the urethra, vagina, and rectum. The pubococcygeus is then inserted in the midline onto the anococcygeal raphe, known as the levator plate, running from the area posterior to the rectum to the coccyx. The levator plate is a midline point of the levator ani fusion. The puborectalis muscle is the most medial U-shaped muscle around the rectum at its junction with the anus. It pulls the anorectal junction forward and contributes to anal continence. The levator ani muscles are innervated from the pudendal nerve on the perineal surface and direct branches of the sacral nerves on the pelvic surface. Barber *et al.* have demonstrated that the levator ani musculature is not innervated by the pudendal nerve but by the "levator ani nerve" originating from the sacral nerve roots (S3–0S5), travelling along the superior surface of the pelvic floor [13].

Functionally, the levator ani exhibits constant baseline tone and can be voluntarily contracted. The muscles contain both slow-twitch (type I) fibers maintaining constant tone and fast-twitch (type II) fibers providing reflex and voluntary contractions [14]. The density of fast-twitch fibers increases in the periurethral and perianal areas [15]. At rest the levator ani maintains closure of the urogenital hiatus. The voluntary contraction of the puborectalis muscle occurs to counteract increased intra-abdominal pressure. A normal voiding mechanism is controlled by contraction of the pubococcygeal muscle as well. Contraction of the pubococcygeal muscle raises the bladder neck; the detrusor and urethral muscles relax, leading to lengthening of the urethra. Finally the internal urethral orifice will narrow and close, and voiding stops [16]. The levator ani provides pelvic floor support, voluntary control of micturition, and fecal continence. Levator ani defects are associated with POP [17, 18], stress urinary incontinence [19], and fecal incontinence [20].

Perineal membrane (urogenital diaphragm)

The "perineal membrane" (or "urogenital diaphragm" in older texts) is a triangular-shaped musculofascial structure covering the anterior pelvic outlet below the pelvic diaphragm. The change in name reflects understanding that it is a sheet of dense connective tissue rather than a two-layered structure with muscles in between. This structure runs between the inferior pubic rami bilaterally and the perineal body posteriorly and is pierced in the midline by the urogenital hiatus. The distal vagina is supported mainly by connection to the perineal membrane anteriorly and the perineal body posteriorly and has a sphincterlike effect to assist in holding them in place. There are two systems holding the urethra in place: [1] the perineal membrane and its attachment to the pubis, and [2] the connective tissue attached between the anterior sulcus and the ATFP. The perineal membrane contributes to urinary continence by attaching to periurethral striated muscles and providing structural support to the distal urethra. The point at which the urethra enters the perineal membrane is the point that urine flow stops and has the highest intraurethral pressure when a women voluntarily contracts her pelvic floor to stop her urine stream [21]. The posterior triangle below the perineal body does not have a supporting diaphragm or membrane. The ischiocavernosus, the bulbocarvernosus, and the superficial transverse perineal muscles are located superficial to the perineal membrane and are considered less supportive.

Perineum

The borders of the perineum are the ischiopubic rami, ischial tuberosities, sacrotuberous ligaments, and coccyx. It is divided into the urogenital triangle anteriorly and the anal triangle posteriorly by using an imaginary line between ischial tuberosities bilaterally as a landmark. The perineal membrane divides the urogenital triangle into a superficial and deep perineal space. The superficial perineal space is composed of the superficial perineal muscles (ischiocavernosus, bulbocarvernosus, and superficial transverse perineal muscles), the erectile tissue of the clitoris, the vestibular bulbs, and Bartholin's glands (Figure 3.3). The deep perineal space is a thin space that is located between the perineal membrane

and the levator ani muscles. It contains the external urethral sphincter, the sphincter urethrovaginalis, compressor urethrae, and deep transverse perineal muscles (Figure 3.3). The perineal body is a pyramidal fibromuscular elastic structure situated in the midline between the rectum and the vagina with the rectovaginal septum ("fascia of Denonvilliers") located superiorly. The perineal body, containing smooth muscle, elastic fibers, and nerve endings, is a merging point of several structures: the superficial and deep transverse perineus muscles, the bulbocarvernosus muscle, the external anal sphincter, levator ani (puborectalis and pubococcygeus muscles), perineal membrane, and the posterior vaginal muscularis. The perineal body plays an important role as distal support of the posterior compartment. DeLancey [22] and Hsu *et al.* [23] have demonstrated the concepts of the posterior compartment support through cadaveric dissection [22] and imaging [23]. Posterior compartment support is contributed by the uterosacral ligaments for the upper portion, the ATFP for the middle portion, and the perineal body for the distal portion. These will be discussed later in the chapter. The perineal body is commonly damaged during labor and delivery. When the perineal body detachment is present, rectocele or fecal or urinary incontinence may occur. In order to correct the defect, the perineal body must be reattached to the posterior vaginal wall and rectovaginal septum to regain the functional capacity of the urinary and fecal continence mechanism [24].

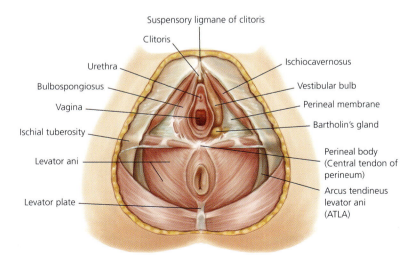

Suspensory ligmane of clitoris
Clitoris
Urethra
Bulbospongiosus
Vagina
Ischial tuberosity
Levator ani
Levator plate
Ischiocavernosus
Vestibular bulb
Perineal membrane
Bartholin's gland
Perineal body (Central tendon of perineum)
Arcus tendineus levator ani (ATLA)

Figure 3.3 Perineal membrane and perineum. Source: Orawee Chinthakanan. Reproduced with permission.

Vascular supply

The internal pudendal artery, a branch of the anterior trunk of the internal iliac artery, is the major arterial supply to the perineal body. The internal pudendal artery travels along with the pudendal nerve through Alcock's canal and is then divided into the perineal, the dorsal artery of the clitoris, and inferior rectal arteries. The perineum is mainly supplied by the transverse branch of the perineal artery and the inferior rectal artery. The middle rectal artery, a branch of the internal iliac artery, provides blood supply to the middle third of the rectum and the superior portion of the perineal body. The superior rectal artery, a branch of the inferior mesenteric artery, also provides minor branches to supply the perineal body.

Somatic innervation

The pudendal nerve innervates the pelvic floor musculature (Figure 3.4). The pudendal nerve originates from the sacral nerve root 2-4 (S2-4), descends between the coccygeus and piriformis muscle, and finally travels under the sacrospinous ligament medial to the ischial spine. The nerve exits the pelvis through the greater sciatic foramen and enters the perineum through the lesser sciatic foramen. It then travels along the lateral wall of the ischioanal fossa within Alcock's canal (pudendal canal) on the medial aspect of the obturator internus muscle before dividing into terminal branches supplying the skin and muscles of the perineum. The inferior rectal nerve branches off as the pudendal nerve wraps around the ischial spine and subsequently supplies the external anal sphincter, which plays an important role in fecal continence and provides sensory innervation to the distal anal canal below the pectinate line. The pudendal nerve is divided into the dorsal nerve of clitoris and the perineal nerve at the level of the superior fascia of the pelvic diaphragm and endopelvic fascia. The perineal nerve then supplies the labia and the perineal body. The external urethral sphincter is supplied by other branches of the perineal nerve and helps maintain urinary continence. The internal anal sphincter is supplied by the uterovaginal portion of the inferior hypogastric plexus, the pelvic splanchnic nerve, and the posterior femoral cutaneous nerve.

External genital anatomy

The female external genitalia (the vulva), from anterior to posterior, is formed by the mons pubis, labia majora, labia minora, vulvar vestibule, external urethral meatus, hymen, ostia of the accessory glands (Bartholin's, Skene's, and vesitubular glands), and the perineum (Figure 3.5). These structures are inferior to the perineal

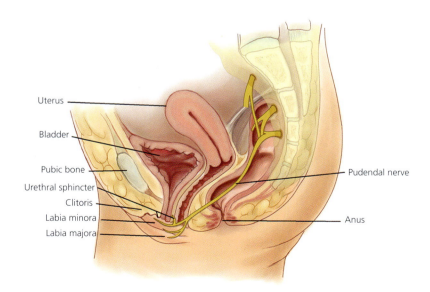

Figure 3.4 The pudendal nerve innervation. Source: Orawee Chinthakanan. Reproduced with permission.

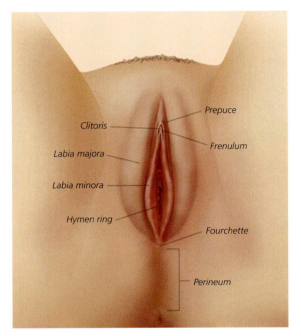

Figure 3.5 Normal external genitalia. Source: Robert D. Moore and John R. Miklos. Reproduced with permission.

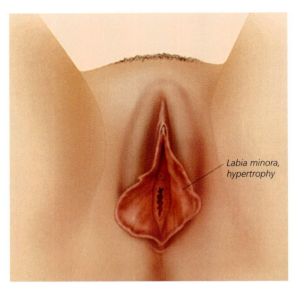

Figure 3.6 Labia minora. Source: Robert D. Moore and John R. Miklos. Reproduced with permission.

membrane. The mons pubis is a fat pad, containing skin appendages with sebaceous and sweat glands, and is located over the pubic bone with a hair-bearing squamous epithelium. A survey conducted in the United State has indicated that 80% of women practice pubic hair grooming regardless of their pubic hair styles [25]. Pubic hair removal is widely performed among diverse ethnic/racial groups. Minor complications of pubic hair removal are folliculitis and abrasion, more likely to occur in obese women [26]. In 82% of women their external genitalia is of a darker complexion than surrounding skin [27].

Labia majora

The labia majora are two prominent cutaneous folds running from the mons pubis, merging at the perineum. They are differentiated from the labioscrotal fold in embryonic development and correspond to the scrotum in men. The normal length of labia majora, measured from the crura of clitoris to the posterior fourchette, is 9.3 cm (range 7–12 cm) [27]. They are separated from the labia minora by a discrete line, the "interlabial fold."

Squamous epithelium covers a fascial layer overlying a fatty layer and a fingerlike fat pad covered by a thin

fascial aponeurosis, Colle's fascia. Not infrequently this layer tears, partially extruding its contents with resultant loss of tension and possible sequelae resulting in laxity and skin folds.

With aging, skin layer relaxation, stretching secondary to pregnancy and involution, weight gain (and loss), and repeated chafing, labial skin can become redundant and protrude [see Figure 8.29(a) and (b), Chapter 8].

Labia minora

The "upper," superior, or cranial portions of the labia minora (see Figure 3.6) begin as one or several folds descending caudally from the prepuce ("hood") and frenulum, eventually coalescing into one relatively thin to broadened fold curtaining the edge of the vulvar vestibule and introitus and ending just above the perineum or continuing as the fourchette, or posterior commisure, in a variable manner onto the perineum, frequently meeting and bonding with the contralateral labum [see Chapter 8, Figures 8.19, 8.21, 8.22, 8.23(a)[1]]. Standing, many women's labia minora are tucked away, not visible from above. Protrusion beyond the labia majora with the thighs abducted is often a cause of significant dissatisfaction for many women [28, 29], often producing a vulvar appearance "which resembles a scrotum" [30] (see Chapter 8, Figure 8.23(a)[2]].

The labia minora (aka "nymphs") are two sometimes thin, oft-times thickened, "corrugated," or redundant skin folds that are located medial to the labia majora and lateral to the vestibule and that "flow down" from the fusion of one or more folds of skin from the frenulum, central to the lateral clitoral hood and more lateral prepuce portion of the clitoral hood (see multiple photographs in Chapter 8 for an array of anatomic variations). They contain no hair follicles and lack subcutaneous fat. They are differentiated from the urogenital fold in embryonic development and are equivalent to the ventral surface of the cavernosa urethra and the corpus spongiosum of the urethra in males. The normal length and width (from the base to the edge) of labia minora are 60.6 (range 20–100) and 21.8 (range 7–50) mm, respectively [27]. Labia minora that protrude from the distal boundary of the labia majora may be of concern to women. This condition can be congenital [31, 32] but often occurs or accentuates with aging and childbearing. There is no formal guideline to indicate when surgical correction is required for "labial hypertrophy" [33]. However, Rouzier *et al.* have reported labial reduction surgery in 163 patients and defined "labial hypertrophy" as a maximum distance from the base to the edge greater than 4 cm [34]. As with size and appearance differentials elsewhere in the body, there are (within reason) few "norms" regarding labial size, contour, or appearance. Individual satisfaction or dissatisfaction is highly subjective.

The labia minora contain sensitive nerve fibers and a generous, albeit delicate, vasculature; during sexual arousal the labia become engorged and contribute to erotic sensation and pleasure. The medial surfaces of the labia minora exhibit a mucosal epithelium within the vulvar vestibule, medial to what has been referred to as "Hart's line," dividing mucosal from squamous epithelium within the vulvar vestibule. The distal vagina, urethral meatus, clitoral complex, prepuce, perineum, vestibule, and labia minora may be considered as a unified structure, as their neurovascular supply is intimately entwined [35].

Two arterial sources supply the labia minora, and it behooves the genital surgeon to understand this vascular anatomy as it may relate to placement of incision lines. Entering more anteriorly is vasculature derived from the external pudendal arteries, the obturator arteries, and the funicular arteries. The posterior supply is dominated by the internal pudendal arteries.

Delicate laterals from these sources run perpendicular to the long axis of the labia, with a confluence beneath the labial edge. The posterior, or lower two-thirds, of each labum is supplied by the internal pudendal, while the anterior or upper portion derives from delicate branches of the external pudendal artery with thin anastomoses in the junction of the upper third/lower two-thirds.

C. A. Georgiou and colleagues from the University of Nice, France, have written an elegant paper ("Arterial Anatomy of Labia Minora: A First Step Towards Evidence-Based Labiaplasty," presently submitted for publication) in which they have outlined in detail the arterial supply to the labia in a series of 10 cadavers, identifying and precisely describing the labial vascular systems via a process of catheterization of the internal and external pudendal arteries utilizing dilute contrast solution and rotational angiography and 3D CT imaging. Arterial molds were made with latex resin to enhance and confirm the precision of the radiologic findings.

For every subject four main arteries were identified. The dominant one was more centrally located and relatively larger than the other arteries. Penetrating the labum at a slightly variable location, it traveled in a perpendicular trajectory to the long axis of the labum, continuing its course in a posterior to anterior direction, fading anteriorly. Two of the four arteries identified by these authors flowed posterior to the more central labial artery and traversed a perpendicular trajectory to the labum's long axis, fading near the labum's edge. The anterior-most of the four arteries identified, and the smallest, flowed anterior to the "central artery," which also had a short perpendicular trajectory to the labia minora's long axis (Figure 3.7).

This refinement in the understanding of labial vasculature may have prospective application in regards to the placement of incision lines when performing a labiaplasty (see Chapter 8). While a curvilinear incision does not interrupt the vascular flow of the remaining labia minora, it may have a disadvantage of disrupting the "normal" appearance of the labial edge. In regards to wedge technique, a more posterior incision, and to some extent central incision, may have the disadvantage of greater interruption in blood supply, leading to a somewhat greater risk of wound dehiscence, while a more anteriorly or centro-anteriorly placed excisional wedge has the advantage of greater preservation of vascular supply, resects what usually is the largest part of the labia, and places the scar

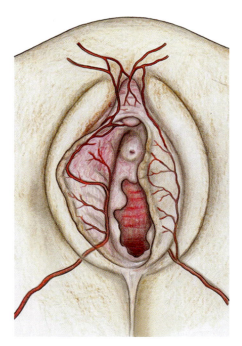

Figure 3.7 Labial vasculature. Source: B. Maes. Reproduced with permission.

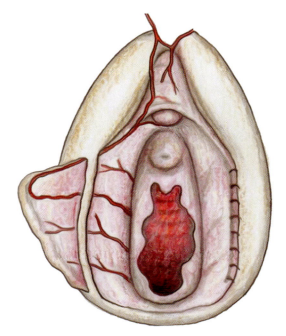

Figure 3.8 Linear resection incision in relation to vasculature. Source: B. Maes. Reproduced with permission.

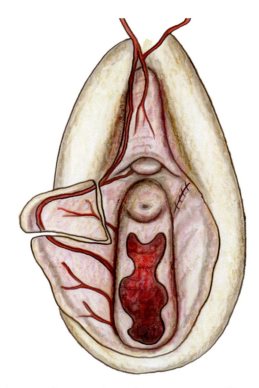

Figure 3.9 Placement of V-wedge incision in area of least vascular interruption. Source: B. Maes. Reproduced with permission.

anteriorly, at the greatest distance from the introitus (Figures 3.8 and 3.9).

Clitoris

The clitoris is composed of three erectile tissue components, the glans, body, and crura [36]. It is derived from the genital tubercle during the embryonic period and corresponds ontologically to the male's penis. The body and glans of the clitoris are covered by the prepuce, or "hood," continuous with the labia minora. The prepuce (hood) acts as a protective cover over the clitoral glans. The clitoral glans may be partially exposed in its resting state or be completely "hooded" by the prepuce, which in normal conditions may be easily exposed by manual retraction or sexual arousal, engorging the clitoral body and glans. Adjacent to the crus (plural, crurae) the vestibular bulbs, also known as the clitoral bulbs, are aggregations of erectile tissue that are an internal part of the clitoris. They can also

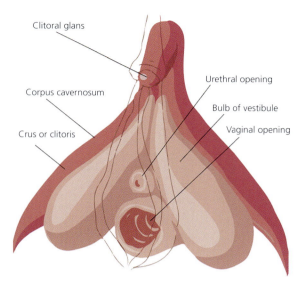

Clitoral glans

Corpus cavernosum

Crus or clitoris

Urethral opening

Bulb of vestibule

Vaginal opening

Figure 3.10 Clitoral anatomy.

be considered as a part the vestibule—next to the clitoral body, clitoral crura, urethra, "urethral sponge," and vagina.

The vestibular bulbs (Figure 3.10) are homologous to the bulb of the penis and adjoining part of the corpus spongiosum of the male and consist of two elongated "bulbs" of erectile tissue, placed one on either side of the vaginal orifice and united to each other in front by a narrow median band termed the *pars intermedia*. Their posterior ends are expanded and are in contact with the greater vestibular glands; their anterior ends are tapered and joined to one another by the pars intermedia; their deep surfaces are in contact with the inferior fascia of the urogenital diaphragm; superficially they are covered by the bulbospongiosus. An average length and width of the clitoris is 19.1 (range 5–35) and 5.5 (range 3–10) mm, respectively, but variations are considerable and normal. The distance between clitoris and urethra is 28.5 mm on average (range 16–45) [27]. The suspensory ligament of clitoris is divided into superficial and deep components [37]. During sexual arousal, the clitoris responds to neuro-transmitter-mediated vascular smooth muscle relaxation; as a result, the clitoris increases in length and diameter from the engorgement. Goldstein and Berman proved that women with vascular impairment of the ilio-hypogastric-pudendal arteries had vasculogenic

female sexual dysfunction manifested as decreasing clitoral sensation and clitoral orgasm [38] (see Chapter 10 for a further discussion of clitoral anatomy and physiology).

The G-spot

Despite controversy over this subject, researchers have found evidence that a sensitive area called the "G-spot", named after Ernst Grafenberg [39], exists in the vaginal canal, typically located 1–2.5 cm from the urethra under the anterior vaginal wall (see also Chapter 11). This has been studied and described as an area that lies beneath the posterior part of the "female prostatic gland" (Skene's glands), typically found 2–3 cm inside the introitus on the anterior vaginal wall in the region of the bladder neck, that when stimulated becomes engorged, enlarged, and sensitive. Orgasm may be produced with stimulation of this area alone. One investigator recently reported to have "found" the G-spot (in a single fresh cadavoric dissection of an 80+ year-old woman), describing it as a well-delineated sac with a wall resembling fibroconnective and erectile tissue, located at 1.6 cm. from the upper part of urethral meatus [40]. Unfortunately, lack of histologic confirmation hampered this case report. Recently, in a study evaluating the thickness of the urethrovaginal space in women with or without vaginal orgasm, it was found that there was a direct correlation of the thickness of this space (i.e., the G-spot) and the presence or absence of vaginal orgasm [41]. Masters and Johnson, on their studies of orgasm, argued that clitoral stimulation was the source of all orgasmic response. They did not deny the possibility of vaginal sensitivity; they merely overlooked it [42] and considered the vagina as merely a passive receptacle for the male organ and ejaculate. Vaginal sensitivity and the possibility of another sensitive spot, in addition to the clitoris, was noted during studies of female ejaculation in the late 1970s. Sevely and Bennett initially described this "female prostatic gland" as the source of fluid that some women expel during orgasm. The area identified by their research subjects as the "trigger point" for their ejaculations was the same area described initially by Grafenberg (see also below, Skene's glands). They confirmed Grafenberg's observation that this sensitive area is located on the anterior vaginal wall, typically midway between the pubic bone and the cervix, on or near the urethra and when stimulated it can lead to orgasm.

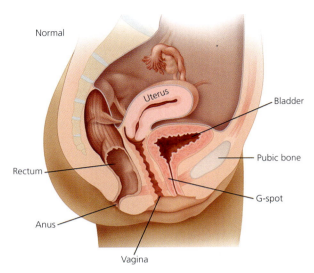

Normal

Uterus

Bladder

Pubic bone

Rectum

G-spot

Anus

Vagina

Figure 3.11 Location of G-spot on the anterior vaginal wall. Source: Robert D. Moore and John R. Miklos. Reproduced with permission.

They trained physicians in their technique, and in a study of 250 women these physicians were able to locate the spot in all 250 patients [43]. Mould confirmed this in several studies by measuring EMG responses in the vaginal canal and the levators during stimulation of this area and subsequent orgasmic response [44]. His and other studies have clearly shown that there is sensation in the vagina itself and a nerve pathway that plays a role in sexual stimulation and satisfaction and that if altered, it may impair sexual function. The surveys found that a majority of women believe a G-spot actually exists, although not all of the women who believed in it were able to locate it [45] (see Chapters 10 and 11 and Figure 3.11).

The vulvar vestibules

The "vestibule," as its name implies, is the "entryway" from the vulva and perineum into the vagina, as "protected" by the hymenal ring. The vulvar vestibule is bordered by the labia minora, posterior fourchette, and hymenal ring. "Hart's line" on its labial boundary separates the vestibule from the remainder of the inner surface of the labum minus and is an important anatomic landmark for the female genital plastic/cosmetic surgeon (see Chapter 8.)

The vestibular bulbs are two erectile organs located between the two labia minora laterally extending medially to the hymenal ring. They join together anteriorly through the pars intermedia (female corpus spongiosum) and extend to the glans base [36]. They are differentiated from an embryological genital tubercle, which is the homologue of the male penile bulbs. During sexual intercourse, the vestibular bulbs create the vaginal orgasmic contractions through rhythmic bulbocavernosus muscle contractions [46].

Bartholin's glands

The Bartholin's glands, or greater vestibular glands, originate from an embryonic urogenital sinus and correspond to the male's Cowper's (bulbourethral gland). They are located in the superficial perineal pouch on either side. They secrete mucus and participate in lubrication during sexual intercourse. Their ducts open into navicular fossa on the vulvar surface. Advancing age diminishes activation.

Skene's glands

Skene's glands, a pair of periurethral glands, are differentiated from urogenital sinus and are a homologue to the prostate gland in males. They lie in the anterior vaginal wall beneath the epithelium proximal to the urethral meatus and are inconsistent structures with egress via ducts exiting unilaterally or bilaterally lateral to the urethral meatus. They have been purported to be the source of "female ejaculation," as distinguished from "squirting," which most likely occurs secondary to pressure-induced incontinence during sexual activities/orgasm [47]. This is undoubtedly the "grape-like" organ with attached ductlike appendages that was dissected by Ostrzenski in his anatomic report on the "G-spot" [40].

Three integrated levels of pelvic floor support

The endopelvic fascia is the most important system that maintains the integrity of the axes supporting the bladder, urethra, uterus, vagina, and rectum in their respective anatomic relationships. This fascia is a network of connective tissue and smooth muscle that constitutes the physical matrix to envelop the pelvic viscera. The endopelvic fascial system extends continuously from the origin of the uterosacral-cardinal ligament complex to the urogenital diaphragm and provides structural support to the vagina and adjacent organs. DeLancey has divided the supports of the vagina into three levels as follows: the upper third of the vagina to the cardinal-uterosacral complex (level I), the middle third of the paravagina to the ATFP (level II), and the lower third of the vagina to the perineal membrane, levator ani muscles, and perineal body (level III) [48] (Figure 3.12).

Level I: apical support
The superior suspension of the vagina to the bony sacrum is provided by the uterosacral-cardinal ligament complex. This complex suspends the uterus and the upper third of vagina in its normal vertical axis. It maintains vaginal length and appears to be the most supportive structure of the apical compartment. This complex is composed of the cardinal ligament and uterosacral ligament. The cardinal ligament envelops the internal iliac vessels and then continues along the uterine artery, merging into the visceral capsule of the cervix, lower uterine segment, and upper vagina. The uterosacral ligament is thicker and more prominent than the cardinal ligament. The uterosacral ligament is fanlike originated from its smallest width at the cervix around the inlet of the pouch of Douglas and inserted at the sacrospinous ligament/coccygeus muscle complex (82%), the sacrum (7%), or the piriformis muscle/the sciatic foramen/the ischial spine (11%) [49]. It divides

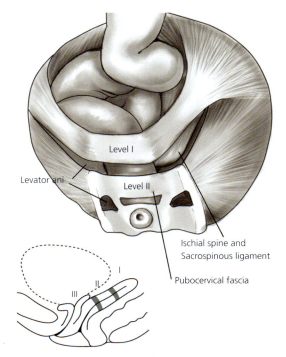

Figure 3.12 Apical (level I) and lateral (level II) support. Source: Robert D. Moore and John R. Miklos. © Chinthakanan. Reproduced with permission.

into three distinct histologic regions [50]. At the anterior third (cervical) attachment, the ligament is made up of closely packed bundles of smooth muscle, generous medium-sized and small blood vessels, and small nerve bundles. The intermediate third of the ligament is composed of predominantly connective tissue and only a few scattered smooth muscle fibers, nerve, and blood vessels. The sacral or posterior third is mainly composed of loose strands of connective tissue and intermingled fat, sparse vessels, nerves, and lymphatics. The mechanical strength of the uterosacral ligaments may also depend on other factors, such as the ability of surrounding cells to degrade extracellular matrix components by expression of matrix metalloproteinases (MMPs), collagen expression, and the aggregate amount of smooth muscle cells. There is evidence that increased MMP-2 [51] and collagen III expression [52] in the uterosacral ligaments is associated with POP. According to the "suture pull out strength test" [53], the most supportive portions of the uterosacral ligaments are the cervical and intermediate parts, which are able to support more than 17 kg weight before failure.

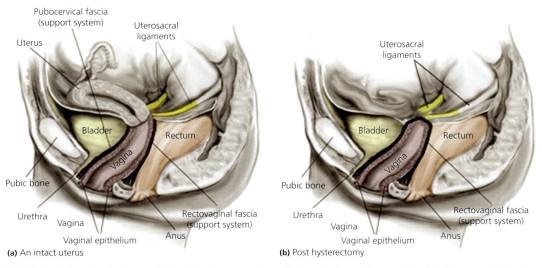

Figure 3.13 Lateral view of apical support (level I) of women with and without uterus. Source: Robert D. Moore and John R. Miklos. Reproduced with permission.

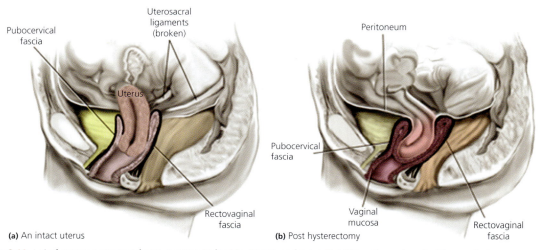

Figure 3.14 Apical compartment prolapse. Source: Robert D. Moore and John R. Miklos. Reproduced with permission.

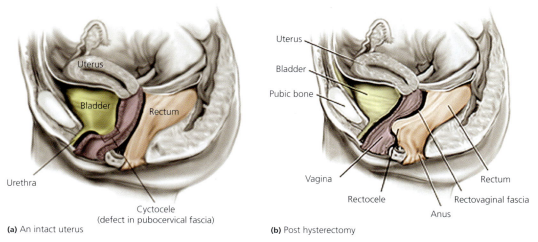

Figure 3.15 Anterior and posterior compartment prolapse. Source: Robert D. Moore and John R. Miklos. Reproduced with permission.

Uterosacral ligament suspension is a procedure performed to correct vaginal vault prolapse by suturing vaginal apex to its original supporting ligaments. The 5-year anatomical success rate of high uterosacral vaginal vault ligament suspension has been reported as 85% [54]. The optimal site for uterosacral ligament suspension is 1 cm posterior to its most anterior palpable margin at the intermediate portion of the ligament [53]. The uterosacral-cardinal ligament complex, pubocervical fascia, and rectovaginal fascia are merged at the vaginal apex forming the pericervical ring. An enterocele is an abnormality of the cul de sac that contains peritoneum and intra-abdominal contents and may involve the apical, anterior, or posterior compartments of the vagina [55]. An enterocele is related to the disruption of the fusion of the apical margin of the pubocervical and rectovaginal fascia. In women with an intact uterus, an enterocele formation can also occur [56].

Level II: lateral support

Level II support or the paravaginal support is the horizontal support of the bladder, upper two thirds of the vagina, and rectum. The uterosacral-cardinal ligament complex continues to the level of ischial spine and provides the level II support. The vaginal wall is supported by its fibromuscular composition, known as fascia. Anterior support suspends the mid-portion of the anterior vaginal wall by the pubocervical fascia (Figures 3.13, 3.15; see also Figure 3.14). The anterior support creates the anterior lateral vaginal sulci. The pubocervical fascia, between the bladder and vagina, is attached to the ATFP bilaterally. Anterior vaginal wall prolapse is descent of the anterior vaginal wall and is commonly due to bladder prolapse (cystocele, either central, paravaginal, or a combination) [56]. Paravaginal defects (Figure 3.16) or detachment of lateral supports cause cystocele. According to DeLancey's study, more than 90% of paravaginal defects occur by detachment of the ATFP from the ischial spine, not from the pubis [57].

The rectovaginal fascia (fascia of Denonvilliers), located between rectum and vagina, provides posterior support. It is attached superiorly to the cardinal-uterosacral complex, laterally to the levator ani fascia, and inferiorly to the perineal body. Detachment of this fascia causes a rectocele [58] (Figures 3.12, 3.15).

Level III: distal support

Level III support maintains the lower vertical axis of the urethra and the distal third of the vagina. The perineal membrane, levator ani muscles, and the perineal body play an important role for the level III support. The vagina fuses with the urethra anteriorly and perineal body posteriorly. The pubourethral ligaments are connective tissue structures that attach the urethra to the pubic bone. An anatomical defect in the pubourethral ligaments might be a contributing factor to urinary stress incontinence in the female [59]. Ashton-Miller and DeLancey clearly describe the mechanism of urinary continence called the "hammock hypothesis." The hammocklike structures are composed of the anterior vaginal wall and the connective tissue that attaches the urethra and bladder neck to the pubic bone (pubovaginal portion of the levator ani muscle, cardinal-uterosacral ligament complex, and the ATFP). These structures provide strong support by compressing the urethra during sudden increase in intra-abdominal pressure [19]. The size of the genital hiatus, especially A-P diameter, is correlated with the degree of POP [60].

Clinical applications

Understanding functional anatomy of the pelvic organs and the mechanism of pelvic floor support is essential to surgically correct POP and incontinence, both urinary and fecal. This knowledge is also very imperative for developing innovative technologies in this field. Normalized pelvic floor support is provided by an interaction between the levator ani muscles and connective tissue attachments. The pelvic floor muscles are the main support of pelvic organs, but these connective tissue attachments are necessary for optimal support from the pelvic muscles. The vagina as well provides support to the bladder, urethra, cervix, and rectum. The levator ani and coccygeus muscles together form the pelvic floor muscle support. In a standing position, the upper two-thirds of the vagina is almost horizontal with a 130-degree angle between the upper and lower axis. There are three levels of connective tissue stabilizing the vagina. The cardinal-uterosacral ligament complex (level I) holds the cervix and upper vagina over the levator plate and away from the genital hiatus. The lateral support (level II) is directly provided by the

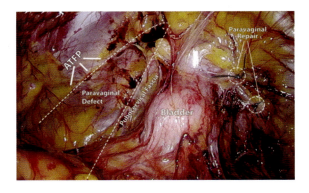

(a) Laparoscopic view

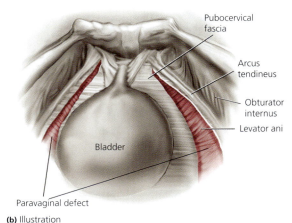

(b) Illustration

Figure 3.16 Paravaginal defect. Source: Robert D. Moore and John R. Miklos. Reproduced with permission.

ATFP. The lower vagina (level III) is supported predominantly by connecting to the perineal membrane anteriorly and the perineal body posteriorly. Identifying an underlying anatomical defect is highly critical to a successful site-specific surgical correction of POP.

Full understanding of the anatomical landmarks is extremely vital for successful surgery. The ATFP is the most prominent landmark of the paravesical space, which is fundamental for anti-incontinence and POP surgeries. The ATLA is another important landmark of an upper margin of the aponeurosis of the ileococcygeus muscle.

The "hammock hypothesis" explains a concept of urethral support during an increase in intra-abdominal pressure as the interaction of fascia and muscles compresses the urethra. In terms of anal continence, the levator ani muscle, especially the puborectalis muscle, helps pulling the anorectal junction forward, contributing to anal continence.

References

1. Wu JM, Kawasaki A, Hundley AF, Dieter AA, Myers ER, Sung VW. Predicting the number of women who will undergo incontinence and prolapse surgery, 2010 to 2050. *Am J Obstet Gynecol* 2011; **205**(3):230–5.
2. Olsen AL, Smith VJ, Bergstrom JO, Colling JC, Clark AL. Epidemiology of surgically managed pelvic organ prolapse and urinary incontinence. *Obstet Gynecol* 1997;**89**(4):501–6.
3. Braun V. In search of (better) sexual pleasure: Female genital "cosmetic" surgery. *Sexualities* 2005;**8**(4):407–24.

4. Handa VL, Pannu HK, Siddique S, Gutman R, VanRooyen J, Cundiff G. Architectural differences in the bony pelvis of women with and without pelvic floor disorders. *Obstet Gynecol* 2003;**102**(6):1283–90.
5. Burch JC. Urethrovaginal fixation to Cooper's ligament for correction of stress incontinence, cystocele, and prolapse. *Am J Obstet Gynecol* 1961;**81**:281.
6. Albright TS, Gehrich AP, Davis GD, Sabi FL, Buller JL. Arcus tendineus fascia pelvis: A further understanding. *Am J Obstet Gynecol* 2005;**193**(3 Pt 1):677–81.
7. Pit MJ, De Ruiter MC, Lycklama À, Nijeholt AAB, Marani E, Zwartendijk J. Anatomy of the arcus tendineus fasciae pelvis in females. *Clin Anat* 2003;**16**(2):131–7.
8. Mostwin JL, Genadry R, Saunders R, Yang A. Stress incontinence observed with real time sonography and dynamic fastscan magnetic resonance imaging—insights into pathophysiology. *Scand J Urol Nephrol* 2001;**35**(207):94–9.
9. Lawson JO. Pelvic anatomy. I. Pelvic floor muscles. *Ann R Coll Surg Engl* 1974;**54**(5):244–52.
10. Kirschner-Hermanns R, Wein B, Niehaus S, Schaefer W, Jakse G. The contribution of magnetic resonance imaging of the pelvic floor to the understanding of urinary incontinence. *Br J Urol* 1993;**72**(5 Pt 2):715–8.
11. Tunn R, Paris S, Fischer W, Hamm B, Kuchinke J. Static magnetic resonance imaging of the pelvic floor muscle morphology in women with stress urinary incontinence and pelvic prolapse. *Neurourol Urodyn* 1998;**17**(6):579–89.
12. DeLancey JO, Kearney R, Chou Q, Speights S, Binno S. The appearance of levator ani muscle abnormalities in magnetic resonance images after vaginal delivery. *Obstet Gynecol* 2003;**101**(1):46–53.
13. Barber MD, Bremer RE, Thor KB, Dolber PC, Kuehl TJ, Coates KW. Innervation of the female levator ani muscles. *Am J Obstet Gynecol* 2002;**187**(1):64–71.

14. Gilpin SA, Gosling JA, Smith AR, Warrell DW. The pathogenesis of genitourinary prolapse and stress incontinence of urine: A histological and histochemical study. *Br J Obstet Gynaecol* 1989;**96**(1):15–23.

15. Gosling JA, Dixon JS, Critchley HO, Thompson SA. A comparative study of the human external sphincter and periurethral levator ani muscles. *Br J Urol* 1981;**53**(1):35–41.

16. Muellner SR. The anatomies of the female urethra: A critical review. *Obstet Gynecol* 1959;**14**:429–34.

17. DeLancey JO, Morgan DM, Fenner DE, et al. Comparison of levator ani muscle defects and function in women with and without pelvic organ prolapse. *Obstet Gynecol* 2007;**109**(2 Pt 1): 295–302.

18. Morgan DM, Larson K, Lewicky-Gaupp C, Fenner DE, DeLancey JO. Vaginal support as determined by levator ani defect status 6 weeks after primary surgery for pelvic organ prolapse. *Int J Gynaecol Obstet* 2011;**114**(2):141–4.

19. Ashton-Miller JA, DeLancey JO. Functional anatomy of the female pelvic floor. *Ann N Y Acad Sci* 2007;**1101**:266–96.

20. Lewicky-Gaupp C, Brincat C, Yousuf A, Patel DA, Delancey JO, Fenner DE. Fecal incontinence in older women: Are levator ani defects a factor? *Am J Obstet Gynecol* 2010;**202**(5):491–6.

21. DeLancey JO. Correlative study of paraurethral anatomy. *Obstet Gynecol* 1986;**68**(1):91–7.

22. DeLancey JO. Structural anatomy of the posterior pelvic compartment as it relates to rectocele. *Am J Obstet Gynecol* 1999;**180**(4):815–23.

23. Hsu Y, Lewicky-Gaupp C, DeLancey JO. Posterior compartment anatomy as seen in magnetic resonance imaging and 3-dimensional reconstruction from asymptomatic nulliparas. *Am J Obstet Gynecol* 2008;**198**(6):651–7.

24. Woodman PJ, Graney DO. Anatomy and physiology of the female perineal body with relevance to obstetrical injury and repair. *Clin Anat* 2002;**15**(5):321–34.

25. Herbenick D, Schick V, Reece M, Sanders S, Fortenberry JD. Pubic hair removal among women in the United States: Prevalence, methods, and characteristics. *J Sex Med* 2010; **7**(10):3322–30.

26. DeMaria AL, Flores M, Hirth JM, Berenson AB. Complications related to pubic hair removal. *Am J Obstet Gynecol* 2014;**210**(6):521–8.

27. Lloyd J, Crouch NS, Minto CL, Liao LM, Creighton SM. Female genital appearance: "normality" unfolds. *BJOG* 2005;**112**(5):643–6.

28. Laube DW. Cosmetic therapies in obstetrics and gynecology practice: Putting a toe in the water? *Obstet Gynecol* 2008;**111**(5):1034–6.

29. Miklos JR, Moore R. Postoperative cosmetic expectations for patients considering labiaplasty surgery: Our experience with 550 patients. *Surg Technol Int* 2011;**1**:170–4.

30. Pappis CH, Hadzihamberis PS. Hypertrophy of the labia minora. *Pediatr Surg Int* 1987;**2**(1):50–1.

31. Capraro VJ. Congenital anomalies. *Clin Obstet Gynecol* 1971;**14**(4):988–1012.

32. Radman HM. Hypertrophy of the labia minora. *Obstet Gynecol* 1976;**48**(1 Suppl):78S–9S.

33. Hailparn TR. What is a girl to do? The problem of adolescent labial hypertrophy. *Obstet Gynecol* 2014;**123** Suppl 1: 124S–5S.

34. Rouzier R, Louis-Sylvestre C, Paniel BJ, Haddad B. Hypertrophy of labia minora: Experience with 163 reductions. *Am J Obstet Gynecol* 2000;**182**(1 Pt 1):35–40.

35. O'Connell HE, Eizenberg N, Rahman M, Cleeve J. The anatomy of the distal vagina: Towards unity. *J Sex Med* 2008;**5**(8):1883–91.

36. Puppo V. Anatomy and physiology of the clitoris, vestibular bulbs, and labia minora with a review of the female orgasm and the prevention of female sexual dysfunction. *Clin Anat* 2013;**26**(1):134–52.

37. Rees MA, O'Connell HE, Plenter RJ, Hutson JM. The suspensory ligament of the clitoris: Connective tissue supports of the erectile tissues of the female urogenital region. *Clin Anat* 2000;**13**(6):397–403.

38. Goldstein I, Berman J. Vasculogenic female sexual dysfunction: Vaginal engorgement and clitoral erectile insufficiency syndromes. *Int J Impot Res* 1998;**10**:S84–90; discussion S98–101.

39. Gräfenberg E. The role of the urethra in female orgasm. *Int J Sexol* 1950;**3**(3):145–8.

40. Ostrzenski A. G-spot anatomy: A new discovery. *J Sex Med* 2012;**9**(5):1355–9.

41. Gravina GL, Brandetti F, Martini P, et al. Measurement of the thickness of the urethrovaginal space in women with or without vaginal orgasm. *J Sex Med* 2008;**5**(3):610–8.

42. Perry JD, Whipple B. Multiple components of the female orgasm. In: *Circumvaginal Musculature and Sexual Function*, pp. 101–14. Basel, Switzerland: S. Karger, 1982.

43. Sevely JL, Bennett J. Concerning female ejaculation and the female prostate. *J Sex Res* 1978;**14**(1):1–20.

44. Mould D, Graber B. Women's orgasm and the muscle spindle. In: *Circumvaginal Musculature and Vaginal Function*, pp. 93–100. Basel, Switzerland: S. Karger, 1982.

45. Kilchevsky A, Vardi Y, Lowenstein L, Gruenwald I. Is the female G-spot truly a distinct anatomic entity? *J Sex Med* 2012;**9**(3):719–26.

46. Puppo V. Embryology and anatomy of the vulva: The female orgasm and women's sexual health. *Eur J Obstet Gynecol Reprod Biol* 2011;**154**(1):3–8.

47. Pastor Z. Female ejaculation orgasm vs. coital incontinence: A systematic review. *J Sex Med* 2013;**10**(7):1682–91.

48. DeLancey JO. Anatomic aspects of vaginal eversion after hysterectomy. *Am J Obstet Gynecol* 1992;**166**(6):1717–28.

49. Umek WH, Morgan DM, Ashton-Miller JA, DeLancey JO. Quantitative analysis of uterosacral ligament origin and insertion points by magnetic resonance imaging. *Obstet Gynecol* 2004;**103**(3):447.

50. Campbell RM. The anatomy and histology of the sacrouterine ligaments. *Am J Obstet Gynecol* 1950;**59**(1):1–12.

51. Gabriel B, Watermann D, Hancke K, et al. Increased expression of matrix metalloproteinase 2 in uterosacral ligaments is associated with pelvic organ prolapse. *Int Urogynecol J* 2006;**17**(5):478–82.

52. Gabriel B, Denschlag D, Göbel H, et al. Uterosacral ligament in postmenopausal women with or without pelvic organ prolapse. *Int Urogynecol J* 2005;**16**(6):475–9.

53. Buller JL, Thompson JR, Cundiff GW, Sullivan LK, Ybarra MAS, Bent AE. Uterosacral ligament: Description of anatomic relationships to optimize surgical safety. *Obstet Gynecol* 2001;**97**(6):873–9.

54. Silva WA, Pauls RN, Segal JL, Rooney CM, Kleeman SD, Karram MM. Uterosacral ligament vault suspension: Five-year outcomes. *Obstet Gynecol* 2006;**108**(2):255–63.

55. Weber A, Abrams P, Brubaker L, et al. The standardization of terminology for researchers in female pelvic floor disorders. *Int Urogynecol J* 2001;**12**(3):178–86.

56. Haylen B, de Ridder D, Freeman R, et al. An International Urogynecological Association (IUGA)/International Continence Society (ICS) joint report on the terminology for female pelvic floor dysfunction. *Int Urogynecol J* 2010;**21**(1):5–26.

57. Delancey JO. Fascial and muscular abnormalities in women with urethral hypermobility and anterior vaginal wall prolapse. *Am J Obstet Gynecol* 2002;**187**(1):93–8.

58. Richardson AC. The rectovaginal septum revisited: Its relationship to rectocele and its importance in rectocele repair. *Clin Obstet Gynecol* 1993;**36**(4):976–83.

59. Milley PS, Nichols DH. The relationship between the pubo-urethral ligaments and the urogenital diaphragm in the human female. *Anat Rec* 1971;**170**(3):281–3.

60. Delancey JO, Hurd WW. Size of the urogenital hiatus in the levator ani muscles in normal women and women with pelvic organ prolapse. *Obstet Gynecol* 1998;**91**(3):364–8.

CHAPTER 4
Definitions

Michael P. Goodman

Caring for Women Wellness Center, Davis, CA, USA

To steal ideas from one person is plagiarism; to steal from many is research.

Steven Wright

A need exists to develop a reasonable nomenclature to replace proprietary terms such as "vaginal rejuvenation" (VRJ), "Designer Laser Vaginoplasty," "revirgination," and so forth, as delightful as they may be, before they become entrenched in the rubric of medical and lay terminology. No one specific term is accepted to describe these procedures, although labiaplasty (LP), labial reduction, vaginoplasty (VP), clitoral unhooding, "intimate operations," and, more encompassing, female genital plastic/cosmetic or plastic/aesthetic surgery (FGPS), female cosmetic genital surgery (FCGS), vulvovaginal aesthetic surgery (VVAS), aesthetic vulvovaginal surgery (AVS), and cosmeto-plastic gynecology (CPG) are among the many utilized. Although all terms are acceptable and descriptive, I have chosen FGPS, and shall use this term throughout the textbook.

FGPS is surgery on the female external genitalia and vagina designed to subjectively improve appearance, diminish discomfort, and/or potentially provide psychological and functional improvement in sexual stimulation and satisfaction.

Labiaplasty involves surgical alteration, usually via reduction, of the size of the labia. Although this usually involves reduction of the labia minora (LP-m) or, less frequently, labia majora (LP-M), occasionally LP involves reconstruction after obstetrical injury or, more rarely, enlargement via injection of bulking agents or autologous fat transfer. The procedure may be performed utilizing sharp dissection with instrumentation including scalpel, stem iris or plastictype fine Metzenbaum scissors,

electrosurgical or radiofrequency needle electrode, or laser (usually via a "touch" fiber). Surgical techniques include V-wedge resection and its modifications, (curvi) linear reduction/resection/excision of the leading edge, excision of the inferior-most portion of the labum, with rotation of the superior flap, Z-plasty, de-epithelization, and other less-utilized techniques (Figures 4.1 and 4.2).

Clitoral hood reduction (RCH or CHR) (aka "clitoriplasty," "clitoral unhooding") involves size reduction of redundant and/or "wrinkly" central hood or redundant lateral prepucial folds for cosmetic reasons or, less commonly, mid-line surgical separation of the female prepuce designed to produce more "exposure" of the clitoral glans in cases of phimosis, theoretically providing improved sexual stimulation. "Unhooding" for exposure of a clitoral glans entirely "trapped" by a phimotic clitoral hood and a reduction procedure designed to reduce aesthetically displeasing redundant folds of the clitoral prepuce are entirely separate procedures, performed for different indications. However, patients report "more feeling" and appear to be quite satisfied after removal of clitoral hood redundancy (author's experience, and personal communication from Drs. Robert Moore and John Miklos; not confirmed by peer-reviewed research). Whether this is secondary to more friction transmitted to the clitoral glans and body or to psychosexual reasons secondary to what this woman considers to be a more pleasing countenance is unknown.

Figures 4.1 and 4.2 are anatomic drawings. Figures 4.3 through 4.5 display anatomy with redundant clitoral

Female Genital Plastic and Cosmetic Surgery, First Edition. Edited by Michael P. Goodman.

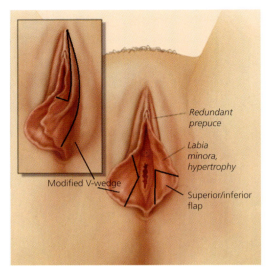

Figure 4.1 V-wedge with reduction clitoral hood; superior-inferior flap procedures. © R. Moore and J. Miklos, modified by M. Goodman. Used with permission.

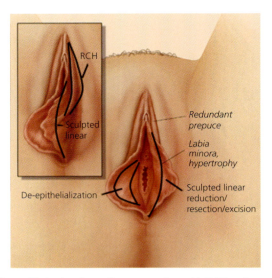

Figure 4.2 Sculpted curvilinear resection with RCH and de-epithelialization. © R. Moore and J. Miklos, modified by M. Goodman. Used with permission.

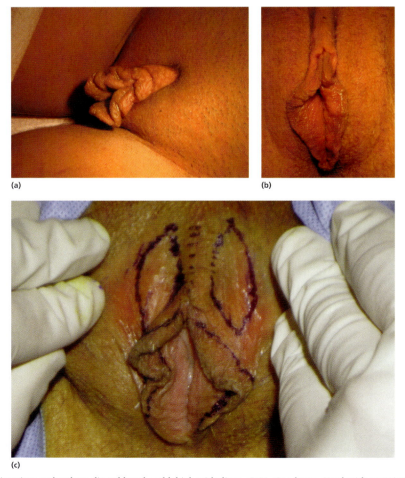

Figure 4.3 (a) Superior view, redundant clitoral hood and labial epithelium. © M. Goodman. Used with permission. (b) Anterior view, redundant clitoral hood and labial epithelium. © M. Goodman. Used with permission. (c) Linear resection and RCH markings. (Hood redundancy is reduced with retraction, which "stretches" the redundancy.) © M. Goodman. Used with permission.

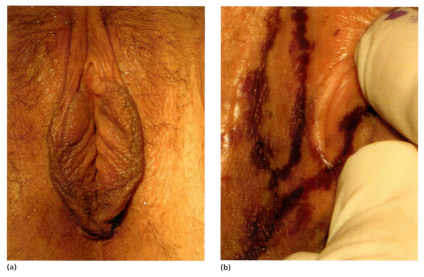

Figure 4.4 (a) Anterior view, redundant clitoral hood and labial epithelium. © M. Goodman. Used with permission. (b) Markings for linear resection plus separate hood redundancy excisional lines. © M. Goodman. Used with permission.

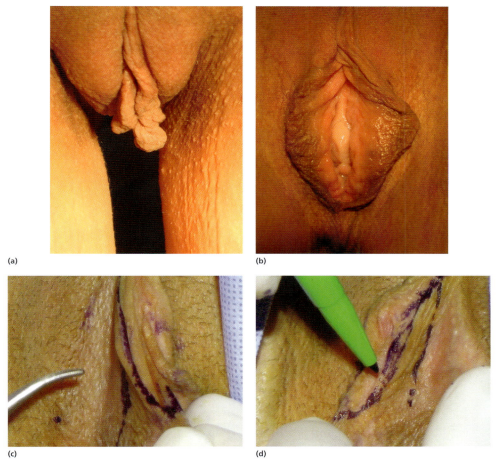

Figure 4.5 (a) Superior view, redundant clitoral hood and labial epithelium. © M. Goodman. Used with permission. (b) Anterior view, redundant clitoral hood and labial epithelium. © M. Goodman. Used with permission. (c) "Y" modification of V-wedge resection to incorporate clitoral hood redundancy, #1. © M. Goodman. Used with permission. (d) "Y" modification of V-wedge resection to incorporate clitoral hood redundancy. Redundancy noted in Figure 4.5(a) reduced by lateral retraction. © M. Goodman. Used with permission.

and labial epithelium, along with placement of incisional lines for LP and RCH. Only superficial epithelium is resected along these lines. The mechanics and performance of labiaplasty and clitoral hood resections will be well reviewed in Chapter 8.

Vaginal rejuvenation originated as a proprietary term first defined and marketed as "Laser Vaginal Rejuvenation" by David Matlock, MD, MBA, and commonly referred to simply as "vaginal rejuvenation." VRJ is a colloquial term that, unfortunately, can mean different (surgical and non-surgical) things to different people. This may prove especially confusing with new non-surgical laser and radiofrequency vaginal tightening techniques presently being tested and brought to market. However, the term is widely utilized in the literature [1,2] and is here to stay. When referring to FGPS, it should be considered an "umbrella term" encompassing an array of elective vaginal tightening procedures designed to tighten the vaginal barrel, provide additional pelvic floor support, and increase friction to the vaginal walls and cervix for reasons of improving sexual pleasure and, potentially, orgasmic function. As such, VRJ is utilized by many surgeons to describe any surgical procedure utilized on either the distal, or both proximal and distal vagina, to produce increased functional tone in order to improve sexual pleasure and facilitate

orgasmic function. The physiology and biomechanics of these procedures and their effects on orgasmic function will be discussed in Chapter 10. As utilized herein, VRJ may include colpoperineoplasty, perineoplasty, and/or vaginoplasty. The procedures themselves will be discussed and dissected in Chapter 9.

Perineoplasty (PP) involves surgical reconstruction of the vulvar vestibule, vaginal introitus, perineum, and perineal body whereby scarred and redundant tissue is excised, any distal posterior compartment defect is repaired, and the superficial transverse perineal musculature is re-approximated in layers in the midline, thus elevating and bulking the perineal body, introitus, and vulvar vestibule. The perineum is re-approximated in an attenuated and carefully anatomic manner (Figures 4.6–4.8).

The term *vaginoplasty*, like "vaginal rejuvenation," is a descriptive but unofficial term, not found in medical nomenclature but present, like VRJ, in patient and marketing vernacular. As defined by genital plastic/cosmetic surgeons, it refers to a general tightening procedure involving the vaginal barrel, from the distal vagina, always up to or proximal to the mid-vagina, and always involving both removal of scarified submucosal tissue and re-approximation of the levator ani musculature. It may or may not involve the proximal vagina, either via a high posterior colporrhaphy, anterior

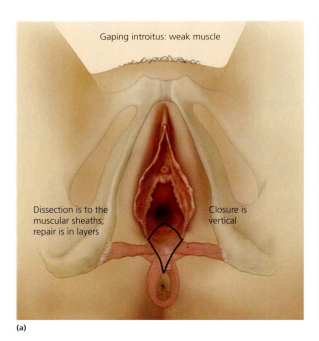

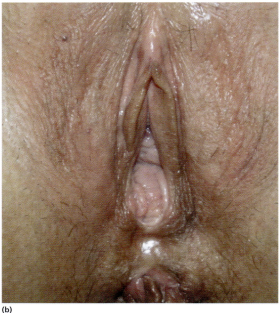

(a)   (b)

Figure 4.6 (a) Perineoplasty incision lines. © J. Miklos and R. Moore, modified by M. Goodman. Used with permission. (b) Gaping introitus with loss of perineal support. © M.P. Goodman. Used with permission.

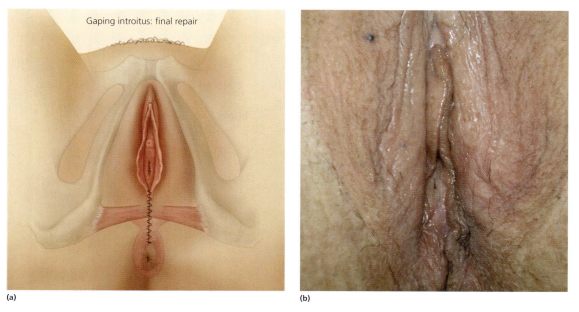

Figure 4.7 (a) Completed perineoplasty repair. © J. Miklos and R. Moore. Used with permission. (b) Post-op perineoplasty. © M.P. Goodman. Used with permission.

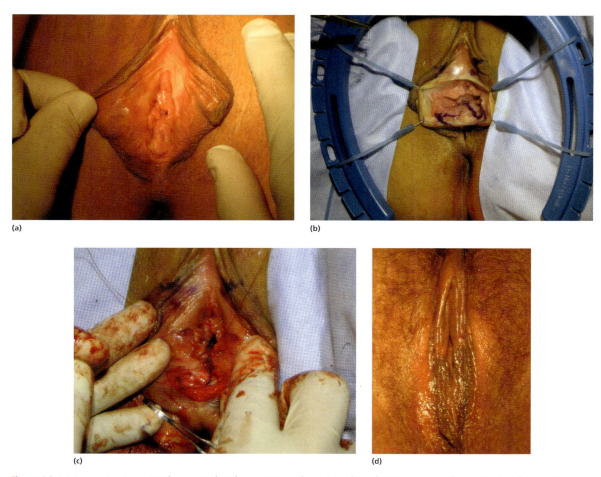

Figure 4.8 (a) Pre-op PP. © M. Goodman. Used with permission. (b) Incision lines for PP. © M. Goodman. Used with permission. (c) Reconstructing introitus. © M. Goodman. Used with permission. (d) Completed LP and PP, 6 weeks post-op. © M. Goodman. Used with permission.

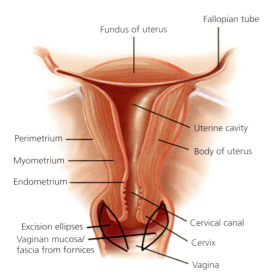

Figure 4.9 Excising elliptical strips of vaginal mucosa from proximal vaginal fornices, occasionally added to vaginoplasty procedures in patients with excessively widened proximal vaginal fornices. From collection of AUA Foundation. Public domain. Modification © M. Goodman. Used with permission.

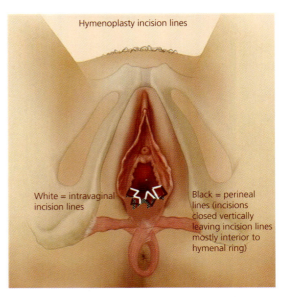

Figure 4.10 Hymenoplasty repair of rents in hymenal ring. White lines are intra-vaginal; black extend slightly into vulvar vestibule. Incisions closed vertically to approximate hymenal aperture. © J. Miklos and R. Moore, modified by M. Goodman. Used with permission.

colporrhaphy, and/or removal of elliptical strips of lateral forniceal mucosa to provide superficial mucosal and fascial approximation (Figure 4.9). A vaginoplasty usually involves a posterior colporrhaphy modified to more tightly re-approximate vaginal walls and strengthen and bulk the posterior vaginal wall utilizing a three- to four-layer closure technique. Tools utilized include scalpel, needle electrode, scissors, laser, or radiofrequency electrode. Site-specific defects are repaired, and fascial defects are re-approximated either horizontally or vertically. The term may be confusing, as it applies to tightening of the vaginal barrel, and can include mid-distal vaginal repair of the pelvic floor, but may incorporate proximal vaginal work as well. In the author's opinion, and in the aesthetic vulvovaginal surgical community, most vaginal tightening procedures take place in the distal half of the vagina. Size-limiting alterations of the proximal vagina may be considered only for those women who have a symptomatic cystourethrocoele and/or significant symptomatic widening of the vaginal fornices.

Colpoperineoplasty (CP) is a rather recent addition to the nomenclature on the subject, first suggested by Jack Pardo S from Chile [3]. It is a valid and descriptive term meant to encompass both VP and PP and will be utilized hereafter to describe the combination of VP and PP procedures.

Hymenoplasty (HP) is a surgical procedure whereby the hymenal ring is surgically altered, frequently via small tightening revisions or denuding/approximation sutures, to produce size minimization of the vaginal aperture, designed to produce temporary introital tightening and facilitate bleeding with subsequent coitus (Figure 4.10). HP is most usually requested as a premarital cultural imperative in a previously sexually active Muslim woman facing an arranged marriage at the consummation of which she is expected (mandated!) to exhibit difficulty with initial penetration and lose a modest quantity of blood upon penetration.

References

1. Kent D, Pelosi III MA. Vaginal rejuvenation: An in-depth look at the history and technical procedure. *Am J Cosmetic Surg* 2012;**29**:89–96.
2. Moore RD, Miklos JR. Vaginal reconstruction and rejuvenation surgery: Is there data to support improved sexual function? *Am J Cosmetic Surgery* 2012;**29**:97–115.
3. Pardo J, Sola V, Ricci P, Guiloff E, Freundlich D. Colpoperineoplasty in women with a sensation of a wide vagina. *Acta Obstet et Gynec* 2006:**85**;1125–7.

CHAPTER 5

Philosophy, rationale, and patient selection

Michael P. Goodman

Caring for Women Wellness Center, Davis, CA, USA

I was going to have cosmetic surgery until I noticed that the doctor's office was full of portraits by Picasso.

Rita Rudner

Cosmetic procedures conducted to alter body shape and contour are realities in our culture; they are opportunities for individuals to make physical changes in their appearance, correct (sometimes self-perceived) "defects," change how they look, address a physical problem of discomfort, enhance their self-esteem, look better in clothes, or improve sexual or orgasmic pleasure.

Those physicians who work with women interested in altering the size, shape, or contour of their external genitalia understand the degree to which extremes of size, dissymmetry, "looseness," or visually self-perceived unattractiveness affect that individual. Protrusion of the labia minora well beyond the confines of the labia majora with cosmetic, self-esteem, hygienic, sexual, and functional (discomfort, hygienic) ramifications are the most common reasons women give as initiators of their surgical request [1] (Figure 5.1). The experiences of many female genital plastic surgeons [1–19] confirm the very real and serious nature of these complaints. Many of these problems have been bothersome for years; these are not decisions hastily made. Physical discomfort and cosmetic concerns are frequently combined (Tables 5.1 and 5.2).

A recent social (pop cultural?) "ideal" appears to be emerging for female genital appearance. The "ideal" is one of absence, of a "clean," petite "slitlike" opening, achieved via removal of pubic hair and through genital plastic/cosmetic surgery. This is an ideal largely created in the media that generates contradictory messages for women [20]. As Lindy McDougall puts it, "female

genitals vary in appearance 'about as much as snow-flakes,' [and] by showing only minimalist clean labia, the implicit message is that women should be worried if their genitals do not match up to this ideal" [20].

Actual quotes from patients speak for themselves: "It's that when you feel bad about your body, especially this part of your body, it's kind of impossible to let your true feelings and passions show." And, "It never bothered my husband, but it was always like 'Yuck!' All I know is that what I had I didn't like" [21]. Additionally, according to Laura Berman, PhD, director of a treatment clinic for female sexual dysfunction, a woman's comfort level with her genitals affects her sexual enjoyment [21]. Of course, any surgical procedure that involves genital intervention has the potential to harm [sexual] function. Dr. Berman goes on to recommend pelvic floor strengthening, advice that finds little argument.

"Plastic surgery was developed to improve quality of life, and vulvovaginal plastic surgery is no different. Having a harmonious vagina makes us feel better with ourselves and with our partner, makes us more comfortable with our intimate life, denotes youth, and increases sexual gratification," according to Lina Triana, MD, of Cali, Colombia, speaking at the 2013 Annual Meeting of the American Society for Aesthetic Plastic Surgery.

For women who wish to have cosmetic reconstruction of the external genitalia, is there any valid reason to deny them this right? Genital reshaping would appear to fall into the same category as other cosmetic alterations

Female Genital Plastic and Cosmetic Surgery, First Edition. Edited by Michael P. Goodman.
© 2016 John Wiley & Sons, Ltd. Published 2016 by John Wiley & Sons, Ltd.

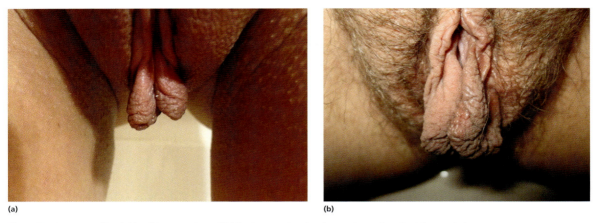

(a)　　　　　　　　　　　　　　　　　　　　　　　　(b)

Figure 5.1 (a) Protruding labia. (b) Protrusion of labia. Source: M. Goodman. Reproduced with permission.

Table 5.1 Patient's indications for labia and/or clitoral hood revision surgery.

Indications Author (reference #) (# patients)	"Aesthetic"	"Self-Esteem" ("Feel more normal")	"Functional" (discomfort with clothes, activities, coitus, etc.)			At Urging of Sexual Partner	Combined Aesthetic and Functional
Rouzier et al. (3) (#163)	87%		Discomfort in clothes 64%	Discomfort with exercise 26%	Entry dyspareunia 43%		
Pardo et al. (15) (#55)							67%
Miklos & Moore (10) (#131)	37%		32% (combination functional complaints)				31%
Goodman et al. (7) (#211)	55.4%	35.5%	75.3% (combination functional complaints)			5.3%	

Table 5.2 Patient's indications for intra-vaginal tightening procedures.

Indications Author (reference #) (# patients)	Diminished Sensation	"Wide vagina"	Unable to Orgasm (previously orgasmic)	Diminished Libido	"Want to tighten"	Wish to Increase Friction &/or Enhance Sexual Pleasure	"Feel loose/ large"	"To enhance partner's sexual pleasure"	At Urging of Sexual Partner
Pardo et al. (4) (#53)	96%	100%	27%	49%	92%	74%			
Goodman et al. (7) (#81)						56.8%	50%	40.7%	4.9%

of the body [22], although care must be taken in regards to sexual health. As in other parts of her body, nature has provided the woman with an enormous diversity in the size, shape, and design of her external genitalia. Because a body part is deemed by others to be "in the normal range," however, does not mean that its form or function is satisfactory to its "wearer." Writers as diverse as Rufus Cartwright, Linda Cardozo, David Matlock, and Alex Simopoulos have contemporaneously weighed in on the subject and find agreement in the fact that effecting a change in her individual genitalia for cosmetic and certainly functional reasons is (and should continue to be) an individual woman's right, not to be legislated or restricted by any third party [23].

Women's sexuality and cosmetic desires have been judged from a male and patriarchal viewpoint (surprisingly, even when judged by female practitioners), as evidenced by comments such as: "Men…do not usually want the size of their genitals reduced for [cosmetic and functional] reasons," and, accordingly, women should "find alternative solutions" [24]. Additionally, very many female physicians and so-called activists wish to force their own definitions of propriety and "normalcy" upon others by denigrating individual women's requests for modification [25–27]. If a woman wishes to enhance her perception of herself or her comfort by breast augmentation or reduction, or by abdominoplasty or blepharoplasty, and asks her practitioner, she will find no argument and will be referred to a competent colleague. Unfortunately, however, if she asks her provider for referral for a vulvovaginal cosmetic/plastic procedure, many times the provider will demur, negating the patient's concern with an officious "why would you want to do that…you're normal" (translation: "I wouldn't do that, and I am an expert [and frequently also female]").

Both functional and cosmetic factors provide motivation for labial reduction and include improvement in self-esteem; diminishment of embarrassment caused by a perception of being large or asymmetrical, with labia minora "peeking out" from between the labia majora; discomfort in clothing; chafing; discomfort when taking part in sports; hygienic difficulties and entry dysparunia via invagination of protuberant tissue [3, 7, 10, 15, 17]. FGPS patients frequently express dissatisfaction with gross protrusion of the labia minora well beyond the confines of the approximated labia majora while visualizing their pudenda from above.

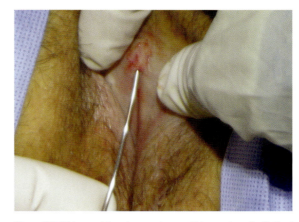

Figure 5.2 Phimosed hood secondary to lichen sclerosis. Patient pre-treated with locally applied clobetasol followed by several months of compounded topically applied estrogen/testosterone. Initial manual separation upper hood noted proximal to probe. Source: M. Goodman. Reproduced with permission.

Women request modification or "tightening" of the vaginal introitus and inner vagina secondary to displeasure and self-consciousness over the appearance of the opening, discomfort secondary to irritation of exophytic vaginal tissue, absent or poor control of pelvic floor musculature, sensation of a "wide vagina," less/lack of "feeling"/friction with sexual relations, diminishment of pleasure and self-esteem, and greater difficulty achieving orgasm [4–7].

Women request revision of their clitoral hoods usually for two reasons. Occasionally, the clitoris is "buried" under an over-abundant prepuce or "trapped" under a tight, phimosed hood, leading to little direct stimulation, regardless of maneuvers attempted (Figure 5.2). Most cases of phimosis are secondary to lichen sclerosis and as such are difficult to adjudicate. A prescribed period of local application of clobetasol and possibly estrogen/testosterone is mandated pre- as well as postoperatively [28].

Much more commonly, as with hypertrophied labia, many women find their generous prepucial folds unsightly, although rarely do their sexual partners find this to be a problem.

Women present for vaginal tightening procedures for enhancement of sexual function. Patients state that their vagina feels "wide" or "open" or "loose and relaxed." They relate less sensation during intercourse, difficulty or inability in achieving coital orgasm as they did before, and requesting a repair in an attempt to return the vagina to a more pre-delivery size and state [6]. Frequently these women have aging male partners, many of whom require greater friction, and the lessening of friction is anathema to satisfying sexual relations. When gynecologists turn these patients away because their only symptom is sexual dysfunction, they are ignoring one of the major aspects of quality of life: sexuality and sexual function.

Women requesting HP make up a very different group, but their issues are certainly compelling [29, 30]. Leaving out a small number of women who seek consultation "to be a virgin again" or as a "gift" to their sexual partner, the bulk of this group seek surgery to conform to religious or ethnic rules on virginity. In many societies, most notably Islamic cultures of the Middle East, eastern Europe, North Africa, and parts of Asia (and their transplanted members around the world), it is imperative that a woman be a virgin upon consummation of her marriage. Virginity is confirmed by evidence of introital tightness and loss of an amount of blood upon penetration. Indeed, women marrying in some Islamic cultures must submit to an examination by an Imam or his representative to assure the clergy and groom's family that the prospective bride is indeed a virgin. Often, the "mother-in-law" awaits confirmation from the blood-stained linen of the marital bed. A lot may be riding on that "intact," tightened introitus, the absence of which may mean familial embarrassment, ostracism, and consequences difficult for the culturally uninitiated to imagine, including death [31, 32].

In the experience of the author, and from an informal poll of other experienced vulvovaginal aesthetic surgeons, women considering FGPS largely fall into two distinct groups: [1] young, usually nulliparous women (age ~16–30 years) seeking labial reduction for reasons of self-consciousness, often with secondary sexual inhibition, diminishment of self-esteem, and/or the functional reasons of discomfort in clothing/sports, hygienic difficulties, and/or invagination of the labia with coitus, or aesthetic concerns frequently precluding the ability to wear bathing suits or thong underwear; or [2] mid-aged (40s, 50s) women who have completed their childbearing and are contemplating renewing themselves during their journey through midlife, frequently with similar complaints as their younger counterparts. Additionally, age, "gravity," genetics, and previous childbirth have conspired to enlarge and

"droop" the labia (minora and majora), gape the introitus, and enlarge and relax the upper vagina and separate and stretch the levator musculature, leading to diminished friction, "gripability," and sexual and orgasmic pleasure. It has been shown that vaginal tone affects vaginal sensation and the ability to reach orgasm [33]. The American Society for Aesthetic Plastic Surgery kept demographic data for VRJ procedures in 2007 and found that of 4,505 procedures noted, 38.1% were in the 19–34 age group and 54.4% aged 35–50 (and 2.4% 18 and under; 5.1% 51 and older) [34], data not dissimilar from that collected by Alter [17] and Goodman *et al.* [7].

Most important as well is the status of the male half of the [hetero]sexual unit. The aesthetic vulvovaginal surgeon must inquire as to the erectile health and constancy of the male partner and, if it is precarious, either work with him or refer to an andrologist in order to improve his erectile quality. Not rarely, surgery has been deferred via a significant improvement in erectile quality.

"Ugly," "floppy," "sticking out," "self-conscious," "loose," "he gets lost in there," "I feel open [and vulnerable]," "more difficult for me to orgasm"—these are among the comments and presenting complaints that FGPS practitioners hear. Very rarely is the patient requesting consultation at the urging of her sexual partner (Tables 5.1 and 5.2). "It doesn't bother him; he says he loves me as I am" is a typical comment. Although not primarily generated by their partners, requests for FGPS procedures appear to be supported by partners, although outside sources (medical organizations, medical pundits, physicians not experienced consulting and working with these women) are frequently a source of discouragement, reflecting an attitude both paternalistic/maternalistic ("you shouldn't be doing this") and "retrofeminist" ("glory in your uniqueness").

Why are cosmetic surgeons seeing the large upturn of interest in these procedures? A variety of factors are involved, including more openness and sharing through social Internet sites including MySpace, YouTube, Facebook, and so forth; more information in the mainstream media; more viewing of pornography, in which models are frequently shaved and usually exhibit "petite" external genitalia (the "Barbie-doll look"); and most especially, in this author's opinion (although no statistics are available), more depilatory activities, diminishing the "cushioning" effects of pubic hair and making more "well-endowed" external genitalia appear prominent.

Herbenick and her colleagues at the University of Indiana have further developed this thesis [35].

Media images tend to reflect pop culture, and viewing genital appearance in both relatively "mainstream" media such as *Playboy* and other magazines, as well as in more pornographic publications notes both the relative emphasis on pudenda in these images, as well as altered genital appearance over time, with women's genitalia certainly over the past 7–8 years appearing more ill defined, noting more of a "genital cleft" or "Barbie-doll look," with labia minora minimized or absent with hairless, undefined genitalia resembling those of a prepubescent female [36].

Increasingly, women are empowered and "taking charge" of their own sexuality. Many studies [37–44] utilizing long-approved instruments such as the Pelvic Organ Prolapse/Urinary Incontinence Sexual Function Questionnaire (PISQ) and/or the Female Sexual Function Index (FSFI), both validated instruments measuring sexual function and dysfunction, make it clear that scores of desire, arousal, orgasm, and overall satisfaction all increase statistically significantly after repairs of pelvic floor defects.

In a revealing but unpublished master's thesis submission ("Ratings of Female Genital Attractiveness Pre- and Post-genital Cosmetic Surgery Differ by Age and Gender"), Pallatto and Meston asked men and women of various ages to rate "attractiveness" of altered and unaltered female genitalia. "The Female Genital Self-Image Scale (FGSIS), the Relational Concern and Personal Concern subscales of the Sexual Satisfaction Scale—Women, and the Female Sexual Functioning Index (FSFI) were administered. Genital self-image was positively correlated with functioning variables including arousal, lubrication, orgasm, satisfaction and pain, and negatively correlated with sexual distress. Men rated unaltered and altered genitalia as more attractive than women; older participants rated unaltered and altered genitalia as more attractive than younger participants, and men and women of all ages found altered genitalia more attractive than unaltered genitalia. Women with positive genital self-image experience higher levels of sexual functioning and lower levels of sexual distress. Female genitalia modified by genital cosmetic surgery are considered more attractive regardless of age and gender."

These are procedures that, for the most part, have improvement in genital appearance and female sexual satisfaction as their primary goal. In a restrictive Judeo-Christian and Islamic cultural heritage, this approaches blasphemy! These are female-empowering (procedures), something that some medical practitioners and religious pundits appear to find "unhealthy." Self-appointed editorialists find the idea of a woman lobbying for her own sexuality anathema to their image of "proper" female sexuality. Sexual health is the "last taboo" [45].

Why do these procedures appear to "work?" The answer for the external vulvar procedures may differ from internal tightening procedures.

For LP and RCH, the reasons appear obvious, and opinions grace the literature [1, 3, 10, 15, 46, 47]. Any procedure that diminishes self-consciousness, improves self-esteem, and diminishes coital discomfort might be expected to, generally, improve sexual pleasure and response.

For vaginal tightening procedures, there appears to be an evidence-proven anatomic justification [48–52]. Evidence in the literature confirms that orgasm and orgasmic intensity may be produced by, and intensified by, pressure on the more intensely innervated anterior vaginal wall [53–55] approximately one-quarter of the way in from the introitus, in the approximate area considered by many to be the "G-spot" or "G-area" [56–65]. Evidence also exists for a similar pressure-produced orgasmic response from the distal one-third to one-half of the posterior vagina [56, 57] and from pressure onto, or manipulation of, the cervix [58, 61, 65, 66] (see also Chapters 10 and 11).

Vaginal tightening operations, whether PP, VP, CP, or anterior/posterior colporrhaphy and/or perineorrhaphy, all serve, to a greater or lesser extent, to both tighten the vaginal barrel and extend and elevate the perineal body, thus both thrusting the penis, during penile-vaginal intercourse, upwards more snugly against the anterior vaginal wall (as well as increasing posterior wall friction) and, by narrowing the available room at the proximal vagina/vaginal fornices, provide for more direct stimulation of the cervix and posterior vagina, all of which are known to improve sexual response by either increasing stretching activity of the bulb of the clitoris, or via direct pressure/autonomic nervous stimulation of erotic areas.

That said, "patient selection" in this, as in all cosmetic, plastic, and other surgical procedures, remains paramount. Who are "good" or "proper" patients for FGPS, and who are more risky choices?

As in all medical procedures, the better educated the patient, the better her recovery and perceived outcome will be. It is equally imperative that your patient understand that, as in other anatomic parts, there naturally is an impressive variation in labial and vaginal size and that, even though she notes room for "improvement," she is quite "normal" and healthy just as she is. She should be informed, and it should be documented, that alternatives to surgical correction would include counseling to enable her to live well in the body that she presently has.

Your patient should have an "isolated complaint" (i.e., limited to the genital area, not just one in a litany of other body image dissatisfactions). The patients themselves, not their sexual partners or glamour magazine ideals, should generate their rationale for a surgical procedure.

It is essential that your patient understands that genital tissue is rarely "smooth and regular" prior to surgery, and that it will not be so after a surgical procedure. She can realistically expect reduction in size, and the cosmetic and functional benefits that may accrue from that, but she cannot expect "perfection," exact symmetry, or a specific outcome. Reasonable expectations are key to successful outcome, and all care and attention must be given to promote your patient's understanding of that fact!

While it is not unexpected that many of our patients may have one or several sexual dissatisfactions, all care must be taken to rule out a sexual dysfunction (see Chapter 18). Because this is typically a strictly *elective* surgery, high-risk patients such as smokers, less-than-well-controlled diabetics, psychologically unstable individuals, and women with serious and/or multiple medical maladies should be screened if complications are to be minimized. Likewise for individuals with body dysmorphia, including eating disorders.

Patient selection, especially in relationship to "reasonable expectations," is crucial. Also of paramount importance, as pointed out by Liao and Creighton [67] is as considered an evaluation of motivations as possible, in an effort to *"primum non nocere."*

References

1. Miklos JP, Moore RD. Postoperative cosmetic expectations for patients considering labiaplasty surgery: Our experience with 550 patients. *Surg Technol Int* 2012;**21**:170–4.

2. Hodgekinson DJ, Hait G. Aesthetic vaginal labiaplasty. *Plast Reconstr Surg* 1984;**74**:414–6.

3. Rouzier R, Louis-Sylvestre C, Paniel BJ, Hadded B. Hypertrophy of the labia minora; experience with 163 reductions *Am J Obstet Gynecol* 2000;**182**:35–40.

4. Pardo J, Sola V, Ricci P, Guiloff E, Freundlich D. Colpoperineoplasty in women with a sensation of a wide vagina. *Acta Obstet et Gynec* 2006;**85**:1125–7.

5. Kent D, Pelosi III MA. Vaginal rejuvenation: An in-depth look at the history and technical procedure. *Am J Cosmetic Surg* 2012;**29**:89–96.

6. Moore RD, Miklos JR. Vaginal reconstruction and rejuvenation surgery: Is there data to support improved sexual function? *Am J Cosmetic Surgery* 2012;**29**:97–115.

7. Goodman MP, Placik OJ, Benson RH III, Miklos JR, Moore RD, Jason RA, Matlock DL, Simopoulos AF, Stern BH, Stanton RA, Kolb SE, Gonzalez F. A large multicenter outcome study of female genital plastic surgery. *J Sex Med* 2010;**7**:1565–77.

8. Girling VR, Salisbury M, Ersek RA. Vaginal labiaplasty. *Plast Reconstr Surg* 2005;**115**:1792–3.

9. Rubayi S. Aesthetic vaginal labiaplasty. *Plast Reconstr Surg* 1985;**75**:608.

10. Miklos JR, Moore RD. Labiaplasty of the labia minora: Patient's indications for pursuing surgery. *J Sex Med* 2008;**5**:1492–5.

11. Alter GJ. A new technique for aesthetic labia minora reduction. *Ann Plastic Surg* 1998;**40**:287–90.

12. DiSaia JP. An unusual staged rejuvenation of the labia. *J Sex Med* 2008;**5**:1263–7.

13. Maas SM, Hage JJ. Functional and aesthetic labia minora reduction. *Plast Reconstr Surg* 2007;**106**:1453–6.

14. Giraldo F, Gonzalez C, deHaro F. Central wedge nymphectomy with a 90-degree Z-plasty for aesthetic reduction of the labia minora. *Plast Reconstr Surg* 2004;**113**:1820–5.

15. Pardo J, Sola P, Ricci P, Guiloff E. Laser labiaplasty of the labia minora. *Int J Gynec Obst* 2005;**93**:38–43.

16. Bramwell R, Morland L, Garland AS. Expectations and experience of labial reduction: A qualitative study. *BJOG* 2007;**1144**:1493–9.

17. Alter GJ. Aesthetic labia minora and clitoral hood reduction using extended central wedge resection. *Plast Reconstr Surg* 2008;**122**:780–9.

18. Jothilakshmi PK, Salvi NR, Hayden BE, Bose-Haider B. Labial reduction in adolescent population—a case series study. *J Pediatr Adolesc Gynecol* 2009;**22**:53–5.

19. Solanki NS, Tejero-Trujeque R, Stevens-King A, Malata CM. (2009) Aesthetic and functional reduction of the labia minora using the Maas and Hage technique *J Plast Reconstr Aesthet Surg* Jul 9 [Epub ahead of print].

20. McDougall LJ. Towards a clean slit: How medicine and notions of normality are shaping female genital aesthetics. *Culture, Health and Sexuality* 2013;**15**:774–87.

21. Berman L, Berman J, Miles M, Pollets D, Powell JA. Genital self-image as a component of sexual health: Relationship

between genital self-image, female sexual function and quality of life measures. *J Sex Marital Ther* 2003;**29**:11–21.

22. Goodman MP, Bachman G, Johnson C, Fourcroy JL, Goldstein A, Goldstein G, Sklar S. Is elective vulvar plastic surgery ever warranted, and what screening should be conducted preoperatively? *J Sex Med* 2007;**4**:269–76.

23. Cartwright R, Cardozo L, Matlock DM, Simopoulos A. BJOG debate: Labiaplasty should be available as a cosmetic procedure. *BJOG* 2014;**121**:767.

24. Berer M. It's female genital mutilation and should be prosecuted. *BMJ* 2007;**334**:1335.

25. Iglesia CB. Cosmetic gynecology and the elusive quest for the "perfect" vagina. *Obstet Gynecol* 2012;**119**:1083–4

26. Tiefer L. Female genital cosmetic surgery: Freakish or inevitable? Analysis from medical marketing, bioethics, and feminist theory. *Feminism & Psychology* 2008;**18**:466–79.

27. Tracy E. Elective vulvoplasty: A bandage that might hurt. *Obstet Gynecol* 2007;**109**:1179–80.

28. Goldstein AT, Burrows L. Clitoral treatment of lichen sclerosis caused by lichen sclerosus. *Am J Obst Gynecol* 2007;**196**:126e1–4.

29. O'Connor M. Reconstructing the hymen: Mutilation or restoration? *J Law Med* 2008;**1**:161–75.

30. Logmans A, Verhoeff A, Bol Raap R, Creighton F, Van Lent M. Ethical dilemma: Should doctors reconstruct the vaginal introitus of adolescent girls to mimic the virginal state? *BMJ* 1998;**346**:459–62.

31. Usta I. Hymenorrhaphy: What happens behind the gynecologist's closed door? *J Med Ethics* 2000;**26**:217–8.

32. Kandela P. Egypt's trade in hymen repair. *Lancet* 1996;**34**:11.

33. Kline G. Case studies of perineometer resistive exercises of orgasmic dysfunction. In: *Circumvaginal Musculature and Sexual Function*, pp. 25–42. Basel, Switzerland: S. Karger, 1982.

34. http://www.surgery.org/download/2007stats.pdf.

35. Herbenick D, Schick V, Reece M, Sanders S, Fortenberry JD. Pubic hair removal among women in the United States: Prevalence, methods, and characteristics. *J Sex Med* 2010;**7**:3322–30.

36. Schick VR, Rima BN, Calabrese SK. Evulvation: The portrayal of women's external genitalia and physique across time and the current Barbie doll ideals. *J Sex Res* 2010;**47**:1–9.

37. Novi JM, Jeronis S, Morgan MA, Arya LA. Sexual function in women with pelvic organ prolapse compared to women without prolapse. *J Urol* 2006;**173**:1669–72.

38. Botros SM, Abramov Y, Miller JJ, Sand PK, Gandhi S, Nickolov A, Goldberg RP. Effect of parity on sexual function: An identical twin study. *Obstet Gynecol* 2006;**107**:756–70.

39. Barber MD, Visco AG, Wyman JF, Fantl JA, Bump RC. Sexual function in women with urinary incontinence and pelvic organ prolapse. *Obstst Gynecol* 2002;**99**:281–89.

40. Rogers GR, Villareal A, Kammerer-Doak D, Qualls C. Sexual function in women with and without urinary incontinence and/or pelvic organ prolapse. *Int Urogynecol J Pelvic Floor Dysfunct* 2001;**12**:361–5.

41. Wehbe KA, Kellogg S, Whitmore K. Urogenital complaints and female sexual dysfunction. Part 2. *J Sex Med* 2010;**7**:2304–17.

42. Azar M, Noohi S, Radfar S, Radfar MH. Sexual function in women after surgery for pelvic organ prolapse. *Int Urogynecol J Pelvic Floor Dysfunct* 2008;**19**:53–7.

43. Rogers RD, Kammerer-Doak D, Darrrow A, Murray K, Qualls C, Olsen A, Barber M. Does sexual function change after surgery for stress urinary incontinence and/or pelvic organ prolapse,? A multicenter prospective study. *Am J Obstet Gynecol* 2006;**195**e:1–4.

44. Thackar R, Chawla S, Scheer I, Barrett G, Sultan AH. Sexual function following pelvic floor surgery. *Int J Gynecael Obstet* 2008;**102**:110–4.

45. Goldstein, S. My turn…finally. *J Sex Med* 2009;**6**:301–2.

46. Goodman MP. Female cosmetic genital surgery. *Obstet Gynecol* 2009;**113**:154–96.

47. Dietz HP, Simpson JM. Levator trauma is associated with pelvic organ prolapse. *BJOG* 2008;**115**:979–84.

48. Kline G. Case studies of perineometer resistive exercises of orgasmic dysfunction. In: *Circumvaginal Musculature and Sexual Function*, pp. 25–42. Basel, Switzerland: S. Karger, 1982.

49. Ozel B, Whiute T, Urwitz-Lane R. The impact of pelvic organ prolapse on sexual function in women with urinary incontinence. *Int Urogynecol J Pelvic Floor Dysfunct* 2006;**17**:14–17.

50. Shek KL, Dietz HP. The effect of childbirth on hiatal dimensions. *Obstet Gynecol* 2009;**113**:1272–8.

51. Sevely JL, Bennett JW. Concerning female ejaculation and the female prostate. *J Sex Res* 1978;**14**:1–20.

52. Mould D. (1982) Women's orgasm and the muscle spindle. In: *Circumvaginal Musculature and Sexual Function*, pp. 93–100. Basel, Switzerland: S. Karger, 1982.

53. Hilliges M, Falconer C, Ekman-Ordeberg G, Johannson O. Innervation of the human vaginal mucosa as revealed by PGP 9.5 immunochemistry. *Acta Anat* 1995;**153**:119–26.

54. Song YB, Hwang K, Kim DJ, Han SH. Innervation of the vagina: Microdissection and immunohistochemical study. *J Sex Marital Ther* 2009;**35**:144–53.

55. Jannini EA, Rubio-Casillas A, Whipple B, Buisson O, Komisaruk BR, Brody S. Female orgasm(s): One, two, several. *J Sex Med* 2012;**4**:956–65.

56. Lavoisier P, Aloui R, Schmidt MH, Watrelot A. Clitoral blood flow increases following vaginal pressure stimulation. *Arch Sex Behav* 1995;**24**:37–45.

57. Buisson O, Foldes P, Jannini E, Mimoun S. Coitus as revealed by ultrasound in one volunteer couple. *J Sex Med* 2010;**7**:2750–4.

58. Shafik A. Vaginocavernosis reflex: Clinical significance and role in sexual act. *Gynecol Obst Invest* 1993;**35**:114–7.

59. Foldes P, Buisson O. The clitoral complex: A dynamic sonographic study. *J Sex Med* 2009;**6**:1223–31.

60. Whipple B, Gerdes C, Komisaruk BR. Sexual response to self-stimulation in women with complete spinal cord injury. *J Sex Res* 1996;**33**:231–41.

61. Komisaruk BR, Gerdes CA, Whipple B. "Complete" spinal cord injury does not block perceptual responses in women. *Arch Neurol* 1997;**54**:1513–20.

62. Darling CA, Davidson JK Sr, Conway-Welch C. Female ejaculation: Perceived origins, the Grafenberg spot/area, and sexual responsiveness. *Arch Sex Behav* 1997;**119**:29–47.

63. Alzate H. Vaginal eroticism: A replication study. *Arch Sex Behav* 1985;**14**:529–37.

64. Levin RJ. Female orgasm: Correlation of objective physical recordings with subjective experience. *Arch Sex Behav* 1998;**37**:279–85.

65. Wimpissinger F, Stifter K, Grin W, Stackl W. The female prostate revisited: Perineal ultrasound and biochemical studies of female ejaculate. *J Sex Med* 2007;**4**:1388–93.

66. Komisaruk BR, Whipple B, Crawford A, Liu WC, Kalnin A, Mosier K. Brain activation during vaginocervical self-stimulation and orgasm in women with complete spinal cord injury: fMRI evidence of mediation by vagus nerves. *Brain Res* 2004;**1024**:77–88.

67. Liao LM, Creighton SM. Requests for cosmetic genitoplasty: How should healthcare providers respond? *BJM* 2007;**334**:1090–2.

CHAPTER 6

Ethical considerations of female genital plastic/cosmetic surgery

Andrew T. Goldstein[1] and Sarah L. Jutrzonka[2]

[1]Department of Obstetrics and Gynecology, The George Washington University School of Medicine, Washington, DC, USA
[2]Pacific Graduate School of Psychology, Palo Alto University, Palo Alto, CA, USA

Women's desire for aesthetic perfection is persistent through the ages and is likely evolutionarily driven. There is a clear biological and reproductive advantage to attracting the opposite sex. There are examples in every culture of women adorning themselves with jewelry, makeup, and clothing in an effort to improve their appearance. Women also use surgeries such as breast augmentations, rhinoplasty, and abdominoplasty to make structural changes and alter their appearances permanently.

Recently, the desire to improve one's physical appearance has resulted in demand for cosmetic procedures aimed at altering the appearance of the genitals. Procedures such as labiaplasty, hymenoplasty, "vaginal rejuvenation," and other female cosmetic genital surgeries may be used to improve one's self-perception and self-confidence (and less commonly for correction of malformations or dysfunction). Motivations for genital cosmetic surgery typically fall into one of three categories: physical, psychological, or sexual. Physical complaints may include dyspareunia, discomfort, chafing, and rubbing. Psychological complaints may include displeasure with one's appearance, embarrassment, and shame. Sexual complaints include decreased sensation, reduced orgasm, and the perception of decreased partner satisfaction.

Awareness of the availability of these procedures has been driven in large part by the Internet and the lay media's fascination with this topic. This has driven demand for these procedures, and with this rise in demand surgeons should reacquaint themselves with the four central tenets of medical ethics, *autonomy*, *nonmaleficence*, *beneficence*, and *justice*, in an effort to confidently offer and perform these procedures.

Autonomy

The principle of autonomy recognizes the right of an individual to self-determination. Autonomy gives a person (e.g., a patient) the right to have, or not have, any medical treatment or procedure. The principle of autonomy is *prima facie* binding over the three other medical ethical principles. However, true autonomy can be quite difficult to achieve. In order for a person to have complete autonomy, she must have a thorough understanding of the risks, benefits, and alternatives of any treatment. In addition, she must be free from outside coercive influences. The best way to confirm a patient's autonomy is by obtaining informed consent. However, the process of obtaining informed consent is much more than having a patient sign a piece of paper prior to receiving a procedure. First, it includes establishing the capacity of the patient to give informed consent. In order for a person to have capacity to make medical decisions, she must thoroughly understand the information provided to her. Barriers to capacity include using overly complicated "medicalese" or discussing the information in a language in which the patient lacks fluency. The easiest way for a surgeon to confirm that a patient has the capacity to give informed consent is for the patient to explain—without significant prompting—the information that has been provided to her.

Female Genital Plastic and Cosmetic Surgery, First Edition. Edited by Michael P. Goodman.

Garrett and Baillie suggest some questions a surgeon may ask his or her patient to determine if the patient meets the minimum suggested requirements for satisfying the demands for informed consent [1]. Through the course of a consultation is the patient able to reflect back:

1 Can she explain the diagnosis?
2 Can she explain the rationale for the proposed treatment?
3 Does she know the risks and benefits of the proposed treatment?
4 Does she know the proposed treatment's success, complication, and failure rates for both the physician and the hospital?
5 Is she able to list alternative treatments?
6 Does she know the prognosis if not treated?

Some psychological disorders can distort a person's view of self and therefore diminish her capacity to give informed consent. Therefore, if a woman exhibits signs or symptoms of one of the disorders listed below, the physician should act ethically by discussing and emphasizing the importance of mental health care prior to a genital cosmetic procedure. If the patient's mental health is in question, a referral to a mental health professional is warranted and the physician should refuse to perform any cosmetic surgery. In addition, no procedure should be performed until the surgeon feels comfortable with the psychological health of the patient. Psychological disorders that a physician should be aware of include but are not limited to depression, body dysmorphic disorder, psychotic disorders, obsessive-compulsive disorder, personality disorders, cognitive disorders such as delirium, neurodegenerative diseases (e.g., Alzheimer's disease), substance abuse, and active intoxication [2] (Table 6.1). In addition, a long history of multiple prior cosmetic procedures should alert the surgeon to the possibility that the patient may have an underlying psychological disorder (e.g., body dysmorphic disorder) that should be addressed prior to the performance of any additional cosmetic surgeries.

Once a patient's competence has been established, the physician must feel confident that the patient is making the decision to proceed with surgery of her own free will. Through the course of the surgical consultation, the surgeon should listen for signs of coercion from romantic partners. This point was illustrated in a large retrospective study in which 5% of women who had genital cosmetic surgery reported that they had surgery at the urging of a sexual partner [3]. Last, sex workers as well as women who work in the adult entertainment industry may also be the victims of coercion.

Also, Goldstein and Goldstein caution that physicians can cause unintentional coercion simply by advertising their expertise [4]. It is important that physicians who choose to advertise do so both honestly and ethically. Terms such as "world-class," "world-famous" and "pioneer" may be misleading and may attract vulnerable populations [5].

In addition, surgeons must adequately inform their prospective patients of their own experience in performing each specific procedure. The old adage "see one, do one, teach one" is an antiquated approach to medical training, and failure by the surgeon to be forthright with regards to his or her limited experience in a specific procedure limits the patient's ability to make an autonomous decision about the procedure and could therefore invalidate any informed consent. This point is particularly noteworthy, as only 31.5% of plastic surgeons have had formal training in genital cosmetic surgery [6]. The percentage of gynecologists who have had formal training in these procedures is presumably much smaller, as this is not part of the core curriculum in gynecology resident training programs. Lastly, a disturbing result in a large retrospective study of 163 women who had labial reduction surgery found that 20% of these women felt that the surgeon inadequately explained either the procedure and/or the expected results of the procedure [7]. For these women, their rights to autonomy were clearly violated as they received inadequate counseling prior to their procedures.

Nonmaleficence

The ethical principle of *nonmaleficence* or first do no harm (*primum non nocere*) is the second-most important medical ethical principle. The basic concept of nonmaleficence is that it is more important to not harm a patient than it is to help her [4]. This ethical principle is especially important when a surgical procedure is elective and is primarily for an aesthetic purpose. While surgical complications are not entirely avoidable, newer procedures typically have higher complication rates than more established procedures [8].

Two large retrospective studies have examined the complication rate of genital cosmetic surgery. Rouzier and

Table 6.1 Common signs, symptoms, and screeners for psychological disorders.

Disorder		Questions to Ask	Screener Questionnaire Examples
Depression*		• Have you been feeling depressed or down most of the day nearly every day for the last 2 weeks? • If yes: Has your mood interfered with your interactions with other people, the law, or at work?	• Patient Health Questionnaire (PHQ) 8 or 9 • Beck Depression Inventory (BDI)-II • Center for Epidemiologic Studies – Depression Scale (CES-D)
Anxiety*		• Do people say that you worry about things too much? • Is it hard for you to control or stop your worrying? • Do you think your worrying/anxiety is unrealistic or excessive?	• Beck Anxiety Inventory (BAI) • Generalized Anxiety Disorder Screener (GAD)-2 or 7 • Anxiety Screening Questionnaire(ASQ)-15
Body dysmorphic disorder		• Do you think that there's something wrong with your appearance, that you are gross, disfigured, or ugly? • If you talk to your friends or family about your concern do they try to convince you that there is nothing wrong with your appearance? • Have you withdrawn from social situations because of your concern about your appearance?	• SCID-I • Psychosocial/clinical interview
Psychotic disorders	Two or more of the following must be present for a significant portion of time during a 1-month period (or less if successfully treated).		
Schizophrenia	1. Delusions 2. Hallucinations 3. Disorganized speech (e.g., frequent derailment or incoherence) 4. Grossly disorganized or catatonic behavior 5. Negative symptoms (e.g., affect the flattening, alogia (impoverishment of thinking, alogia, a restriction name on the spontaneous speech, brief and concrete plans to questions), or avolition (the inability to initiate and persist in goal-directed activities)		
Delusions		• Do you notice that the TV, newspaper, or strangers are referring to you, or that there are special messages intended specifically for you? • Do you ever think of something so strongly that people can hear your thoughts or people are able to read your mind and know what you are thinking? • Are your thoughts ever taken out of your head or have you had thoughts put in your head? • Do you think you have special talents, abilities, or powers? • Do you ever get the feeling you're being controlled by some outside force or power?	• SCID-I • Psychosocial/clinical interview
Hallucinations		• Have you seen visions or things that other people don't see? • Have you heard noises, or sounds, or voices that other people didn't here?	

Continued

Table 6.1 Continued

Disorder	Questions to Ask	Screener Questionnaire Examples
Obsessive compulsive disorder	• Have you ever been bothered by thoughts that didn't make sense and kept coming back to you even when you tried not to have them? • Have you ever had to do something over and over again and couldn't resist doing, like washing your hands again and again, counting up to a certain number, or checking something several times to make sure you got it right?	• SCID-I • Psychosocial/clinical interview
Cognitive disorders Neurocognitive diseases Alzheimer's type	Are they oriented to: • Place? • Date? • Location (e.g., city, state, or location of clinic or floor of the building)? • Reason for visit? • Current events (e.g., Who is the current president?)	• Mental Status Exam • Mini Mental Status Exam • MOCA Mental Status Exam • SLUMS Mental Status Exam
Alcohol abuse/ dependence	• What are your drinking habits like? • Has anyone in your family, friends, a doctor, or anyone else ever said that you drink too much?	• Audit • Audit-C
Drug abuse/ dependence	• How often do you use street drugs? • How many times have you taken more of a prescription medication than what was prescribed?	• The Drug Abuse Screening Test (DAST)

*Only detrimental when debilitating/severe.

colleagues described a group of 163 women who had labial reduction surgery (labiaplasty) [7]. They report that 7% of the women had a wound dehiscence requiring a second procedure. In addition, 23% reported dyspareunia lasting 3–90 days, 45% of the women complained of significant post-operative discomfort, and, in retrospect, 4% of women would choose not to undergo the procedure again.

Goodman and colleagues performed a large retrospective study of genital cosmetic surgery and examined 258 women who underwent 341 separate procedures: 104 labiaplasties, 24 clitoral hood reductions, 49 combined labiaplasty/clitoral hood reductions, 47 vaginoplasties and/or perineoplasties, and 34 combined labiaplasty and/or clitoral hood plus vaginoplasty/perineoplasty [3]. This multicenter study showed that 17% of women who had labiaplasty/clitoral hood reductions and 7.9% of vaginoplasty/perineoplasty patients found the results of surgery to be unsatisfactory. Complications were reported in 8.5% of women who underwent labiaplasty and/or clitoral hood reductions, in 16.6% of women who underwent vaginoplasty/perineoplasty, and in 18.2% of women who underwent a combination of procedures. These complications included problems with healing, dyspareunia, and excessive post-operative bleeding. It should be noted, however, that in this same study, >95% of women with vulvar and >87% of women with vaginal procedures were ultimately "satisfied" with overall results, suggesting that the majority of "complications" did not affect overall results.

Given the results of the two large retrospective studies discussed above, it is not clear that the complication rates of genital cosmetic surgery are low enough to overcome the burden of nonmaleficence. Clearly, prospective randomized controlled trials are warranted to answer this question more clearly. However, until the results of prospective trials are available, surgeons who perform these surgeries must be aware that they are operating in an ethically questionable area and they must redouble their efforts to counsel their patients as to the true complication rates of these procedure and to not minimize the potential for long-term or possibly permanent harm [9].

Beneficence

Healthcare providers are ethically bound to try to help relieve their patients' suffering. This is the ethical principle of beneficence. However, as mentioned previously,

the desire, or obligation, to help is still secondary to principles of autonomy and nonmaleficence. In order to determine whether or not a cosmetic genital surgery is ultimately beneficial, the surgeon must discover the motivation of the patient. As mentioned previously, motives for seeking a particular procedure may include cosmetic concerns in which a woman perceives part or all of her vulva to be aesthetically unpleasing, functional reasons such as discomfort in clothes or while participating in activities (e.g., walking, running, etc.), psychologically based reasons (to improve self-esteem), or to increase sexual satisfaction or function. A woman's motives for seeking a procedure can be single or a combination of these reasons. Given the wide disparity in motivations for cosmetic genital surgery, as well as the many different types and combinations of surgery (as illustrated by Goodman's study), it not surprising that there are few studies that examine the potential benefits of each type of surgery. However, Goodman and colleagues did attempt to compare the satisfaction of two different surgical techniques of labiaplasty: modified wedge and the linear resection, finding an overall satisfaction of 95.2% and 95.7%, respectively. Seventy percent of patients reported "mild to significant" enhancement of sexual function with the modified wedge technique versus 56% with linear resection [3]. Rouzier and colleagues reported that 83% of their patients were satisfied with the results of their labiaplasty surgery [7].

However, there are very significant limitations to these papers that call into question the apparently high satisfaction rate. First, they were retrospective studies. Second, in the Rouzier study 40% of the patients were lost to follow-up or did not respond to the study questionnaire. In the Goodman study, 45.5% of patients either refused to answer the study questionnaire or did not answer the questionnaire after agreeing to do so. It is certainly possible that women who were dissatisfied with the results of their surgery were less likely to respond to post-operative questionnaires, thereby falsely inflating the satisfaction rate of these procedures [9].

Last, as there are such limited data regarding the long-term satisfaction with cosmetic genital surgery, it is worthwhile to examine the long-term satisfaction of other cosmetic procedures. While cosmetic genital surgery and breast augmentation are clearly different procedures with different potential complications, they both affect sexual organs and self-perception of sexuality. Holmich and colleagues report that there is only a

60% long-term satisfaction with the results of breast augmentation [10]. Given this high long-term dissatisfaction rate with breast augmentation, and the limitation of the two retrospective studies previously discussed, it is not clear that genital cosmetic procedures meet the ethical burden of beneficence. As such, surgeons who offer these procedures must emphasize to their patients that it cannot be guaranteed, with any certainty, that they will be pleased with the outcome of the procedure, even if proper surgical techniques are used. In addition, it should be specifically mentioned that improved sexual satisfaction may not be a benefit from the proposed surgery. Although all studies that looked at sexual functioning found overall enhancement of function for both external vulvar procedures [65% in Goodman et al. [3] and 71% in Alter's [11] studies of labiaplasty] and vaginal tightening operations [90% in Pardo et al.'s [12] and 89% [3] in Goodman et al.], follow-up was not ideal, and none of these studies were prospective in design.

Justice

The principle of *justice* states that in societies where there are limited medical resources, these resources should be distributed to benefit the greatest number of members of that society.

Goldstein and Goldstein point out that when female genital cosmetic surgery is performed for aesthetic reasons, in countries where the cost is covered by the patient—such as in the United States—the principle of justice is less of an ethical consideration than the three medical principles already discussed [4]. However, an argument could be made that surgical training *is a limited resource that is paid for, in part, by taxpayers' dollars.* Therefore, trained surgeons should be ethically obligated to use their skills in ways that society finds more beneficial than cosmetic genital surgery. In addition, Goldstein and Goldstein point out that insurance companies should not be asked to pay for these types of surgeries unless there is deformity that causes significant dysfunction such as dyspareunia. Justice, however, does apply in countries where medical resources are rationed, such as in Canada or the United Kingdom. In these countries, given the paucity of data showing long-term benefit of these procedures, it is improbable that an argument could be made that limited resources should be used for cosmetic genital surgery.

Conclusion

After reviewing genital cosmetic surgery through the lens of the medical ethical principles of *autonomy, nonmaleficence, beneficence,* and *justice*, it is clear that data is insufficient at this time to conclude that genital cosmetic surgery is always ethical or always unethical. Therefore, it is the responsibility of the surgeon to adequately counsel prospective surgery patients. In addition, it is the responsibility of these surgeons to gather prospective data to further clarify the true risks and benefits of these procedures.

References

1. Garrett TM, Baillie HW. *Health Care Ethics: Principles and Problems,* 2nd ed. Upper Saddle River, NJ: Prentice Hall, 1993.
2. American Psychological Association. American Psychological Association ethical principles of psychologists and code of conduct, 2010. Available at: http://apa.org/ethics/code/index.aspx?item=1 (accessed December 1, 2013).
3. Goodman MP, Placik OJ, Benson RH III, Miklos JR, Moore RD, Jason RA, Matlock DL, Simopoulos AF, Stern BH, Stanton RA, Kolb SE, Gonzalez F. A large multicenter outcome study of female genital plastic surgery. *J Sex Med* 2010;**7**:1565–77.
4. Goodman MP, Bachmann G, Johnson C, Fourcroy JL, Goldstein A, Goldstein G, Sklar S. Is elective vulvar plastic surgery ever warranted, and what screening should be done preoperatively? *J Sex Med* 2007;**4**:269–76.
5. ACOG Committee Opinion No. 341. Ethical ways for physicians to market a practice. *Obstet Gynecol* 2006;**108**: 239–42.
6. Mirzabeigi MD, Moore JH, Mericli AF, Bucciarelli P, Jandali S, Valeiro IL. Current trends in vaginal labiaplasty: A survey of plastic surgeons. *Ann Plast Surg* 2012;**68**:125–34.
7. Rouzier R, Louis-Sylvester C, Paniel BJ, Haddad B. Hypertrophy of labia minora: Experience with 163 reductions. *Am J Obstet Gynecol* 2000;**182**:35–40
8. Iglesia C, Yuteri-Kaplan L, Alinsod R. Female genital cosmetic surgery: A review of technique and outcomes. *Int Urogynecol J* 2013;**24**:1997–2009.
9. Goodman MP. Female genital cosmetic and plastic surgery: A review. *J Sex Med* 2011;**8**(6):1813–25.
10. Hölmich LR, Breiting VB, Fryzek JP, Brandt B, Wolthers MS, Kjøller K, McLaughlin JK, Friis S Long-term cosmetic outcome after breast implantation. *Ann Plast Surg* 2007;**59**(6):597–604.
11. Alter GJ. A new technique for aesthetic labia minora reduction. *Ann Plast Surg* 1998;**40**:287–90.
12. Pardo J, Sola V, Ricci P, Guiloff E, Freundlich D. Colpoperineoplasty in women with a sensation of a wide vagina. *Acta Obstet Gynecol Scand* 2006;**85**:1125–8.

CHAPTER 7

Patient protection and pre-operative assessment

Michael P. Goodman

Caring for Women Wellness Center, Davis, CA, USA

The early bird might get the worm, but the second mouse gets the cheese.

Ernst Berg—or Steven Wright

In addition to expecting the application of the ethical principles previously discussed, patients have the right to expect that their surgeon has the proper level of training and experience to perform the agreed-upon procedure (see also Chapter 21). Patients should be counseled that they are not "abnormal" and should know the expected outcomes of their procedure. They should understand the alternative surgical and non-surgical techniques available, expected complications, and rates of (mal)occurrence, so as to be able to choose what they wish done based on a knowledge of the procedure, alternatives, and known complication rates [1]. They should be well informed so their expectations are reasonable.

Some risks (e.g., over- or underremoval of tissue, post-surgical irregularity of labial edges, incisional opening and healing by secondary intention, sexual pain, over-tightening of the introitus with perineoplasty, risks of bowel or bladder entry [with possibility of fistula formation] or risk of producing incontinence by alterations of the anterior or posterior compartments in colpoperineoplasty, infection, delayed wound healing, etc.) are known and must be discussed with the patient. As these procedures are relatively new and the literature investigating outcomes and risks is not yet robust, the possibility of other untoward outcomes must be candidly discussed. The patient should be informed that these are serious surgical procedures, that recovery may be protracted, and that potentially significant risks exist. The physician must be clear regarding expected downtime. Equally importantly, the surgeon's inability to guarantee a specific outcome or results meeting a patient's expectations must be explained.

Many patients seeking aesthetic genital surgery perceive themselves as abnormal, unattractive, deformed, and so forth. Clear and direct information must be provided to each patient regarding the wide range of anatomic variation and that they fall within this normal range. Given this, they still may reasonably wish to alter their appearance.

Keep in mind that these are elective surgical procedures. Patients at higher risk for medical or surgical complications and poor wound healing should be excluded or very carefully evaluated. These procedures should not be performed on the smoker, the diabetic (unless meticulously controlled), the poorly controlled hypertensive, those with significant pulmonary, renal, neurological or cardiovascular disease, or patients with undiagnosed vulvar dystrophic disorders or history of vulvar or vaginal area radiation. A full medical history is an essential part of the pre-operative process.

- Special situations—smokers: Any person smoking over 1–2 cigarettes/day should be informed of the increased risk for wound disruption. The author, like virtually all plastic/cosmetic surgeons, refuses to perform elective cosmetic surgery on any smoker unless a withdrawal from tobacco products for 3–6 weeks prior to and 3–6 weeks post-surgery (depending

Female Genital Plastic and Cosmetic Surgery, First Edition. Edited by Michael P. Goodman.

on length of time on tobacco products and intensity of use) is guaranteed in writing by the patient.

- Special situations—abnormal glucose tolerance: Diabetics heal poorly. Elective vulvovaginal plastic/cosmetic surgery should not be performed on anyone whose HgbA1C has not been in the range of 8 or lower (many surgeons would reasonably require 6.5–7.5), verified by repeated lab analysis, in the full month prior to surgery. Likewise, fasting blood sugars, upon multiple analyses in the pre-operative month, should not be regularly >100; certainly nor regularly >120. These values are not absolute; however, diabetic patients should receive careful pre- and post-operative attention to reduce the risk of complication.
- Special situations—recurrent herpes genitalis: A herpes recurrence in the early post-operative period is a serious complication. Patients should be asked directly regarding any history of genital herpes. Any woman with a history of recurrent herpes should take prophylaxis with 400 mg acyclovir or 1,000 mg valcyclovir daily for 2–3 days prior to and 10–14 days subsequent to surgery.

Each patient seeking a cosmetic genital procedure should be evaluated either by the use of an approved instrument, for example, the Arizona Sexual Experience Questionnaire (ASEX), Female Sexual Function Index (FSFI) short or long form, and so forth, or by a general set of uncovering questions. Patients with sexual dysfunction should be further evaluated either by the operating surgeon if she or he is trained in this evaluation or by referral to a qualified sexual medicine practitioner. Patients with serious sexual dysfunction should not undergo these procedures; however, many patients avoid sex secondary to embarrassment or lack of "feeling." These patients do not necessarily have a sexual dysfunction and are likely to be helped by FGPS. Although it is reasonable to expect that there may be positive effects on sexual function, this result should not be touted nor guaranteed.

A detailed and personalized consent form should be part of the pre-operative process and should include information about the procedure, short- and long-term recovery protocols, known and potential complications (emphasizing the surgeon's inability to guarantee an "expected outcome"), as well as a disclaimer regarding inability to guarantee beneficial effects on sexual functioning and enjoyment. An example of informed consent documents for both external (vulvar) and internal (vaginal/perineal) procedures is reproduced here (Figures 7.1

and 7.2). The patient is instructed to initial each statement, showing that it has been read and understood.

Adequate time should be given to pre-operative preparations (Figure 7.3). Does your patient have help at home? Many stairs to negotiate? Is her vehicle a manual or automatic transmission? What are her return to school/work plans and are they realistic to her recovery? She should be advised to discontinue the use of aspirin and NSAID products 2 weeks prior to surgery. Her postoperative instructions should be initially reviewed preoperatively, to adequately ensure understanding and preparation for the necessary restrictions on her activities that these procedures mandate.

As previously noted, patients have the right to expect that their surgeon has a sufficient level of training and experience. Patients can reasonably expect that if their surgeon has completed an approved OB/GYN residency program, she or he is experienced in vaginal and perineal surgery and fully understands the anatomy of the pelvis. If the surgeon has not completed an OB/GYN residency, for example, a general, urological, or plastic surgeon, it is important for these physicians to be adequately trained in vulvar and vaginal anatomy and the intended surgical procedure(s), and patients should be informed of their professional training and background [1].

In any case, a surgeon embarking upon a procedure should have specific expertise in the operation he or she will perform, either secondary to previous performance of an "adequate" number of cases or completion of a legitimate training course, ideally followed by proctoring. The makeup of such courses, the number of hours required, and the course content are not something we as a profession can necessarily legislate; however, it is helpful that the VVAS practitioner also have sexual medicine training sufficient to evaluate the sexual health of his/her patient and to be able to uncover sexual dysfunction that may masquerade as a surgical request. If the surgeon has not participated in such training, a referral to a sexual medicine practitioner may be warranted. For gynecologic surgeons, a modicum of training in and understanding of plastic surgery techniques is valuable. Additionally, and of utmost importance for patient protection, is the requirement that any gynecologic surgeon performing vulvovaginal aesthetic surgery and/or vaginal surgery for the specific purpose of tightening for enhancement of sexual function be able to show evidence of training both in plastic technique and training specifically for

Informed Consent for Cosmetic Surgery

I have elected to have _____, M.D., perform a "labiaplasty/labial reduction" and/or reduction of the size of my clitoral hood and/or hymenaplasty/hymenal repair on me in order to reduce the size of my labia and/or clitoral hood or to repair the hymen. I have come in voluntarily either because I would like the hymen reconstructed or I find my labial and/or clitoral hood size to be "excessive," which causes me difficulties.

I understand:

1. _____The risks of the surgery include: incomplete or prolonged healing, opening of the incision, irregularity, scarring, or dissymmetry of the size of the labia after surgery, infection, painful sexual relations, delayed bleeding after surgery, increased or decreased sensation, and other rare events.

2. _____The surgical area will be swollen, uneven in appearance, and discolored in the weeks after surgery. It will take 4-6 weeks before I am completely healed and a full 3-4 months before I can truly assess the results of my surgery.

3. _____I may need a second ("two-stage") surgery to fully reduce the size to my liking.

4. _____I will need to limit my activities during the recovery time as outlined on my post-operative instruction sheet.

5. _____I understand that Dr. _____ will do his/her best to perform surgery to my specifications but that exact results cannot be guaranteed. Although good results are expected, it is possible that the result might not live up to the expectations or goals that I have established.

6. _____It is possible that a second procedure may be necessary to revise results to my liking, and there may be a charge for that procedure.

7. _____Smokers are recognized to have a significantly higher risk of post operative wound healing problems with a subsequently higher potential of infection as well as operative and post operative bleeding. **If you are a smoker you should completely discontinue smoking for a minimum of three weeks before and three weeks after surgery.** Although it helps to stop smoking before and after surgery, this does not completely eliminate the increased risks resulting from long-term smoking. Smoking also has a long term adverse effect on the skin and aging process.

8. _____Other information related specifically to me: _____
_____

9. _____I certify that I fully informed Dr. _____ correctly and to the best of my knowledge of my full medical history and status. I understand that withholding medical information could lead to complications or problems that may have been prevented if that information were known prior to my surgery.

10. In my own words, this is what I expect Dr._____ to do:_____
_____

I certify that I have met with Dr. _____ on two or more occasions and that (s)he has discussed the operation/s with me to my satisfaction. This form has been fully explained to me; I have read it and understand its contents. I understand the procedure, its risks, and the recovery involved. I agree to follow the instructions given to me by Dr. _____ to the best of my ability before, during and after the above mentioned surgical procedure, and will notify Dr. _____ of any problems following my surgery.

I hereby accept that the essential information necessary to make an informed decision has been given to me. All questions have been answered to my satisfaction.

_____ Additionally, I hereby give Dr. _____ permission to take "before and after" photographs. I may receive a copy of these upon my request.

_____	_____	_____	_____
Patient Signature	Date	(Physician signature)	Date

_____   _____
(Parent or Guardian)   Date

Figure 7.1 Suggested informed consent document, vulvar plastic/cosmetic procedures.

aesthetic vulvovaginal procedures, not simply training in general vulvovaginal surgery.

FGPS is decidedly not a "see one, do one, teach one" discipline. Experienced surgeons are aware of the significant differences in anatomy from one patient to the next, and also between contralateral sides in the same patient. This is decidedly not the place for a "one size fits all" surgery, and any surgeon approaching FGPS should understand alternate surgical approaches.

Your patient must be individually assessed pre-operatively. This surgery is elective and should not be performed on medically or psychologically unstable individuals, or on someone who is not prepared to closely follow your post-operative instructions (see Chapter 12). This author suggests at least two evaluations prior to surgery, although the second may be a pre-operative assessment, so long as a second complete exam with discussion of procedure, post-operative care,

**INFORMED CONSENT FOR VAGINAL AESTHETIC SURGERY
("VAGINAL REJUVENATION," "VAGINOPLASTY," "PERINEOPLASTY," AND/OR
INTROITAL RECONSTRUCTION)**

I have elected to have vaginal aesthetic surgery and/or pelvic support surgery for the following reasons (patient: write in your own words here):

_____

Procedures scheduled for me are:

1._____

2._____

3._____

I understand that these procedures are designed to help control urinary incontinence and/or eliminate symptomatic "bulges" from the vagina, and/or improve the appearance and/or "size" and "tone" of the vagina.

In all likelihood my goals will be accomplished. However, I understand that the following may be unexpected outcomes of my procedure(s):

1. _____ Complications including but not limited to: 1. infection, 2. hematoma, abscess, 3. injury to an adjacent organ which could produce a "fistula,"or excessive loss of blood which may lead to the necessity for other procedures to control bleeding and/or repair the injury, 5. delayed or incomplete healing, 6. excessive or prolonged postoperative pain, or other rare events.

2. _____ Under-tightening ("...still too loose...") or over-tightening, leading to the necessity of several weeks or longer "stretching" the vagina prior to being able to engage in vaginal intercourse..

3. _____ Results inadequate to control the problem.

4. _____ Cosmetic results not up to my expectations.

I understand that Dr. _____ will perform surgery carefully and make every effort for results up to or exceeding my expectations, but that these results cannot be guaranteed.

In my own words, this is what I expect Dr. _____ to do:_____

_____

I understand the above and elect to have the surgery performed.

_____ Additionally, I hereby give Dr. _____ permission to take "before and after" photographs. I may receive a copy of these upon my request.

_____
Patient

_____   _____
Witness   *Date*

Figure 7.2 Suggested informed consent document, vaginal tightening procedures.

and assessment of the patient's understanding and psychological health are included. The surgeon should be prepared to cancel surgery if any physical or psychological obstacle is encountered.

The author's second (pre-operative) consultation begins with a genital evaluation where he reviews the patient's anatomy as she holds a mirror and observes, either confirming or revising our initial operative plan. Again, the patient is encouraged to participate in the decision-making process as it relates to technique and

procedure choice. Short- and long-term recovery protocols are then reviewed, and written instructions are given. Informed consent is given (see above), pre-op medications are given, and any additional questions from the patient or her family are answered. This is a good time to mention to the patient that she may experience some diversion of her urinary stream. Educate her that, although your surgery is nowhere near her urethra, the act of removing what previously may have been "curtains" deflecting the urinary stream will, for

PRE OPERATIVE PREPARATION FOR LABIAPLASTY, PERINEOPLASTY & VAGINOPLASTY PLASTIC SURGERY

1. No smoking for 3–4 WEEKS prior to **and** 3–4 weeks after surgery.
2. No Aspirin, Ibuprofen, "Aleve", etc. for two weeks prior to surgery. Tylenol is okay.
3. You will need to have adequate help around the house for at least 3–7 days after surgery and minimize your activities.
4. Prior to surgery, wash the entire genital area well trim your hair short. (Please use scissors or an electric razor/buzzer, DO NOT shave or wax closer than 1 week prior to surgery.
5. Wear loose fitting/comfortable, dark clothing the day of your surgery. (No loose jewelry please)
6. **For office Perineoplasty/Vaginoplasty only** – start taking your antibiotics as directed two days prior to the procedure up until two days after.
7. **If you have a history of recurrent Herpes, make sure you tell your doctor well prior to surgery

Before leaving our office you will be given:
1. A bottle of Arnica tablets- This is a homeopathic remedy, not a medication, and is a gentle anti-inflammatory that works very well in reducing swelling.
2. A "peri-bottle" (a plastic squirt bottle) – used to cleanse/rinse yourself after you use the restroom.
3. Cu-3 intensive hydrating gel (**for Labiaplasty/hood reduction only**) – This is a tissue repair cream with a soothing base, used to enhance healing immediately post-procedure. It helps prevent the formation of
4. An inflatable "donut" cushion- This will make your ride home, your recovery and your first few days back at work or school more comfortable.

You will need to have/purchase:
1. Tucks Medicated Pads/Wipes (commonly used for hemorrhoids) – These help cool and soothe itching, burning and irritation. (Or you may get something similar that contains Witch Hazel. *Keeping them in the refrigerator provides an added cooling effect.)
2. Dermaplast™ Spray- This is an anesthetic pain and itch relieving spray. It contains aloe and lanolin which moisturizes the skin and aids in healing.
3. Sanitary napkins/maxi pads – Enough for approximately 5 days.
4. Ibuprofen (Motrin) 200 mg – take two along with your Vicodin prescription (or tale 3–4 in place of your hydrocodone if pain is minimal).

For in-office procedures ONLY:
1. You must have either someone to drive you the day of surgery or have local hotel and taxi accommodations. (*Our office can help you with this.)
2. Eat a light, non-greasy meal before your surgery. (i.e.: cereal, muffin, toast, fruit, yogurt, soup, half sandwich, etc…).
3. You will be given one Lorazepam (or substitution) 30 minutes prior to surgery and, if needed a second lorazepam under your tongue 15 minutes before surgery. Bring your hydrocodone pills (or substitute) with you to the office; we will give you one to take with a light post-op meal prior to your returning home.
(*If your pre-op appointment is the same day as your surgery, please bring your pain medication with you; the Lorazepam will be given to you at the office.)

For Hospital Procedures:
1. You must have either someone to drive you the day of surgery or have medical transport arrangements.
2. You may not have anything to eat or drink for 6 hours prior to the time you are supposed to arrive at the hospital. If you take medication that you cannot skip, you may take it with a minimum amount of water.
3. You may wish to bring a book or magazine to read while you wait.

Figure 7.3 Pre-operative instructions.

better or worse, no longer be present, and she may have to re-adjust her position on the toilet to re-direct the stream.

In the author's office, pre-op medication consist of 1 mg oral lorazepam given with a granola bar and a large bottle of Gatorade or similar hydration/electrolyte solution ~30 minutes prior to entry to the procedure room. The RN is given authority to administer another 1 mg lorazepam sub-lingually if she or the patient feels additional sedation would be helpful. Although the author's patients are instructed to hydrate and eat a small meal prior to coming to the office, they often arrive "un-watered and un-fed," which does not sit well with 1–2.5 hours in leg rests, lorazepam, stress of surgery, and re-assumption of an upright posture. Hydrocodone with acetaminophen 5–10 mg/325 mg is given with a small meal post-procedure.

Remember, this is elective surgery! Your exceptionally anxious patient, the woman who may have sexual dysfunction, the one who may have difficulty following recovery instructions, the one to whom a particular, specific appearance is important, the diabetic, the hypertensive, the smoker…may not be an acceptable surgical candidate and may certainly warrant additional evaluations prior to scheduling a surgical procedure. Proper patient selection, appropriate pre- and post-operative education, meticulous surgical technique, and close follow-up are all essential to a successful outcome.

Reference

1. Goodman MP. Female cosmetic genital surgery. *Obstet Gynecol* 2009;**113**:154–96.

CHAPTER 8

Surgical procedures I: vulva and mons pubis

Michael P. Goodman

Caring for Women Wellness Center, Davis, CA, USA

With contributions from David Matlock, Alex Simopoulos, Bernard H. Stern, and Otto J. Placik

How I do it: curvilinear reduction of labia minora and excess prepuce, by David Matlock and Alex Simopoulos
How I do it: stem-iris scissors technique, by Bernard Stern
How I do it: linear reduction labiaplasty by radiofrequency, by Michael P. Goodman
How I do it: the V-wedge and "Y" modification, by Michael P. Goodman
How I do it: LP-M (labia majora), by Michael P. Goodman
How I do it: mons pubis reduction, by Otto J. Placik

Standing in an operating room doesn't make you a surgeon any more than standing in a garage makes you a car.

Michael P. Goodman (adapted)

Labiaplasty, labia minora (LP-m)

Several techniques have been described to effect cosmetic alteration of the labia minora; each has its acolytes and rationale. It is interesting to note, however, that the only study to compare labiaplasty (LP) outcome based on surgical technique found little difference in satisfaction or complications between the linear reduction/resection and modified V-wedge approaches [1] (Table 8.1). This author's personal experience reviewing medical-legal actions and the literature [2] seem to agree that procedures removing a more liberal portion of labial and clitoral hood epithelium fare considerably poorer than more conservative "adjustments."

As we will discuss as this chapter progresses, several different labial reduction techniques have been described in the literature. These include primarily linear resection/linear reduction and the V-wedge and its modifications, including the "Y" extension of Alter's V-wedge technique in order to include hood redundancies, perfected by

Goodman and other surgeons as natural progressions along their learning curves. Lesser-utilized techniques include de-epithelialization, superior-inferior flap techniques, and Z-plasty, the latter two actually modifications of V-wedge. In the right hands and correct application, all can give superior results, but since the great bulk of practitioners utilize either linear or V-wedge techniques, and virtually all anatomic variables may be approached with one of these two approaches, only these two will be described in detail in this chapter (see Figures 4.1 and 4.2). Of paramount importance is the mantra "The Right Procedure for the Right Patient for the Right Reasons."

Prior to discussing the procedures themselves, a few words must be said about pre-operative "artwork." Whether LP, clitoral hood reduction (RCH), or perineoplasty (PP), the drawing of incision lines on the patient's genitalia is one of the most important parts of the procedure. This must be done on dry skin, with a sterile marking pen at the beginning of the case, prior to injection of any local anesthesia, utilizing only the most gentle

Female Genital Plastic and Cosmetic Surgery, First Edition. Edited by Michael P. Goodman.
© 2016 John Wiley & Sons, Ltd. Published 2016 by John Wiley & Sons, Ltd.

Table 8.1 Outcome by labiaplasty surgical technique.

Method of Labiaplasty	Linear Excision (N = 83) No. (%)	Modified Wedge (N = 70) No. (%)
Overall patient Satisfaction: "Yes"	80 (96.4)	67 (95.7)
Satisfaction: "No"	3 (3.6)	3 (4.3)
Patient perception of Complication: "None"	76 (91.6)	65 (92.9)
Perception of complication: "Yes"	7 (8.4)	5 (7.1)
Enhancement of sexual function:	(N = 81)	(N = 67)
"None"	36 (44.5)	20 (29.9)
"Mild-significant enhancement"	45 (55.6)	47 (70.1)

Source: Goodman et al. 2009 (1). Reproduced with permission of Wiley.

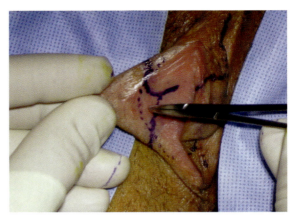

Figure 8.2 Mucosal surface. Dotted line, linear resection marking; solid line, V-wedge marking with mucosal orientation "tail." Instrument points to (difficult to visualize) "Harts Line." In V-wedge, mucosal incision may barely penetrate Hart's Line, but not >1 cm. Line continuing medially on mucosal surface for orientation during repair. Source: M. Goodman. Reproduced with permission.

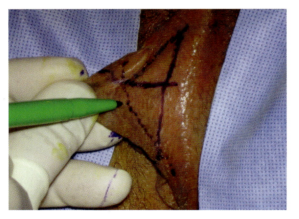

Figure 8.1 Marking, lateral surface of labum. Dotted line, linear resection; solid line, V-wedge marking, continuing cephalad for "Y" modification. Source: M. Goodman. Reproduced with permission.

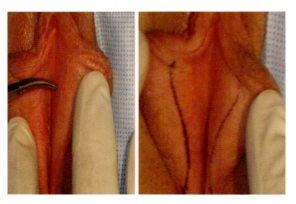

Figure 8.3 Linear resection; marking mucosal surface right side; "kissing" transfer to contralateral side. NB: Hart's line 2–3 mm beyond tip of instrument. Source: M. Goodman. Reproduced with permission.

traction to allow drawing without distortion of this so-elastic tissue (Figures 8.1–8.3). "Dots" may be used rather than drawing a "line" in the presence of skin redundancy. This is a time for quiet contemplation, sitting at the perineum, carefully drawing (and revising as necessary) appropriate incision lines. It is advisable to be conservative, especially when outlining a linear resection, as labial tissue retracts significantly, frequently leaving far less remaining labum than expected. Lines should be carefully drawn on both mucosal and lateral surfaces, taking care mucosally to stay lateral to Hart's line, and on the

lateral labial surface to be at least 1/2–1 cm medial to the inter-labial fold in a linear resection procedure, to take care not to stray too deeply into the mucosa medially in a V-wedge, and to be sure to "up-curve" the lateral V-wedge incision line to avoid "dog-ears."

Sculpted linear resection [3–7]: In this technique, a cutting tool such as a focused or "touch" laser, plastic surgery scissors (baby Metzenbaum, Keye), electrosurgery needle electrode with cutting current, or radiofrequency (RF) shielded wire cutting device is utilized to linearly

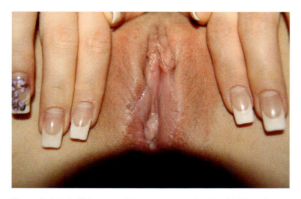

Figure 8.4 Injudicious excision ("amputation") of labia minora. Source: M. Goodman. Reproduced with permission.

sculpt and excise a portion of labum, removing as much or as little redundant tissue as desired, taking great care to be conservative and to stay well outside of Hart's line on the mucosal surface and to not trespass too far laterally on the lateral surface so as to put tension medially and draw the mucosal surface outward. Since tissue tone of squamous epithelium is greater than mucosa, if a too-generous amount of labum is excised, especially if the mucosal incision is medial to Hart's line and the lateral incision is at or beyond the inter-labial fold, little or no labum will remain and mucosa will be retracted outward, producing both discomfort and a far less-than-pleasing appearance also known as "amputation" (Figure 8.4). Equally problematic is the fact that sutures may tear from mucosa when under tension, resulting in wound dehiscence, discomfort, and a displeasing appearance.

After excision, bleeders are controlled, preferably using suture ties for arterial bleeders, cautery for light bleeding points. An absorbable mono- or polyfilament (never chromic) sub-cutaneous suture line is utilized to diminish dead space and provide additional support. Monofilament is less reactive and is preferred, although more difficult to work with. Many surgeons like a fine, rapidly absorbable suture for the skin closure layer. The resected edge is approximated (not strangulated!) with fine sub-cuticular or through-and-through interrupted sutures. A continuous suture line should not be used on the labial edge. Advantages include small, relatively straight, and "even" labia, which can be made relatively flush with the labia majora, frequently exhibiting a lighter colored ("pinker") edge, as well as a shorter surgeon's learning curve. Disadvantages of this technique may include a more scalloped appearance if the edge is closed by running or too

tightly placed sutures (occasionally exhibiting scarring and disfigurement if care is not used), hypersensitivity of the edge, and, if resection is performed close to the frenulum or clitoris, pain with genital engorgement/excitation. If there is a color discrepancy between the mucosal and lateral surfaces of the labum, a "color line" will be present along the line of resection. Usually this fades and merges within a year. Specific linear resection techniques will be discussed in detail by experienced practitioners as this chapter progresses.

Modified V-wedge [8,9]: A technique, first described by Gary Alter, MD [8], whereby a modified V-shaped "wedge" of redundant labum is excised, the superior edge beginning inferior to the fold flowing from the clitoral hood; the inferior edge beginning well above the posterior commissure (Figures 4.1, 8.1, and 8.2). Either a Z-plasty (rarely used) or "hockey-stick" curvature is utilized laterally to take up redundancy and prevent "dog-ears." Sub-cutaneous "anchoring" sutures of fine 3-0 to 5-0 synthetic delayed absorbable suture are utilized to provide initial re-approximation, taking tension off of the skin suture lines and diminishing "dead space." Skin closure is effected usually with interrupted small-caliber (4-0 to 6-0) absorbable sutures. Some surgeons utilize a running suture line, but this risks separation via "unraveling." A sub-cuticular suture line is difficult for V-wedge closure and also risks separation. If using interrupted sutures, care must be taken to avoid inward rolling of the edges. Periodic mattress sutures will minimize this risk. Resection of redundant clitoral hood skin may be accomplished at the same time by modifying the "V" to a "Y" incision to include the hood redundancy (Figure 8.1). The operative procedure will be discussed in greater detail later in the chapter.

Advantages of V-wedge techniques are a more "natural"-looking leading edge, potentially less interruption of edge nerve supply, and better aesthetic capability of working with women with a large, redundant, multi-folded clitoral hood. Disadvantages include a longer learning curve, greater risk of wound dehiscence, more careful initial post-operative care on the part of the patient, and a greater potentiality for removing less tissue than desired. As in curvilinear resection, a "two-toned appearance" may be noted if the superior and inferior leaves are of different color. Because of this, every effort should be made, when choosing resection sites, to consider color match.

Inferior wedge resection with superior pedicle flap rotation [10,11]: In this variation of wedge resection, the inferior portion of the labum (posterior commissure) is amputated, and the superior portion brought down as a pedicle flap and anchored to the denuded inferior edge (Figure 4.1). Sub-cutaneous and skin suturing are as described above for V-wedge.

De-epithelialized reduction labiaplasty [12]: In this procedure, the contour and anatomy of the labum is preserved by reducing its central width via bi-sided de-epithelialization and re-approximation of the central portion with (hopefully) preservation of neurovascular supply to the edge (Figure 4.1). Closure procedure and sutures are a variation of those described above. This procedure is little utilized by all but a handful of accomplished genital aesthetic surgeons.

Z-plasty (aka "W-plasty") reductional labiaplasty [13,14]: Another refinement in the wedge procedure, this technique involves removing a central wedge of labum via a "Z"- (or "W"-) shaped incision, with a classic Z-plasty type repair with fine sutures, as previously described for V-wedge.

The several techniques each have their advantages, disadvantages, and most certainly their proponents. The linear reduction/resection, modified wedge, and rotational techniques appear to be the most widely utilized. Potential advantages of contoured linear resection include easier recovery, smaller, more "flush" and linear labia and, usually, lightening of the frequently darkened-edge labia. Dissatisfaction with occasional scalloping and scarring/discomfort via over-vigorous amputation, plus the occasional incidence of hypersensitivity of the edges, led to the development [8] of the various wedge/flap procedures, each of which may provide a more "natural"-looking labial edge with rare encounters with scarring and hypersensitivity. Approximation of skin edges with fine absorbable sutures carefully placed so as to avoid "bunching" and the generous use of everting mattress sutures appears to obviate most risks of edge hypersensitivity. Unknown at this time is the very important issue of the performance of these altered labia during childbirth, and whether one technique fares better than another. Although the literature is silent regarding this issue, neither this author, nor several other high-volume genital surgeons polled (whose total case volume exceeds 5,000 cases) has been made aware of dehiscence of previously performed LP attendant with childbirth.

Most courses and a majority of novice genital plastic/cosmetic surgeons utilize a linear excision technique, as it presents a shorter learning curve and, if strict surgical principles are followed, a more reproducible result. Disadvantages include greater potential for poor cosmetic results, excessive tissue removal, and dissymmetry in difficult anatomic environments.

Following are narrations of their techniques by some of the world's most experienced genital plastic/cosmetic surgeons.

How I do it: curvilinear reduction of labia minora and excess prepuce

David Matlock and Alex Simopoulos

Introduction: We describe the reduction of the labia minora and excess prepuce using the 980 nm laser in a curvilinear fashion. The majority of these procedures also entail reducing the excess prepuce to further enhance the aesthetic appearance of these vulvar structures. The technique was devised and modified after consideration of what our patients informed us regarding how they wanted these structures to appear. Patients generally do not want the labia minora to protrude far past the labia majora; they want them to appear symmetric in the process and, if they are overly thick, make them thinner. In addition, patients have expressed that they want the prepuce to neatly drape over the clitoral shaft by reducing a portion of this tissue if redundant.

Many of these procedures, while elective, are not merely limited to aesthetic goals. The majority of patients seeking LP-m also have a concomitant functional issue, whether it be discomfort wearing tight garments, "chafing" with physical activities, hygiene difficulties, or dyspareunia [5].

The procedure described here uses the FDA-approved PhotoMedex LaserPro 980 nm. This contact laser in our experience is precise and effective for incising with simultaneous cauterization and ablation. We find this as an added benefit given the vascular nature of vulvar tissues. Because the laser fiber is applied directly to labial tissue tactile feedback is not sacrificed as may be the case with non-contact lasers.

Relevant anatomy: Proper identification of anatomy is fundamental to success with the procedure. Any individual patient variation should be noted. The labia minora split anteriorly to run over and under the glans of the clitoris. The more anterior folds form the hood-shaped prepuce of the clitoris and the posterior folds insert into the underside of the glans as the frenulum. It is important to note that the prepuce is the fold of skin surrounding the clitoris but with an insertion point that can be noted on the lateral aspect of the labia minora. Noting this during the reduction of excess prepuce will prevent leaving redundant prepuce after the excision. Figure 8.5(a), (b), and (c), respectively, illustrate prepuce, frenulum, and hood of the clitoris.

We have routinely encountered patients with a glans clitoris not only deviated from the midline but attenuated to a point where differentiation from the frenulum has been challenging. Our approach to the reduction of prepuce is to be superficial and lateral to the shaft of the clitoris. The dorsal nerve of the clitoris (DNC) is bilateral and lies on the anterolateral surface of the body of the clitoris. The two cords

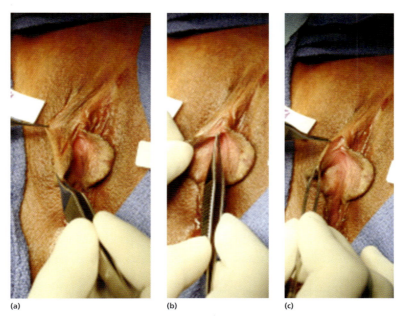

(a)   (b)   (c)

Figure 8.5 (a) Prepuce of clitoral hood. (b) Frenulum. (c) Clitoral hood. Source: D. Matlock and A. Simopoulos. Reproduced with permission.

of the DNC terminate 1 cm short of the glans of the clitoris. A thorough understanding of this anatomy is necessary to avoid iatrogenic injury. The shaft of the clitoris is medial to where we perform our excision of excess prepuce and is deeper relative to our superficial work.

Patient selection and preparation: At times patients express the desire for a very aggressive excision of the labia minora but the goal should be not an amputation but a sculpting so as not to appear as prominent. It is acceptable to tailor your surgical plan based on the patient's desires, but a degree of conservatism is required given the nature of the labia minora and how they will heal during the post-operative period as will be discussed. At no time should complete removal of labia minora be entertained. Patient selection is of utmost importance and is fully discussed in Chapter 7.

Full disclosure of risks and complications should be discussed with patients. We have provided a carefully constructed and inclusive list of potential complications that we discuss with our patients. (*See Chapters 7 and 14 for full discussion of risks.*) Of high concern to the patient is the potential loss of sensation to the clitoral region. We have not encountered this. In addition, in our hands we have not encountered significant change in the texture and feel of the labia minora once the healing phase has been completed (3–6 months), although this certainly has been reported in untrained hands. While we choose to perform our procedures under general anesthesia, we are well aware that other experienced competent surgeons utilize local or pudendal block alone for anesthesia.

Technique: We advise pre-operative pictures taken prior to the procedure. Findings relevant to the individual patient should also be noted. The vaginal area and vulva are prepared with Betadine solution and the patient is draped in the dorsal lithotomy position. For post-operative pain control a pudendal block of 5 cc of 0.5% Marcaine with epinephrine is placed bilaterally prior to starting the laser surgical procedure. (*Editor's note: local infiltration along resection lines may also be utilized.*) A surgical laser nurse is in attendance and in charge of laser safety and laser operation. The patient and all OR personnel are appropriately protected with eye garments.

Care is taken to assess the labia minora, lining both of them up to determine the aesthetic approach that would yield the desired aesthetic result. It is vital to note how the labia minora are aligned with each other in their natural state without artificial manipulation or tension by the surgeon. When the medial aspects of the labia minora are placed together it can be determined whether they are equal in length or one labum is longer or shorter than the other.

A surgical marking pen is then used to make the desired aesthetic surgical mark on the medial aspect of the right labum minus [Figure 8.6(a)]. The superior mark of the outline starts approximately 1–1.5 cm from the frenulum, extending inferiorly just enough to provide the desired aesthetic result. If the frenulum is encroached with marking and then subsequent laser excision, this invariably will lead to over-resection of labial tissue; the labia will retract during the healing phase and this could lead to an overly attenuated

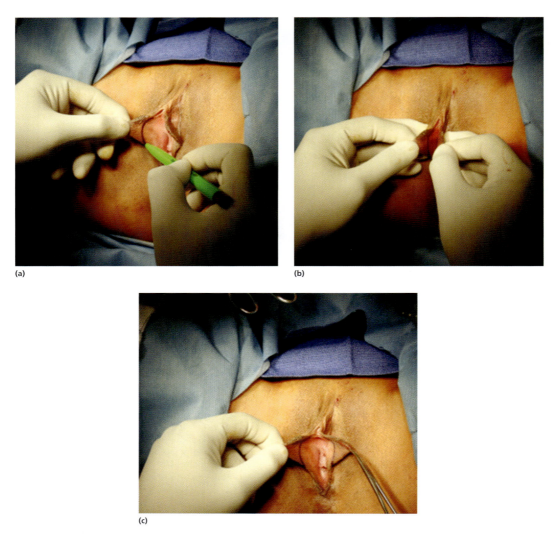

(a)   (b)

(c)

Figure 8.6 (a) Marking the labia for excision. (b) Realignment of labia minora to transfer mark. (c) Transfer of ink to contralateral labia minora. Source: D. Matlock and A. Simopoulos. Reproduced with permission.

and almost nonexistent residual labia minora. As illustrated, a curvilinear mark best maintains and preserves the natural curved contour of the labia minora after excess length is removed with the laser. Conservative excision of excess tissue is preferred. "A little is a lot" when it comes to reducing the labia minora. The surgeon must endeavor to operate on squamous epithelium lateral to Hart's line at all times.

The initial careful assessment of length by placing the medial aspects of the labia minora together is now repeated [Figure 8.6(b)], and the surgical marking is transferred to the contralateral side [Figure 8.6(c)]. This lends precision in determining the correct amount to be excised from the contralateral labia. When done correctly, the labia minora will be equal in length after both have undergone excision.

The labia minora are then infiltrated at the base with approximately 1–2 cc of 0.25% Marcaine with epinephrine. Wet 4 × 4 gauze are then placed behind the labia minora prior to laser usage to provide an extender of the labia minora and prevent excess heat transfer to surrounding tissue.

The LaserPro 980 nm laser general surgery handpiece is used with 12 watts of power and a continuous wave. Starting superiorly approximately 1 cm from the frenulum and distal to the outlining mark, the laser is directed in a 90-degree angle to the labia minora [Figure 8.7(a)].

Meticulous hemostasis is assured with a needle point electrocautery. The exact same procedure is carried out on the contralateral side. Prior to closure of the labial edges, thickness can effectively be reduced by excising small of

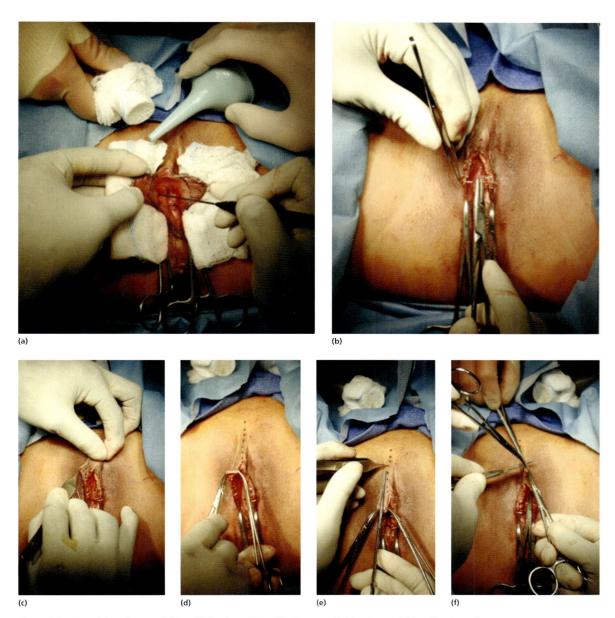

(a)

(b)

(c)   (d)   (e)   (f)

Figure 8.7 (a) Excision of excess labia utilizing laser fiber. (b) Closure of labia edges. (c) Identification of excess prepuce. (d) Creation of "triangle" of prepuce. (e) Clamping of excess prepuce. (f) Excision of excess prepuce. (g) and (h) Sub-cutaneous and sub-cuticular closure. (i) Placement of memory sutures. (j) Completed procedure. Source: D. Matlock and A. Simopoulos. Reproduced with permission.

amounts of interstitial tissue between the medial and lateral edges of the labia minora. If debulking is performed, it should be done throughout the entire length of the labum to ensure uniform reduction of thickness. We use 4-0 Vicryl to approximate the skin edges with horizontal mattress sutures [Figure 8.7(b)].

After three-quarters of the labia are re-approximated attention is then turned to the identification of excess prepuce with the extension to the lateral side of the labia minora [Figure 8.8(c)]. We find that reduction of excess prepuce is required in >90% of cases. A mosquito clamp is placed on the inferior edge of the frenulum >1 cm from the

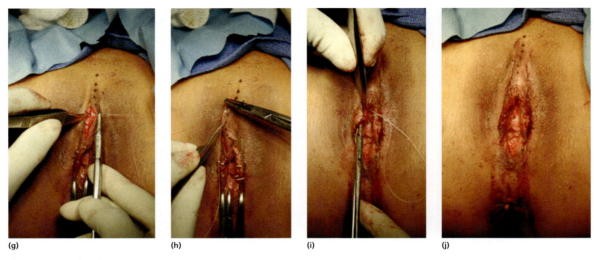

(g)   (h)   (i)   (j)

Figure 8.7 (*Continued*).

glans to aid in identification of the end of the clitoral hood. A second clamp is placed on the inferior edge of the hood. The mosquito on the inferior aspect of the frenulum is then removed and placed on the apex of the proximal edge of the excess skin at the lateral minorum edge, thereby creating a triangle with the base along the lateral edge of the minorum [Figure 8.7(d)].

A small amount of 0.25% Marcaine with epinephrine is injected at the base of the prepuce for hemostasis and initial post-operative pain relief, and a long thin Kelly is placed at the base of the excess skin and prepuce, ensuring that the prepuce edges at the base are aligned [Figure 8.7(e)]. A #11 blade is then used to resect excess skin [Figure 8.7(f)]. Cut edges are gently opened and any bleeding areas are cauterized. Interstitial tissue sutures are placed using 4-0 Vicryl in simple interrupted fashion [Figure 8.7(g)]. The skin edges are then closed via a sub-cuticular suture of 4-0 Vicryl [Figure 8.7(h)]. The remainder of the superior aspect of the labum is then closed using interrupted mattress sutures of 4-0 Vicryl. Baby Metzenbaum scissors are used to gently sculpt the frenulum if needed. Hemostasis is assured with point cautery and 4-0 Vicryl interrupted mattress sutures. The same procedure is carried out on the contralateral side. A few "memory sutures" are placed along the base, intermediate, and superficial aspects of the labia minora using 4-0 Vicryl in horizontal mattress fashion [Figure 8.7(i)]. The end result is seen with completion of contralateral side in Figure 8.7(j).

Post-operative care: It is uncommon for patients to have significant post-operative pain. Patients will uniformly experience some degree of swelling or bruising that is frequently asymmetric. One of the main goals in the post-operative period is to reduce edema as soon as possible.

Persisting edema may result in wound dehiscence by placing excess tension on wound closures and may compromise aesthetic results, promoting a degree of hypertrophy that could remain asymmetric. Along with meticulous hemostasis and respect for the delicate nature of the labial tissue during the intraoperative phase, we have patients begin Arnica Montana and Bromolein 2–3 days prior to surgery followed by continuation for several more days after surgery for the mitigation of inflammation. We begin icing the labia while in the recovery room immediately in the post-operative period. Patients are instructed to continue icing 15–20 minutes of every hour for the initial 48–72 hours after surgery. Patients are instructed to only wear loose-fitting clothing and no tight undergarments. Patients may shower the following morning and are encouraged to avoid touching the operative area with fingers when possible to decrease risk of infection. They are also counseled to refrain from sexual intercourse and placing anything in the vagina and only to shower (no submersion) for a period of 6 weeks. Post-operative visits should be regularly scheduled to monitor residual swelling. If a patient is found to have persisting swelling, we routinely encourage oral ibuprofen 200 mg taken 2–3 times with meals for a period of 7 days and have seen excellent reduction of swelling with this measure. This is contraindicated in patients with known ulcer disease. Patients should expect pruritus upon suture hydrolysis. Once candida has been excluded, reassuring the patient that this situation is temporary and counseling that she may take an antihistamine to ease these symptoms is helpful. (*Editor's note: a sample post-op instruction sheet may be found in Chapter 12.*)

Following are a small collection of our pre- and post-operative documentation (Figs 8.8–8.11):

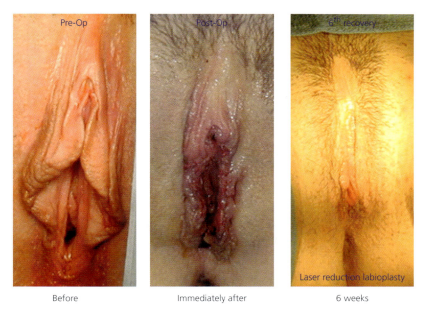

Before   Immediately after   6 weeks

Figure 8.8 Source: D. Matlock and A. Simopoulos. Reproduced with permission.

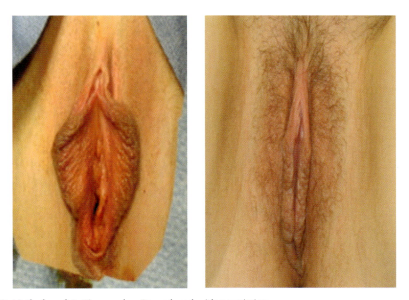

Figure 8.9 Source: D. Matlock and A. Simopoulos. Reproduced with permission.

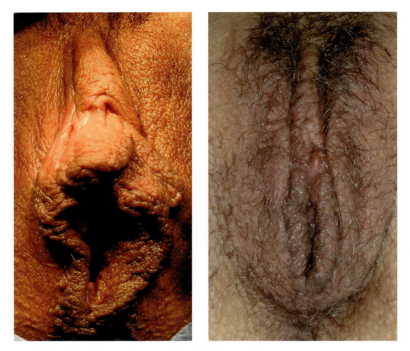

Figure 8.10   Source: D. Matlock and A. Simopoulos. Reproduced with permission.

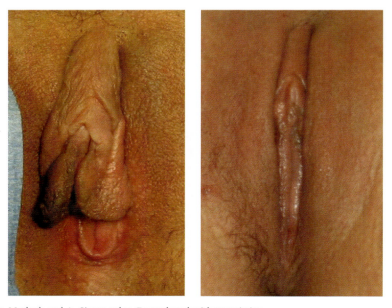

Figure 8.11   Source: D. Matlock and A. Simopoulos. Reproduced with permission.

How I do it: stem-iris scissors technique

Bernard Stern

The common denominator of the thousands of women I have had the pleasure of consulting with over the years has always been to achieve or restore what each individual patient believes to be "normal" or enhancing it toward some aesthetic and functional ideal. This is achieved by careful leading edge reduction of asymmetrical, thick, dark, and often very large and uncomfortable labia minora. The final result is to achieve "natural"-appearing labia minora that look as if the labia were always that way (Figures 8.12–8.14).

For me, achieving consistent pleasing results is dependent on multiple digital and computer-generated imaging, pre-operative "marking," fine blepharoplasty delicate instruments,

4-0 and 5-0 "eye" sutures, exacting suturing techniques, meticulous attention to detail during surgery, and explicit post-operative care by patients with training and teaching prior to surgery.

My hood resection technique will not be covered in detail as it is very similar to that of others with prepuce resection and Z-plasty where the hood meets the crura (crus) and resected labial edge.

Technique

Anesthesia: I select local, conscious sedation, or general anesthesia pending patient choice. "Local" is a mixture of 1% xylocaine with epinephrine 50/50 with 1% Marcaine plain, buffered with sodium bicarbonate, 0.1–0.2 ml/10 my anesthetic. Using any more local than is necessary to achieve

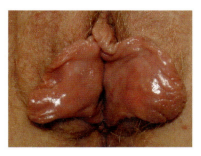
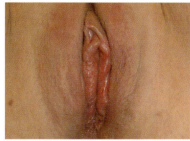

Figure 8.12 Stem-iris linear LP technique. Source: B. Stern. Reproduced with permission.

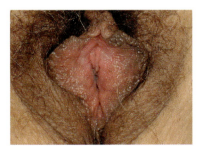
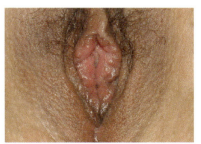

Figure 8.13 Source: B. Stern. Reproduced with permission.

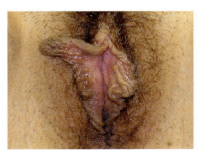
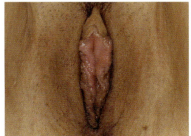

Figure 8.14 Source: B. Stern. Reproduced with permission.

anesthesia, tissue plane dissection, and small vessel hemostasis will distort and/or disrupt the surgical site. No more than 4–8 ml total is usually sufficient to achieve desired effects.

All injections are done medial to proposed lines of dissection. This will minimally distort proposed surgical dissection lines yet will provide anesthesia, hemostasis, and tissue planes. Occasionally at the termination of a procedure additional local is injected especially for the patient who may have a longer travel time.

Instruments

1 Kaye serrated supercut scissors, 4 1/2" curved (*Black and Black Instruments*) (Figure 8.15).
2 Castroviejo Diamond Dust Onyx Forceps, 4" (10 cm,) 5 mm tip.
3 Castroviejo curved flat handle needle holder, tungsten carbide, curved 5 1/2" 7000 jaw. (*Editor's note: fine Adson-type forceps may also be utilized.*)
4 Mosquito clamps; Allis clamps.

Handling, cutting, re-approximating tissue with absolute minimal trauma is one of the major keys to success.

Meticulous attention to hemostasis is imperative to a beautiful outcome. A hematoma in the surgical repair, even a small one, can stretch the immediate area surrounding the repair and compromise surgical outcome. Pinpoint hemostasis with an "eye cautery" often is sufficient to edge oozing or elsewhere. However, arteriolar bleeders should always be isolated and tied off. The common venous edge bleeders in the inferior portion of the labia minora usually are controlled with skin sutures, locking where necessary

Conservative trimming: The most common complication [of linear sculpting] is unintentionally taking too much if not completely removing a labum minus. This occurs because often the attachment of the labia minora laterally (inter-labial fold) is far shorter than may be imagined viewing the labum from only the mucosal aspect. Also, less skilled surgeons may pull on the labia (which in some cases are very elastic), thus further distorting the anatomy. Cutting with only a medial (mucosal) view, without marking and straying

interior to Hart's line medially can lead to disastrous outcomes. Marking the lateral side, without tension 1/2–1 cm from the inter-labial fold and having your assistant continually advising you while you are excising will avoid resecting too much tissue.

I prefer to do the larger, more difficult side first then match the smaller side to the larger one. When marking, measure, measure, measure! Also when in doubt, take less off rather than more. You can always "trim" later.

Meticulous closure: The key to closure (other than total hemostasis) is eliminating all dead space, taking tension off edge closure, everting the edge, and closing with 5-0 Vicryl, tiny needle interrupted close vertical mattress sutures.

Explicit post-op instructions: Patients are given all postoperative (as well as pre-operative) instructions verbally (from patient care coordinator and RN and well as by me) and in written form, which they read pre-operatively and *sign*. Q-tip instructions are given for first 48 hours with Neosporin or peroxide to keep "tips" or labia edges from sticking to each other, as well as showering instructions, allowing soaping water to "drip" and how to pat dry. I advise application of local estradiol cream (0.01–0.02%) in addition to, or mixed with a copper peptide cream such as *Cu-3* (if not allergic to copper), applied sparingly to edges for patients who are pre-/peri-menopausal (over 42/43 years old). I advise patients to not frequently look at the surgical area and to never pull up to visualize. Ice, ice, ice first 48–72 hours. Icing can continue if necessary and it gives physical comfort, but heat is advised after 72 hours if swelling. No running, jumping, aerobics, lower body exercising, or swimming for 3 weeks. Tampax use is discouraged until 28 days. Soaking is OK after day 21. Sexual activity is not advised for 5–6 weeks.

Post-op contact and follow-up: Every patient has my cellular number to call, text, or send pictures. Local patients often see me at 1 week. Out-of-town patients either text or email pictures. A 5–6 week follow-up visit is encouraged and advised for all patients within reasonable distance. Pictures and phone visits with all out-of-town, out-of-country patients are performed at ~6 weeks.

The aesthetic and functional results achieved by this evolving and continuously refined technique are remarkable. In over 2,300 female cosmetic genital surgeries in my practice, the "touch-up" rate was less than 6% with 92% overall satisfaction. The totally natural-looking results are based on my individual surgical skills utilizing the inexpensive and easily obtainable instruments, sutures, and techniques delineated above (Figure 8.16). The technique is reproducible and, in properly trained hands, similar results can be expected.

How I do it: linear reduction labiaplasty by radiofrequency
Michael P. Goodman

The basic techniques, with refinements and specific pearls, have been discussed earlier in this chapter. As the reader will have undoubtedly surmised both in the overall description and directed "How I do its" above, the technique is the same,

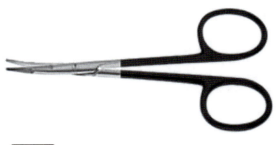

Figure 8.15 Kaye serrated Supercut scissors.

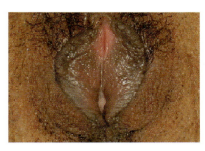 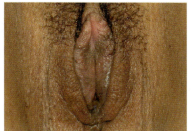

Figure 8.16 Source: B. Stern. Reproduced with permission.

only the tools are changed. I shall direct a few comments in this section toward specifically the use of radiofrequency (RF) energy to accomplish desired results when performing a curvilinear resection and add additional useful "pearls." Of course, the same equipment may be utilized for V-wedge procedures, described later in the chapter.

For current usage, RF energy is power delivered at a characteristic wavelength via a handheld wand with inter-changeable tips designed for focusing or de-focusing this energy. The waveform is different, but the concept is not at all dissimilar to that of the use of lightwave energy in laser applications. Like laser, RF energy may be focused (e.g., at the tip of a thin-gauge wire) or diffused (e.g., dispersed via larger diameter tip.) Focused RF energy, like laser, produces a fine-line cutting appliance, capable of "scrolling" and meticulously producing "cut-outs" along a carefully drawn roadmap. Like laser, very little heat is produced at its acutely fine-tipped edge, with negligible dispersal into tissue. It is a hand-held fiber wand device, controlled by a knowledge-able, steady touch. Power is supplied by a commercially available generator. Interchangeable tips are available. The fine wire cutting tip is available both straight and 30-degree curved, and ceramically shielded or unshielded (Figure 8.17). This is a "touch" instrument with cutting produced via touch of the wire tip with the tissue, providing cutting with minimal heat conduction.

I will not be redundant and re-describe technique. I agree with the basic tenets put forward by Drs. Simopoulos, Matlock, and Stern: proper patient choice, staying outside Hart's line on the mucosal surface and well medial to the inter-labial fold on the lateral surface. Take great care to not put the labum on stretch when drawing lines, remember to curve the line, leaving perhaps more tissue in situ at the cephalad portion of the incision line than your eyes may tell you. Bevel the line into the descending clitoral hood fold, or incorporate that fold into the incision line on a case-by-case basis (Figure 8.18). A step-by-step depiction of a curvilinear reduction, in my hands, is shown in Figure 8.19.

Please understand: RF energy is simply a tool. The sur-gical concepts remain the same with scissors, laser, or RF. Where RF and laser find their unique application is the "sculpting" and control possible when adding reduction of redundant clitoral hood epithelium to the procedure. See Figure 8.20.

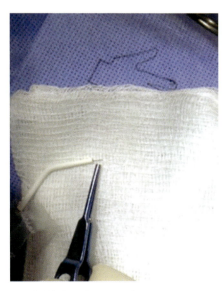

Figure 8.17 Shielded 30-degree RF fine wire tip. Forceps point to tip. Source: M. Goodman. Reproduced with permission.

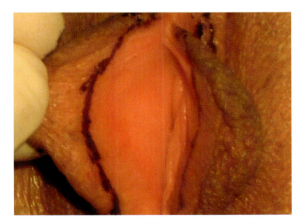

Figure 8.18 Mucosal incision line. Note surgeon pulls excessively on labum; best to let it "lie" while drawing. Source: M. Goodman. Reproduced with permission.

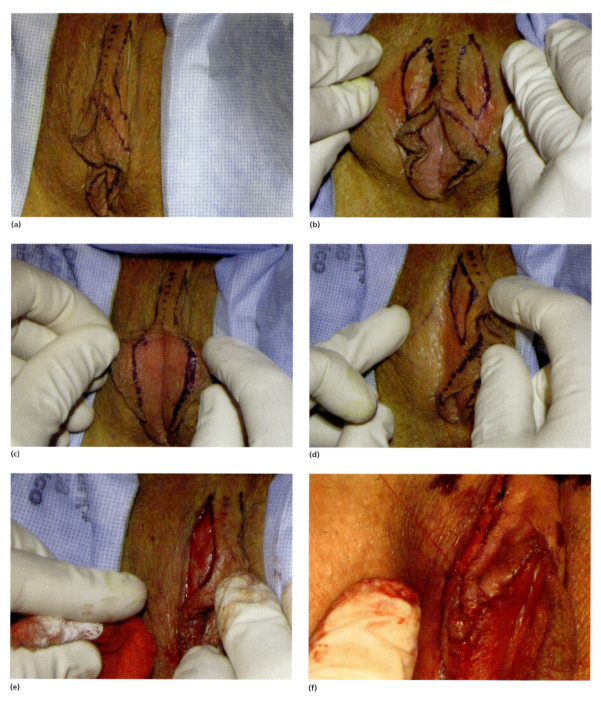

Figure 8.19 (a) Pre-op LP, RCH, with markings. Midline dotted line delineates the midline of the clitoral hood. Labia are marked for linear resection; hood hypertrophy will be separately diminished via the use of bilateral elliptical excisions. (b) All incision lines. Lateral hood folds (prepuce) "disappear" when put on stretch. It is this redundancy that is superficially resected. (c) Incision line, mucosal surface. (d) Lateral view. RF needle facilitates incisions. (e) Clitoral hood incision via RF. (f) Completing sub-cuticular line with 5-0 Vicryl Rapide. Source: M. Goodman. Reproduced with permission.

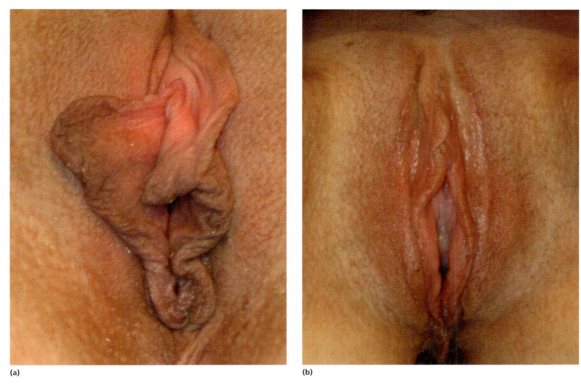

(a)   (b)

Figure 8.20 (a) Pre LP-m, RCH, LP-M via RF energy. (b) Six weeks post-op linear LP-m, RCH, LP-M utilizing RF energy. Source: M. Goodman. Reproduced with permission.

Clitoral hoods "flow down" into the labia in ways varying from individual to individual, and from side to side in the same woman. When the labum "flows" directly from one fold only, be it from the lateral aspect of the clitoral hood, frenulum, or prepucial fold, the procedure is straightforward, and the sculpted excisional line proceeds directly, encompassing the labum and hood fold, beveling at both cephalad and caudad portions, taking care to not remove excessive epithelium, especially at the posterior commissure, and to stray no closer than 1 cm from the clitoral glans or immediate central hood. Difficulty, however, will be encountered when, as it frequently does, the labia contain components from various portions of the hood, with different insertions and dissymmetry bilaterally. It is in this frequent eventuality where RF energy and a maneuverable micro-fine-tipped handpiece are elegant. If removal of non-continuous hood folds is aesthetically appropriate, this may be accomplished with the use of elliptical-shaped separate excisions, taking care to leave at least 5 mm (the more the better) between incision lines, avoiding any "T-ing" or lines, with resultant increased risk of wound separation at the junction.

How I do it: the V-wedge and "Y" modification

Michael P. Goodman

This technique, first described by Gary Alter, MD [8], and others [9], excises a modified V-shaped "wedge" of redundant labum, the superior edge beginning inferior to the fold flowing from the clitoral hood; the inferior edge beginning at or above the posterior commissure (Figure 8.21). Either a Z-plasty (rarely used) or an upwards oriented "hockey-stick" curvature is utilized laterally to take up redundancy and prevent a "dog-ear." If lateral hood or prepucial fold redundancy producing a "pseudo-hypertrophic" and protruding hood is an issue for the patient, the lateral labial incision line is continued cephalad in a "Y-shaped" manner to incorporate this epithelial redundancy.

"*If all you have is a hammer, everything looks like a nail.*" The wedge technique and its cousins, superior/inferior flap and Z-plasty modification for labial size and redundancy reduction, are simply alternatives to produce reduction/modification of functionally and/or cosmetically displeasurable labia minora and/or clitoral hood epithelium.

Individual women have vastly different anatomy, and in no area is this more evident than in their vulvar structures, where appearance may radically differ from both person to person, and from side to side in the same individual. Thus, it is helpful for the genital plastic/cosmetic surgeon to have alternate surgical techniques at his/her disposal to better manage disparate anatomy.

While it is impossible for a textbook to instruct the student on procedural choice for an individual surgical candidate, suffice it to state that wedge procedures fit nicely into the armamentarium of the genital surgeon, managing certain

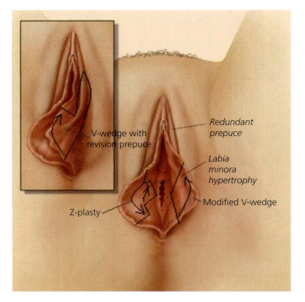

Figure 8.21 V-wedge; Z-plasty. Inset photo shows "Y" modification that is utilized as a continuous incision line to trim excess prepuce. Source: R. Moore and J. Miklos. Reproduced with permission.

anatomical realities better than a linear resection procedure and, importantly, adding an element of individual patient choice to these essentially elective surgical procedures.

In a wedge procedure, the cephalad or "upper" labial incision is made a minimum of 1 cm distal to the intersection of the glans clitoris, proximal frenulum, and central-most clitoral hood. As the labum minus "flows" distally from one to several folds flowing "down" from the more cephalad and frequently multi-folded clitoral hood, the "upper" incision is made distal, or "below" the confluence of frenular and central hood fold(s). The "lower" or more caudad incision of the "V" is made above the labial reflection of the posterior commissure; the exact locations of these "arms" of the "V" depend on individual anatomy and the particular desires of the patient in regards to the amount of labial tissue she wishes remaining framing her introitus. With greater recent understanding of labial vascularity (Chapter 3), placement of the "V" incision more cephalad may improve healing opportunities and diminish dehiscence rate by providing a more intact post-operative vascular supply.

Choice of procedure: Any labum may be reduced via linear resection; any labum may be reduced via a V-wedge modification. How to decide? As this author performs both linear resection and V-wedge procedures, with modifications of both basic techniques, pre-surgical evaluation takes into account both patient anatomy and her choice of procedure after viewing "before and after" LP-m photos of women with labia similar to her anatomy performed via alternative techniques. Additionally important is the surgeon's estimation of his/her patient's ability to follow recovery protocols, as a linear resection procedure may be more "forgiving" in

the early post-operative period than a V-wedge, which is on greater tension and exhibits a greater risk of wound disruption when confronted with inappropriate early recovery activities.

Instruments and setup: A labial reduction procedure lends itself to in-office performance under a local anesthetic, and presently virtually all of the author's labiaplasties are performed in-office in a small surgical suite. The exam/surgical table with knee rests or Allen-type stirrups is mid-room, allowing adequate space at the head and one side of the table for the circulating RN and a member of the patient's family, should she desire. An RF generator and electrocautery unit occupy the other side of the table. A shelf pulls out 1–2 feet from the end of the table for instruments and as a surface on which the surgeon may rest forearms during the procedure (Figure 8.22).

Operative procedure (see Figure 8.23)

1 *Marking*:   The labum is dried to allow for drawing [Figure 8.23(a)]. Utilizing a sterile marking pen, incision lines are drawn, taking into account the patient's desires and individual anatomy [Figure 8.23(b)]. Not infrequently, my patient will hold a mirror and observe this portion of her procedure. The carpenter's adage, *"Measure twice; cut once"* certainly applies here!

2 *Local anesthesia*: Although a number of methods have been described to "numb" the labum pre-injection (application of 5% lidocaine ointment for 1+ hours pre-injection; ethyl chloride; benzocaine spray, etc.), and this author has tried them all, they are time-consuming and, in my opinion, do not appreciably diminish discomfort of the injection. Through years of trial and error, the author does the following:

   (a) Injection solution: 0.5% (0.25% may be utilized) bupivacaine with epinephrine (unless patient is sensitive), buffered for minimization of injection discomfort with ~0.15–0.2 ml sodium bicarbonate/10 ml anesthetic. A 1.5-inch 25–27 ga. needle is utilized; volume varies between ~6 and 10 ml total for both sides, depending on size and inclusion of clitoral hood and/or posterior commissure reduction.

   (b) Injection technique: Initial injection is a skin wheal at base of incision line. All subsequent needle entries are via this wheal, or into previously anesthetized areas. Injection is slow, "laying down" a minimum ribbon of anesthetic just inside of incision lines [Figure 8.23(c)]. Test anesthetic effect with forceps prior to commencing incision.

3 *Incision*: Incision may be effected with electrosurgical needle electrode, fine plastic scissors (petite Metzenbaums, Kaye, etc.), laser or RF needle electrode. The author utilizes either scissors or RF method and utilizes a ceramic shielded 30-degree angled RF needle electrode or plastic scissors described above [Figure 8.23(d) and (e)]. Incision follows pre-drawn lines, and great care is taken to avoid excess removal of sub-cutaneous tissue, which can result in invagination of fine epithelial edges and surface overlap. An exception may be made for women with bulky, thickened labia, but this (debulking) method of removal should be reserved for accomplished surgeons.

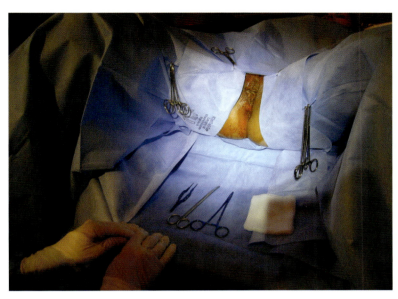

Figure 8.22 Office setup. Instruments (L to R): Mosquito clamps X2, clamped to drape; fine forceps; Metzenbaum (or Kaye) scissors; needle holder; Allis clamps X2, clamped to drape. Towel clips on top. Base of table pulled out for elbow rest, instruments. Source: M. Goodman. Reproduced with permission

4 *Excision and bleeders*: Excision may be effected with either dissecting scissors, laser, RF, or electrical current. All venous bleeders must be cauterized in as localized manner as possible; arterial bleeders are best suture ligated, but minor ones may be grasped with a forceps and fulgurated. It is important to leave a dry field and avoid "spray" hemostasis [Figure 8.23(f)].

5 *Closure and "adjustments"*: Most valuable is a centrally placed layer of ~2–4 interrupted sub-cutaneous sutures (bury knots) to both securely re-approximate the arms of the "V" and eliminate dead space. An additional 1–3 sutures may be utilized sub-cutaneously along the lateral arm of the incision to further modify "dead space" [Figure 8.23(g)].

Sub-Q suture material must be relatively non-reactive and of small caliber. 4-0 or 5-0 multifiber or monofiber absorbable sutures may be utilized. I have recently switched from 4-0 Vicryl to 5-0 Monocryl. I, and others, have had rare cases of patients exteriorizing the sub-Q multifilament sutures, resulting in fistulae or suture line separations. Although elegant, 5-0 Monocryl is difficult to see and work with; PDS may be substituted, either 4-0 or 5-0, but the 5-0 comes only on a needle that is a bit small for the job.

After the sub-cutaneous layer is placed, the surgeon can get an idea of the size and aesthetics of the "finished product" and may wish to trim an additional small amount of skin from the lateral surface to avoid "dog-ears." Great care must be taken not to be over-aggressive and stray significantly into the inter-labial fold. Trim may be performed with a scissors, but laser or RF is elegant for this task.

6 *Adding RCH to the LP*: For patients with symptomatic redundancy of their central and/or lateral/prepucial portions of their hoods, an RCH may be added either separately to the "V," or by extending the "V" at its nadir into a "Y-shaped" excision, extending the tail to encompass the redundant mid-lateral/lateral folds. A sub-Q layer of either interrupted or continuous sutures is placed to well approximate the cut edges of redundant hood epithelium. If the excision of redundant hood epithelium is to be done separately, it is performed via an elliptical excision, staying superficial, taking care to not "T" the incision lines if possible, and utilizing a layer of sub-cutaneous sutures prior to skin closure.

7 *Skin closure*: Although a sub-cuticular closure may work well for a linear technique, it is technically difficult for a V-wedge, and I utilize a series of interrupted 5-0 Vicryl Rapide sutures placed ~2–3 mm apart, with *generous* use of mattress sutures to prevent edge inversion. As the epithelium may be redundant and pliable, especially if one was overly generous in excision of sub-cutaneous tissue, the edges tend to imbricate.

Most surgeons utilize 4-0 or 5-0 mono- or multifilament suture for skin closure. If closure is to be "through and through," I like the Vicryl Rapide as it dissolves in 10–14 days, which is satisfactory so long as a supportive sub-cutaneous layer is utilized, and it is not as "stiff" and irritating as monofilament [Figure 8.23(h) and (i)].

8 *Dressing*: The incision is coated with mupericin ointment and covered with a non-stick dressing (Telfa, etc.), gauze, and disposable panties. Care is taken with immediate post-operative ambulation, and it is done slowly and in stages to

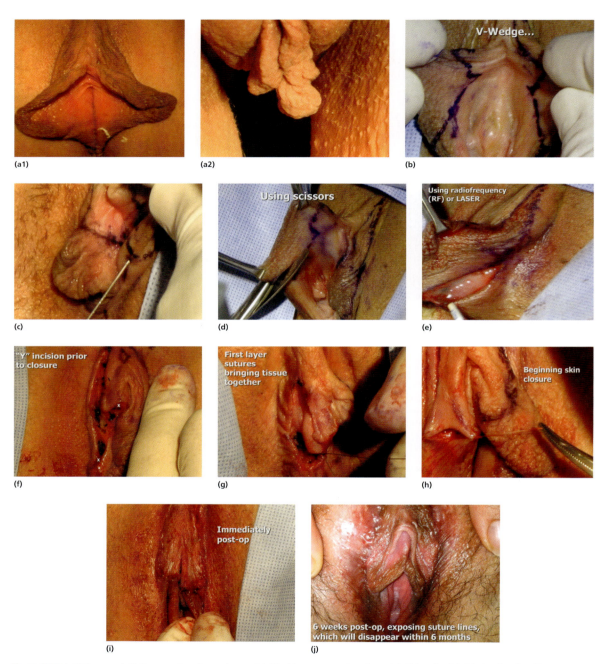

Figure 8.23 (a1) Pre-op. (a2) Pre-op view from above. (b) Marking, mucosal surface. (c) Skin wheal initiation local infiltration. (d) Initial incision. (e) Initial incision, using RF. (f) The "Xs" denote the upper and lower edges of the "V," to be approximated by sub-cutaneous sutures prior to skin closure. (g) Sub-Q layer. (h) Apex and nadir sutures, lateral surface. (i) Procedure completed. (j) Six weeks post-op. Source: M. Goodman. Reproduced with permission.

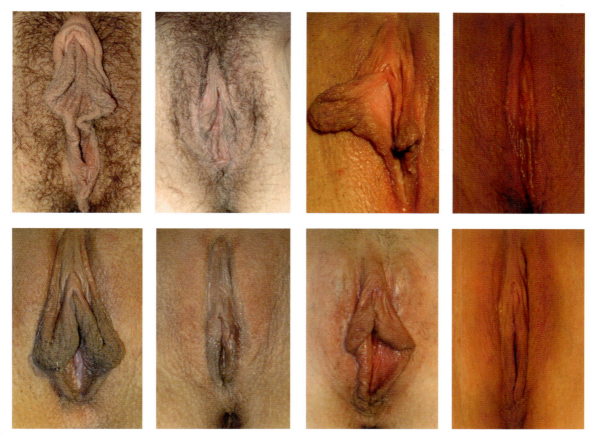

Figure 8.24 Typical modified V-wedge results. Source: M. Goodman. Reproduced with permission.

avoid hypotension in a premedicated patient who has been in dorsal lithotomy for 1–2.5 hours.

At 4–6 weeks initial results may be appreciated, and full activities, including sexual activities, may be resumed [Figure 8.23(j)]. However, it will be 3–6 months before final results are manifested.

Below (Figure 8.24) are several "before and afters" of V-wedge LPs performed by the author. Note disparate anatomy and variety of aesthetic results. Post-op photos are ~6–12 weeks after procedures.

LP, labia majora (LP-M)

A less-utilized procedure than reduction of labia minora, LP-M is performed in situations where large, wrinkled, and redundant labia majora are cosmetically unappealing to the patient (1,15). Majora reduction is effected by a vertical excision of an ellipsis of labial

dermis, with or without (usually *without*, to avoid "puckering" via loss of adipose support) a portion of underlying adipose tissue within Colles' fascia, with repair via sub-cutaneous imbricating sutures, utilizing either non-reactive synthetic, preferably monofilament 3-0 to 5-0 sub-cuticular sutures, or interrupted nylon skin closure. If found to be torn, Colles' fascia surrounding the underlying adipose "finger" may be repaired with fine synthetic non-reactive absorbable sutures. Frequently, the suture line may be partially hidden in the inter-labial fold if adequate redundancy exists to allow this. LP-M may also be accomplished by injection of autologous fat transplantation or synthetic bulking agents. Most recently, Dr. Red Alinsod (personal communication) has utilized RF energy off-label, supplied via wand with a 15–20 mm "paddle" to heat and potentially "denature" underlying collagen, providing collagen "shrinkage" and modest minimization of redundancy for cases with only modest redundancy. Treatment time is ~20 minutes for both sides and should be repeated X 2 at monthly intervals. While ongoing data is unavailable, Dr. Alinsod presently recommends re-treatment ~every 18 months (personal communication).

How I do it: LP-M (labia majora)

Michael P. Goodman

As with the labia minora and other parts of the vulva, there are individual anatomic differences. Labia may be flattened or robust. With pregnancy, age, significant weight loss, and/or genetics, the labia majora may become redundant, and the skin may "sag" or appear excessively prominent, causing an embarrassing perineal fullness while erect that women pejoratively term "camel toe," most noticeable upon wearing tight fitting clothing.

Women request size modification of their labia majora for a variety of reasons. A common personal reason is the appearance of "bulging," usually found in healthy younger women with robustly full labia. This is in no way "abnormal," but, as with many requests for cosmetic alteration, stems from a feeling of "fullness," a desire to be "trim," or the appearance of "camel toe" described above. Another common reason, usually in multiparous or "older" women, is the redundancy and "saggy" appearance produced by loss of skin tone, pregnancy-related stretch, or other weight reduction.

Surgical Technique

The surgical technique is relatively straightforward. Success stems from clearly understanding the patient's purpose for the intended surgery, a frank discussion of possible/probable results, and an honest pictorial review of results in women who have previously undergone the procedure.

LP-M may be performed both in-office and in a surgical center or other outpatient facility. Anesthesia choices mirror other labial aesthetic procedures (see Chapter 14). Surgery may be performed under conduction, general endo-tracheal, and local infiltration techniques. Following are the general tenets of the procedure, with "advisories" as indicated.

1 *Preparation/setup/anesthesia*: This is a hair-baring area. Any trimming, shaving, or other hair removal technique should be performed >1 week prior to surgery, or immediately pre-op to avoid an operative field possibly contaminated by folliculitis. The patient is placed in the dorsal lithotomy position with legs abducted, after evaluation in the adducted position to ascertain the anatomical situation. If surgery will exceed 1.5 hours (e.g., performed along with another genital plastic surgery), the use of support hose or SCDs is encouraged. After appropriate skin prep, the labia majora are dried and incision lines are drawn with a sterile marking pen [Figures 8.25 and 8.26(b)]. If local anesthesia, I utilize 0.25–0.5% bupivacaine. I prefer 0.5% but have an absolute limit of 30 ml of 0.5% bupivacaine total per case in order to avoid bupivacaine toxicity. If other procedures have or will be performed at the same time, the anesthetic concentration may be diluted to 0.375 or 0.25% (see Chapter 14).

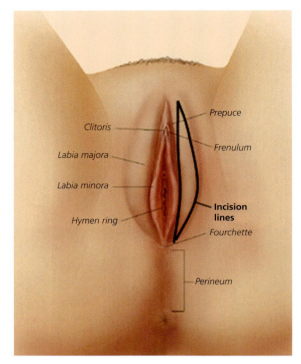

Figure 8.25 Labia majoraplasty. Source: R. Moore and J. Miklos. Reproduced with permission.

I perform virtually all my labial surgery, LP-m and LP-M, in-office and utilize bupivacaine buffered with 0.15–0.2 ml sodium bicarbonate/10 ml anesthetic, administered with a 1.5 inch 25 ga. needle, beginning with a skin wheal at the nadir of the incisional ellipse, proceeding with a small ribbon of anesthetic just outside of the incision lines. One must remember that the epithelium in this area is relatively fibrous and has a rich nerve supply (anesthetic injection hurts!)

2 *Incision and excision*: As with other genital aesthetic procedures, care in drawing incision lines is imperative. I start medially, placing the "inner" line almost vertically at the junction of the hair-bearing and hairless area just lateral to the inter-labial fold. The outer portion of the incision line, depending on the anatomy, patient desires, and skin elasticity, extends in a curvilinear manner to include a majority of redundant labial epithelium, which will appear "flattened" in abduction. As it is not infrequent that the most dependent ("lowest") portion of the labum will be additionally redundant, take care to extend the incision line around this area in a "teardrop"-like manner so as to include this redundancy and avoid the appearance of "festoons" after healing. Skin incision may be effected by a scalpel, needle electrode (cutting power), laser, or RF energy. The touch laser fiber and RF are elegant and easy to use. I start the incision line at the bottom, progressing to the top, to avoid blood flow from obscuring incision lines. The incision need not be greater

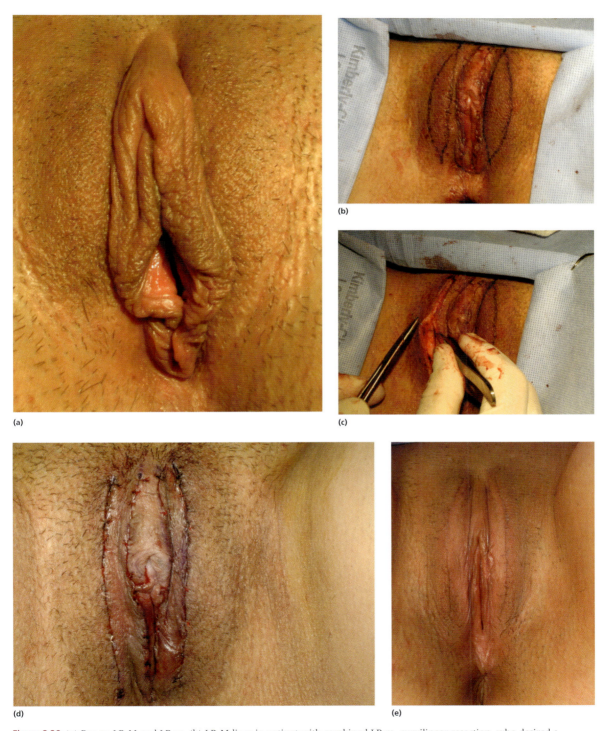

Figure 8.26 (a) Pre-op LP-M and LP-m. (b) LP-M lines in patient with combined LP-m, curvilinear resection, who desired a "flattened look." Clitoral hood edema secondary to tumescent anesthesia. (c) Placing sub-cutaneous layer. Note intact fat pad beneath subcutaneous suture line. (d) Finished LP-m and LP-M. Sub-cuticular 5-0 Monocryl with occasional interrupted 5-0 Vicryl Rapide sutures to eliminate any "gaps." (e) Six weeks post-op. Source: M. Goodman. Reproduced with permission.

than 2–3 mm in depth. Superficial skin removal may be with dissection scissors or surgical fiber on fulguration or hemostatic wave form. **Take care when excising epithelium to not violate Colles' fascia.

3   *Repair*: As with minoraplasty hemostasis is mandatory. Small venous and tiny arterial bleeders may be controlled with focal electrocautery; larger vessels and most all arterial bleeders deserve suture ligation with 4-0 or 5-0 multi- or monofilament delayed absorbable suture material. Carefully inspect Colles' fascia for any rents; these should be repaired with small-caliber absorbable suture. I place a careful sub-cutaneous approximating layer with either an interrupted or continuous 4-0 braided or monofilament inverting suture line, taking care to include the sub-epithelial fascia and little or none of the fatty layer [Figure 8.26(c)]. This will provide a tension-free approximation as well as minimizing "dead space," making a sub-cuticular closure safe and aesthetic. I have tried various skin closure techniques and have settled on either a 5-0 Monocryl sub-cuticular line or interrupted 5-0 nylon mattress sutures, with removal in 7–10 days. If utilizing a sub-cuticular closure, I place occasional interrupted 5-0 Vicryl Rapide skin sutures to approximate any "gaps" that may appear in the sub-cuticular line [Figure 8.26(d)]. Another option is to utilize Steri-Strips or a skin closure product such as Dermabond.

Activity restriction is similar to that of minoraplasty (see Chapter 12). Full activities may be resumed at 1 month; it will take 6–12 months before the incision line is aesthetically mostly undetectable [Figures 8.26(e), 8.27(b), 8.28(c), and 8.29(b)].

How I do it: mons pubis reduction

Otto J. Placik

The mons pubis (MP) is also referred to as the mons veneris or the suprapubic region [16]. Overgrowth or excessive size has been termed hypertrophy and may be associated with laxity and/or ptosis [17]. Treatment may be described as a monsplasty but others have called this "rejuvenation." [18] Good results are most commonly achieved using mons reduction and/or suspension techniques.

The mons has vague anatomic boundaries roughly defined as the top of the hair-bearing pubic area and laterally to the inguinal crease ending inferiorly at the apex of the vulvar crease (also referred to as the anterior labial commissure) and the labia majora. These borders are not obviously fixed and require interpretation in some individuals. It is generally convex with an outward bulge created by a superficial fatty deposit that thins at the vulvar cleft (anterior labial commissure) and is separated by the superficial fascial system (SFS), which continues on as Colles' fascia containing the deeper adipose tissue layer into the labia majora as discussed above. The MP is predominantly innervated by branches of the ilioinguinal nerve. The vascular supply is from both the inferior epigastric artery as well as collateral branches of the external pudendal artery supplying the labia majora from below.

Pregnancy as well as weight gain will produce an increase in size, and resulting weight loss and natural involutional changes following delivery or with age will commonly result in unpredictable degrees of skin laxity and ptosis.

Some patients are made acutely aware of the condition because it may become even more obvious following abdominoplasty when the veiling panniculus has been removed [17,18]. Patients have reported difficulties with maintaining hygiene, and intertrigo, erythema, or candidiasis may become problematic [15,16]. Descriptions of altered sexual function have been cited [15,16] Discomfort in pants and swimsuits is not an infrequent complaint [15].

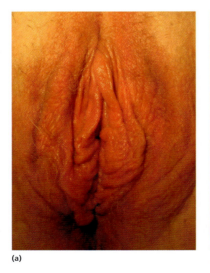

(a)

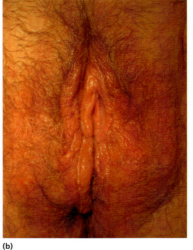

(b)

Figure 8.27 (a) Sixty-one-year-old woman, in new relationship, felt "old and saggy." (b) One month post-op modified V-wedge/Y procedure, combined minora/majora excision. Source: M. Goodman. Reproduced with permission.

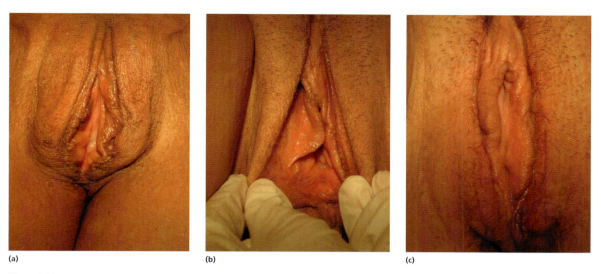

Figure 8.28 (a) Pre-op LP-M. Labia minora not an issue for this patient. Note dependent "sag." (b) Pre-op. (c) One month post-op LP-M and PP. No LP-m performed. Note healing LP-M lines. Source: M. Goodman. Reproduced with permission.

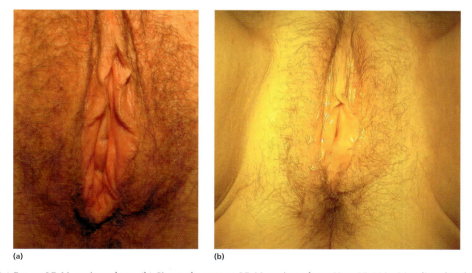

Figure 8.29 (a) Pre-op LP-M, perineoplasty. (b) Six weeks post-op LP-M, perineoplasty. Note LP-M incision lines barely perceptible vertically mid-labum. Source: M. Goodman. Reproduced with permission.

In the event of good skin laxity, interventions may range from simple volume reduction with lipectomy, most commonly performed with suction-assisted lipectomy, with or without combinations of ultrasound-assisted lipoplasty [19], laser-assisted lipolysis, and external or internal RF-assisted lipolysis. In the following text, the aforementioned may be collectively referred to as "liposuction" and is a commonly used option for management of the mons in combination with abdominal dermolipectomy procedures or may be used with labia majora procedures discussed elsewhere in this chapter. Although often performed at the time of abdomino-plasty, mons reduction may be performed on a staged basis. Given the ability to conceal a horizontal scar, this is generally preferred by most surgeons.

Treatment goals are to accomplish a smooth transition from the abdomen to the pubic region.

Satisfactory outcomes are acquired via a learning curve. Important points and technical pearls that will be addressed below include:

1 Examining the patient in the standing position with the mons retracted superiorly as well as the lithotomy with the legs abducted if performing combined procedures (thigh lift or labia majoria reduction).
2 The area is prone to prolonged edema.
3 The area is prone to prolonged ecchymosis.
4 Meticulous hemostasis is important due to the large vessels in this area (especially following weight loss).
5 Permanent SFS sutures may result in suture granuloma.
6 Liposuction alone is insufficient if ptosis is present.
7 SFS repair is essential.
8 Lymphatics are predominantly in the deeper tissues.
9 Monsplasty with labia majora can be combined but the monsplasty is to be performed first to assess labia majora distortion.
10 Avoid over-resection of fat of mons or labia majora with attention to matching thickness to abdominal panniculus. Keep thinning cepahalad to symphysis pubis.
11 Ultrasonic-assisted lipoplasty is commonly associated with dysesthesias.
12 Aggressive suction-assisted lipectomy of deep fat may result in an increased incidence of seroma.
13 The horizontal incision should come to lie 5–8 cm above the vulvar cleft.
14 The width of the mons pubis ranges from 8 to 16 cm.

Surgical technique
Case study: mons reduction and suspension following massive weight loss
The surgical technique is commonly performed in combination with an abdominoplasty but may be carried out

as an isolated procedure. A favorable outcome is more likely if the patient has been educated and has realistic expectations of the scar with a review of both good and bad results. Ancillary procedures such as liposuction, labia majora reduction, abdominoplasty, thigh dermolipectomy, and laser hair removal may be considered as part of the overall aesthetic planning.

Mons procedures, especially when performed in combination with an abdominoplasty or body contouring procedure, are commonly carried out under general anesthesia in an outpatient facility or hospital. Isolated liposuction or limited lifts may be completed using local or regional anesthesia with sedation as needed and in an office setting. Local tumescent anesthesia may be utilized in an office setting.

Preparation/marking: Smoking is stopped for a minimum of 4 weeks. Aspirin and non-steroidal medications are discontinued 2 weeks pre-operatively. If patients have had a history of intertrigo with fungal infections along the crease, they are asked to apply a topical over-the-counter anti-fungal agent, such as 1% clotrimazole cream twice a day for 1 week prior to surgery with 150 mg ketoconazole orally the night prior to surgery.

The day of surgery, the patient is examined with a garment and the level indicating the highest possible location for the incision to be concealed beneath the waistband is delineated (Figure 8.30). The patient is asked to adjust this keeping in mind different types of anticipated postoperative clothing.

The patient is asked to then aggressively lift the abdominal panniculus cephalad to simulate the effects of the abdominoplasty (Figure 8.31). The fullness and ptosis/laxity of the mons is then assessed. Four factors are taken into account: [1] a minimum of 5 cm of skin between the inci-

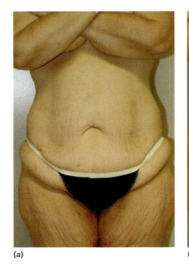 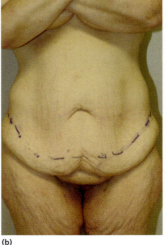

(a)　　　　　　　　　　　　(b)

Figure 8.30 (a) and (b) Pre-op. Massive weight loss patient undergoing extended abdominoplasty, thigh dermolipectomy, and mons reduction with suspension. Patient is allowed to adjust waistband to desired level; incision must lie under or below this. Source: O. Placik. Reproduced with permission.

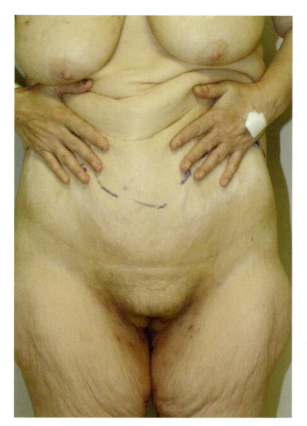

Figure 8.31 The patient is asked to put the abdominal flap on traction pulling the flap upward. Persistent ptosis and fullness of the mons is noted even with aggressive upward skin displacement. Source: O. Placik. Reproduced with permission.

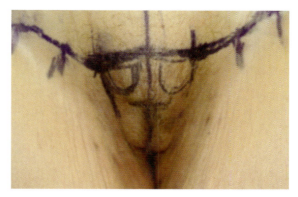

Figure 8.32 With the panniculus on upward traction, markings of the mons are completed. Source: O. Placik. Reproduced with permission.

sion and the apex of the vulvar cleft should remain; [2] the apex of the vulvar cleft should come to lie over the symphysis pubis (cephalad shift); [3] the anticipated level of the abdominoplasty incision, which is a minimum of 10 cm below the umbilicus; and [4] attention to any potential distortion of the labia majora. In the presented case, given the marked laxity, the lowest possible horizontal line was drawn 5 cm above the vulvar cleft with the skin on tension and the desired area of the residual mons to be debulked was marked (Figure 8.32).

The necessity of placing all structures on tension is illustrated in the panels in Figures 8.33 and 8.34 by relieving the traction on the skin. The incisions are completely concealed in the standing position (Figure 8.35).

Set-up/anesthesia: Depilation is to be avoided in the week before surgery. Patients should be cautioned that shaving, in particular, the week or day before surgery may lead to an increased incidence of wound infection. Shaving or trimming, in order to facilitate wound closure, is accomplished immediately prior to the prep. The patient is most

commonly placed in the supine position but lithotomy may be preferred when simultaneous labia majora or other vulvar procedures are also planned. Thromboembolic prevention is usually indicated for all cases under general or spinal anesthesia in the form of mechanical prophylaxis with graduated compression stockings or sequential compression devices. Chemoprophylaxis is prescribed for higher risk individuals. If surgery will exceed 1.5 hours (e.g., performed along with another genital plastic surgery), the use of support hose or SCDs is encouraged. If local anesthesia, I use 10 cc of 1% lidocaine with epinephrine for the incisions administered with a 27 g needle followed by a dilute solution for "tumescent" infiltration prepared by 50 cc of 1% lidocaine with epinephrine to 1 liter of normal saline or Ringer's lactate. Approximately 150–250 cc are infiltrated throughout the superficial and deep fat layers with either a 19 g spinal needle or infiltration cannula/pump for larger reductions. If general anesthesia, the local anesthetic described above is still used once induction is complete. The sterile prep is conducted after the local anesthetic to allow time for vascoconstriction to take effect (7–10 minutes).

Traditionally, the vulva is then prepped with povidone-iodine or chlorhexidine gluconate solution. Following surgical prep, the measurements and markings are confirmed and refreshed. Hash marks are made every 4–5 cm on the superior and inferior flaps to minimize malalignment and "dog-ear" formation. In larger resections, where the marks may wear off during the case, they are "tagged" with staples (Figure 8.35).

Small reductions are performed with liposuction (various techniques) and can be carried out under local anesthesia in tolerant patients or with sedation in an office setting. Mons reductions or suspensions following an unfavorable cosmetic result after a Pfannenstiel incision can be performed under similar conditions (Figure 8.36). However, I do prefer general anesthesia in the majority of patients as was done in this example.

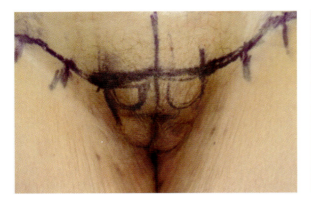
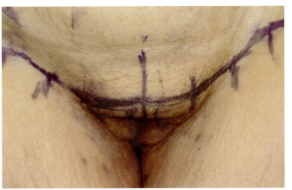
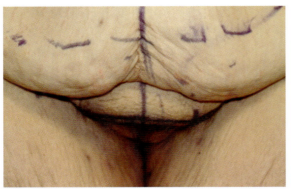

Figure 8.33 By lessening cephalad tension on the abdominal flap, the mons becomes more ptotic and overlying abdominal panniculus conceals the underlying incisions lines. Source: O. Placik. Reproduced with permission.

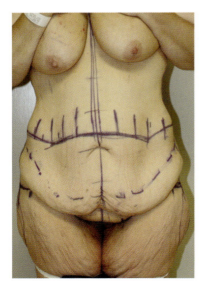
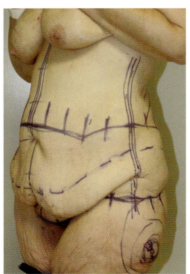
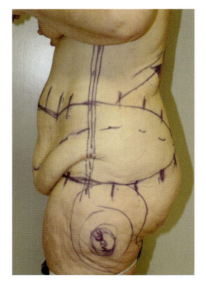

Figure 8.34 Traditional pre-operative of views once marking is complete. The mons resection is not visible without retracting the overlying panniculus. Source: O. Placik. Reproduced with permission.

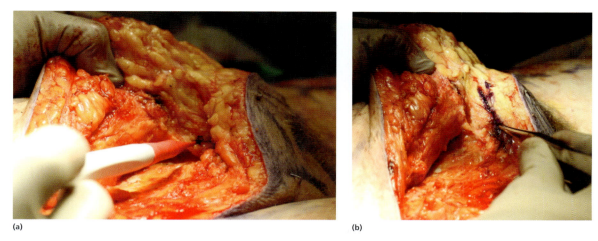

(a)   (b)

Figure 8.35 (a) and (b) Mons incision viewed from the right side of patient. (a) As dissection proceeds the SFS is visible and indicated by electrocautery pencil tip. Staples placed over hash marks. (b) Traction on SFS, now marked in purple ink, confirms ability to suspend mons. Source: O. Placik. Reproduced with permission.

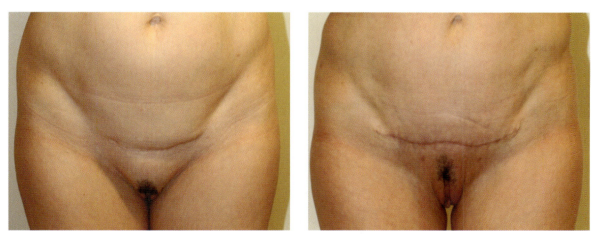

Figure 8.36 Pre- (left) and post- (right) op result at 3 months following mons elevation via liposuction of abdomen/mons, fat resection, and suspension. Source: O. Placik. Reproduced with permission.

Incision and excision: The incision may be accomplished with a scalpel, electrocautery, laser, or RF. I most commonly use a 10 or 20 blade (for larger incisions) followed by electrocautery for hemostasis and cutting of deeper layers. The SFS is now identified [Figure 8.37(a) and (b)]. I will complete the "more sterile" portions of the procedure such as the abdominal/hip/thigh dermolipectomy prior to addressing the mons or vulvar structures. Here the abdominoplasty has been completed and the views are from the head of the bed looking down on the incision (Figures 8.37 and 8.38).

Mons reduction: Resection of the pubic fat is commenced and illustrated in Figure 8.37. The fat deep to the SFS is approached first beginning at the edge of the SFS and beveling toward the symphysis pubis using electrocautery.

Large vessels may be encountered and hemostasis must be meticulous with electrocautuery or suture ligation. Subsequent to this, the fullness of the labia majora is assessed externally and, if moderate fullness exists and no external separate incision, labia majora reduction is planned, the fat of the labia majora can be conservatively resected from above. This is the fat contained by the Colles' fascia. The thickness of the mons is repeatedly assessed throughout each step. If the mons remains excessively protruberant, I cautiously excise additional superficial fat with attention to preserve the integrity of the SFS. On occasion, I will use a 2 or 3 mm cannulae with an open liposuction technique to accomplish further fine adjustments in thickness at this step or as needed throughout the subsequent closure process.

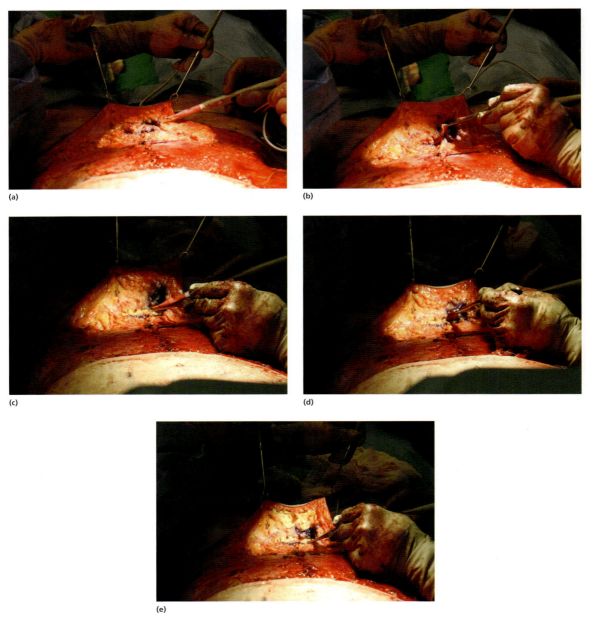

Figure 8.37 (a) Steps for fat resection. View of surgical field from head of the bed looking downward following completion of abdominoplasty. Retractors are on pubic skin. Electrocautery points to SFS of mons marked in purple. (b) Electrocautery resection of the deep fat between SFS and symphysis pubis. Forceps hold fat. The area has a rich lymphatic supply. (c) Following resection of deep fat, the forceps point to the symphysis pubis. The undersurface of SFS is colored in purple ink. (d) Following removal of deep fat, the labia majora may be conservatively debulked from above. Forceps grab fat of labia majora prior to resection. Following treatment of deep fat and labia majora, the fat superficial to the SFS may be conservatively resected so that the thickness of the mons matches the abdominal flap. This can also be accomplished with liposuction. (e) Dissection is complete. Forceps point to the marked symphysis pubis and overlying deep fat and toward the patient's right labia majora. Source: O. Placik. Reproduced with permission.

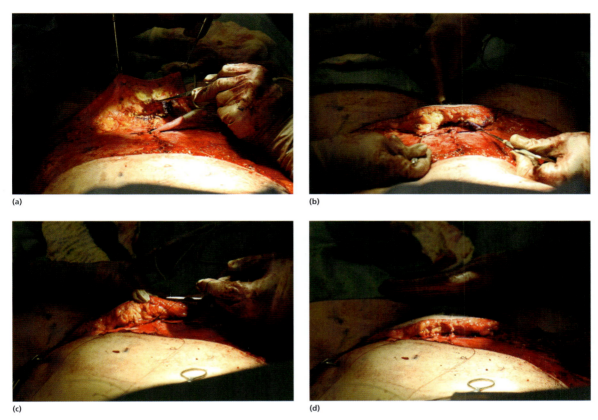

(a)   (b)

(c)   (d)

Figure 8.38 (a) Steps for mons suspension. Forceps grab SFS and electrocautery points to level of proposed suspension on rectus fascia located at least 5 cm above symphysis pubis and at least 10 cm below umbilicus. (b) Skin hooks placed on SFS exert tension and simulate elevation to level of proposed suspension on rectus fascia. Upper finger points to mons to assess effects on labia majora and vulvar cleft distortion as well as thickness relative to abdominal flap. (c) Suture fixation of SFS to rectus fascia is completed with several interrupted 0 PDS sutures. Assistant's hand relieves tension on mons flap. (d) Overall contour of mons is assessed as well as labia majora and external vulvar structures. Minor adjustments are completed. Open liposuction may be used to further thin remaining superficial fat to match thickness of abdominal panniculus. Source: O. Placik. Reproduced with permission.

Mons suspension: Figure 8.37 demonstrates the dissection and Figure 8.38 the suspension procedure. I will select a point for suspension of the SFS to the rectus fascia at a location that is a minimum of 5 cm above the symphysis and at least 10 cm below the umbilicus. This may require some adjustment depending on the body type of the patient. This is first simulated by placing traction on the SFS and lifting it to the level of the proposed fixation while assessing the effects on the mons and external genitalia. Adjustments in the level of fixation are made at this point, if necessary. The fascia is approximated with several interrupted 0 PDS™ sutures as the assistant relieves tension on the flap. As with LP, hemostasis is mandatory.

Repair: Approximation of the abdominal flap to the mons and the remaining flaps lateral to the mons is completed with additional 0 PDS™ interrupted sutures typically placed in the SFS every 2.5–5.0 cm. If significant dead space exists, I will follow this with a barbed-type suture (No. 2 Quill™ or No. 1 Stratafix™). I have traditionally used deep dermal buried interrupted 2-0 Vicryl™ sutures placed every 1–2 cm. However, I have increasingly found that patients seem to spit these sutures. I prefer the holding strength of the Vicryl™ but have decreased their use to every 5 cm interspersed with 3-0 Monocryl™ deep dermal buried interrupted sutures placed every centimeter. I subsequently perform a sub-cuticular running closure with either a 3-0 Monocryl™ (here) or 2-0 Monoderm™. Wounds are then covered with Xeroform™ gauze reinforced with staples placed every 5 cm to reinforce the wound and hold the Xeroform™ in place because the wound may ooze for the first 48 hours.

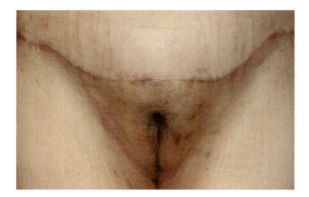

Figure 8.39 Abdominoplasty and resection MP; post-op result at 3 months. Source: O. Placik. Reproduced with permission.

Dressing and immediate post-op care: Typically the wound is covered with absorbent ABD pads or Topifoam™ gauze with a gentle abdominal compression band. Mesh underwear and ice compresses are advised. Compression over the mons area is difficult to achieve. The Xeroform™ and staples are removed at 3–5 days followed by Steri-Strips left on for 2 weeks followed by Micropore™ for 2–3 months. Abdominal compression is continued for 3 weeks post-operatively followed by commercially available compression garments (i.e., Spanx™) for a total of 6 weeks post-operatively. Patients are typically seen at 3 days (see above), 10 days (seroma check), 3 weeks (discontinuation of compression), occasionally at 6 weeks (lifting of activity restrictions), and at 3 and 6 months for longer-term follow-up and photographs (Figures 8.39–8.41).

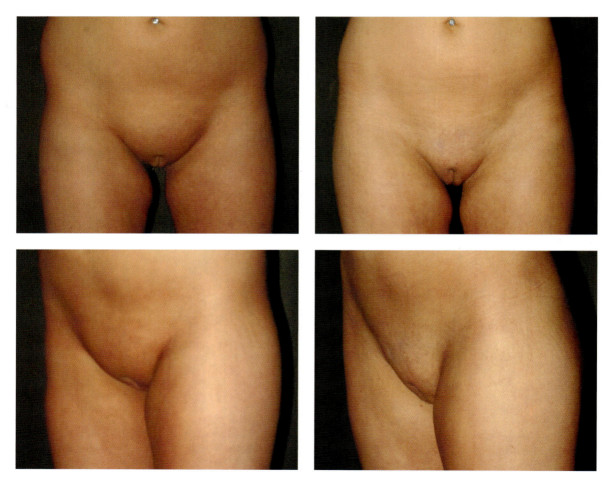

Figure 8.40 Pre- (left) and post- (right) op results at 3 months following liposuction of mons and abdomen. Source: O. Placik. Reproduced with permission.

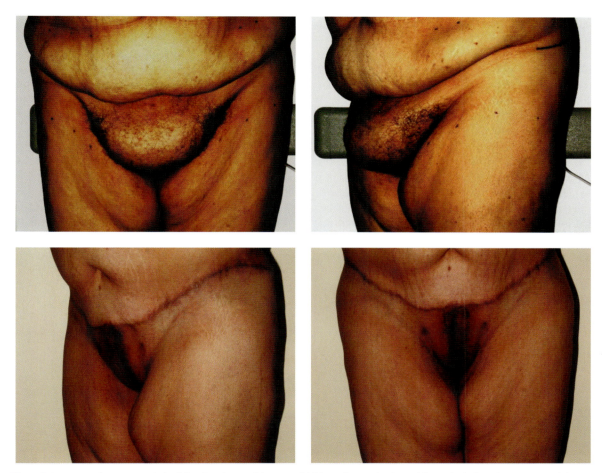

Figure 8.41 Pre- and post-op "mini" abdominoplasty with MP and labia majora reduction with marked elevation (<5 cm) of the vulvar cleft. Paramedian vertical scars lateral to the vulvar cleft were employed. Source: O. Placik. Reproduced with permission.

RCH ("clitoral unhooding")

Clitoral hood reduction (CHR) or reduction of clitoral hood (RCH) procedures are most often performed concomitantly with a reduction of labial size. As the labia minora "begin" superiorly, "flowing down" from one or more of the varying folds of epithelium making up the central, (frenulum. central hood), medial (lateral folds of the central hood), and lateral (prepucial) folds of the "clitoral hood," these hood folds are frequently a part of the "tissue protrusion" that is bothersome to the patient. Only occasionally are hood size reductions performed solo, without labial reduction. As noted in the anatomic descriptions of labial reductions and in many photographs and diagrams above, hood reduction is either continuous with the labial excision line, or separate, if the anatomic area of hood hypertrophy does not connect directly with the area of labial reduction.

If performed for redundant prepucial tissue, the redundancy is excised unilaterally or bilaterally as indicated, but well lateral to the underlying clitoral body, and in a vertical elliptical manner, with great care taken to remain superficial, so as to avoid damage to the clitoral nerve that enters laterally ~mid-clitoral body, traveling deep to the overlying mobile skin. Laterally, an easy tissue plane exists, as the skin overlies loose areolar tissue. Medially, however, around the area of the central clitoral hood, the skin is more densely adherent to the underlying fascia, and dissection is difficult. It is best to avoid vigorous dissection in this nerve-rich area. Care must be taken, whether accomplishing the dissection with scalpel, scissors, laser, RF, or cautery (cutting current) needle, to remain superficial with the skin incision. Remove only stretchable, loose/redundant skin. Surface epithelium may be removed with scissors, laser, electrocautery, or RF. This is an area where the use of laser or RF-related focused energy source is elegant.

It is best not to make incision lines over the central hood, unless absolutely necessary, and to dissect laterally, removing redundancy and, if the anatomy requires, stretching excess central epithelium laterally, repairing the defect as laterally as possible with a two-layer closure (sub-Q and skin) with fine absorbable suture either in a sub-cuticular or interrupted manner (Figure 8.42).

However, if redundant clitoral hood prolapses well over the clitoral glans and proves difficult to retract, a "clitoripexy" may be effected by making a very superficial diamond-shaped incision over the upper central hood, with closure horizontally so as to elevate the redundancy. As this suture line is under significant tension, careful sub-cutaneous approximation must precede surface closure. See also Figure 8.43.

If performed for a phimotic prepuce, restricting clitoral emergence (and, theoretically, sensitivity), the tightened hood is undermined with a lacrimal duct probe, #1 or #2 Hegar dilator, or equivalent. The hood is separated in the midline with scissors, laser, RF, or electrocautery (shielding the glans), with a fine repair of the

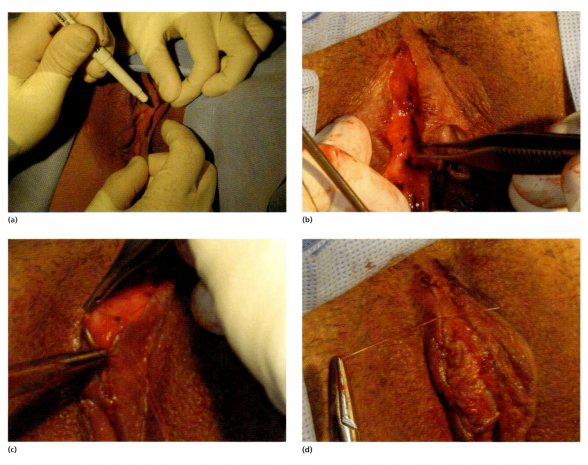

(a)   (b)

(c)   (d)

Figure 8.42 (a) Marking hood reduction portion of straightforward linear resection LP where labum "flows" directly from lateral portion of central hood. (b) Excision complete to depth of 2~3 mm, bleeders cauterized. Putting in sub-cutaneous layer. (c) Placing sub-cuticular layer. (d) Sub-cuticular layer completed. Placing occasional interrupted 5-0 Vicryl Rapide interrupted sutures to secure line. Source: M. Goodman. Reproduced with permission.

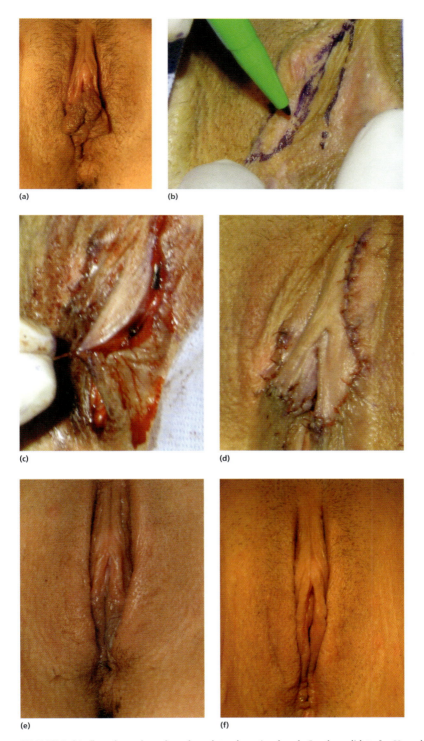

Figure 8.43 (a) Pre-op LP, RCH. Labia flow down from frenulum, lateral portion hood. Good candidate for V-wedge, "Y" modification to include hood that patient considered hypertrophic and desired reduction along with labia. (b) Bringing nadir of V-wedge incision line up to encompass redundant hood ("stretched" and decompressed in this photo). (c) "Y"'d portion of incision; redundant hood resected. (d) Incision line completed with interrupted 5-0 Vicryl Rapide suture line. (e) One month post-op. (f) Six months post-op. Source: M. Goodman. Reproduced with permission.

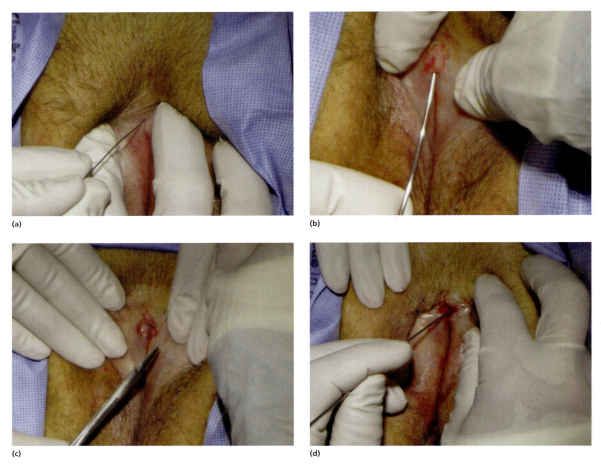

(a)

(b)

(c)

(d)

Figure 8.44 (a) Location of "dimple" in markedly atrophic and phimotic anterior commissure/clitoral hood. (b) Superficial separation of phimotic central hood. (c) Glans is exposed after hood separation. Cut edges sutured with 5-0 Vicryl Rapide. 6-0 Vicryl may also be used. (d) 5-0 nylon sutures have been used to widely "curtain" the repair and prevent agglutination. Sutures will be removed in 5–10 days. Testosterone + clobetasol ointment is utilized q.d- q.o.d. X 3 months post-op. Source: M. Goodman. Reproduced with permission.

edges. The resultant flaps are temporarily pulled aside, curtainlike, and anchored laterally with 1 or 2 fine-grade nylon sutures per side, allowing for edge healing for ~7–10 days prior to suture removal. Figure 8.44 depicts this procedure on a patient with long-standing lichen sclerosis who has been pre-treated for 6 months with estradiol/testosterone transdermal gel. Careful post-operative care, post-op testosterone with or without clobetasol, and frequent sexual activity will improve the chances of success, but even with surgery and adjuncts, the chances of ongoing exposure are not outstanding.

Hymenoplasty

Hymenoplasty, a "plastic" repair/reconstruction of the hymenal ring, is usually sought as a cultural imperative by Muslim women with (an "arranged") marriage on the horizon, who have previously been sexually active and fear a telltale lack of "tightness" and loss of blood upon consummation. Rarely, the procedure is requested by Western women as a "revirgination" procedure sought as a "gift" for their sexual partner.

Most often, hymenal reconstruction is sought for the express purpose of well-tightening the hymenal ring to produce difficult entry with probable tearing and the concomitant loss of a small amount of blood. While it may be difficult for a westerner to understand, the cultural imperative is stringent, and the repercussions of lack of blood loss and/or laxity are real and may be devastating.

The Procedure

Utilizing two to several small, diamond-shaped excisions similar to those utilized for a PP, with the maximal width of the diamond just inside the hymenal ring and the external apex barely onto the vestibule (Figure 8.45), each incision is closed vertically with fine absorbable sutures, producing a size-compromised aperture (Figure 8.46). An alternative method, utilized by Dr. Alinsod (personal communication), is to denude portions of hymenal ring anteriorly and posteriorly, approximating these areas to purposefully produce synechiae that bleed with resultant coitus. This method, however, is less anatomically "pure" and may not pass the potential pre-nuptial "inspection" that some young Islamic women must undergo prior to marriage.

Multiple procedures

Not rarely, surgery planning includes >1 procedure, not including the frequent combination of LP-m and RCH. Following are several observations and pearls regarding bundling more than one procedure:

1 Do you have the stamina for it?
2 Look carefully at the total amount of anesthesia and anesthetic percentage; watch out for toxicity. For bupivacaine, usually my choice, and I routinely utilize 0.5% solution, I know that with amounts (of 0.5% bupivacaine) >30 ml 0.5% I may flirt with toxicity. For 0.25%, potential for toxicity begins at >60 ml. Toxicity of course fluctuates with weight, but the figures quoted here are for a small (~110–120#) woman. Calculate the amount you are likely to require before the case so you know what percentage (0.5, 0.25, or a mixture of both to produce 0.375% solution) solution you will require. Bupivacaine toxicity is particularly nasty!
3 Remember to utilize some sort of lower extremity compression device to prevent venous pooling in longer cases (usually >2 hours, but dependent on patient's age and lower extremity vascular status.)

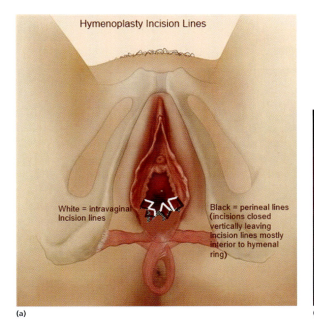

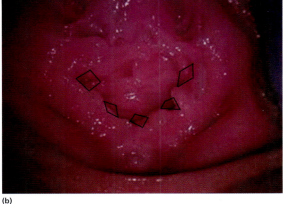

(a)   (b)

Figure 8.45 (a) Schematic of hymenoplasty incisions. Source: R. Moore and J. Miklos. Reproduced with permission. (b) Potential hymenoplasty incisions.

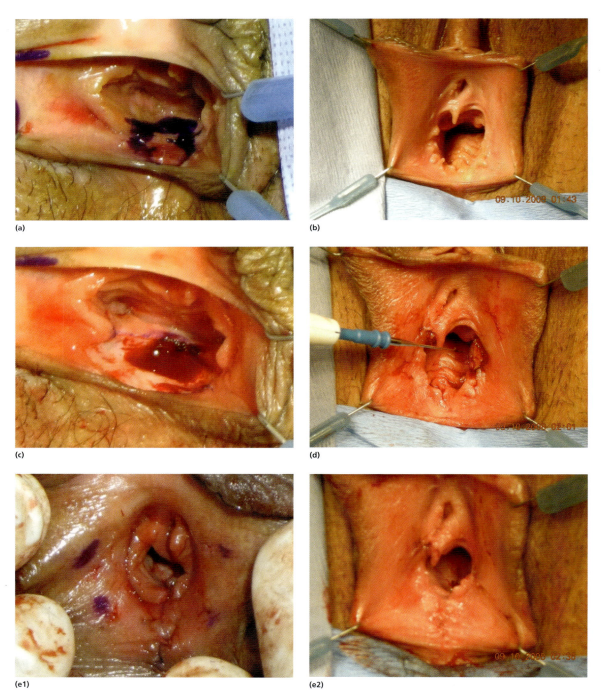

Figure 8.46 (a) Case #1, repair area inked. (b) Case #2 pre-op. Areas to be approximated are at 2/3 o'clock., 6 o'clock, and 9/10 o'clock. (c) Case #1, incision @ 6 o'clock. (d) Case #2, making 2/3 o'clock incision. (e) Completed hymenoplasties (case #1 left; #2 right) with attenuated introitus. Source: M. Goodman. Reproduced with permission.

4 Labiaplasty with vaginal tightening procedure: Do the perineoplasty first. Although it would seem intuitive to perform the "clean" LP prior to the "dirty" PP, edema from the local anesthetic utilized, especially if the labial resection is performed via curvilinear incision and if the patient has a prominent posterior commissure, plus surgical edema can make aesthetic dissection of the posterior commissure, vulvar vestibule, and/or perineum more difficult than anticipated. When combining labiaplasty minora with majora, personal preference will decide. In the author's experience, there is no advantage proceeding with one over the other.

5 Remember, multiple procedures require greater healing time and are more harsh on the constitution, requiring more downtime and resulting in greater edema and fatigue as the body adjusts. Make sure your patient allows for this!

Final note

It is the authors' hope that this chapter will give the aspiring vulvar genital plastic/cosmetic surgeon a strong foundation with which to begin practice of these procedures. The authors wish to convey that hands-on, practical experience is also required prior to actively practicing this surgical discipline.

References

1. Goodman MP, Placik OJ, Benson RH III, Miklos JR, Moore RD, Jason RA, Matlock DL, Simopoulos AF, Stern BH, Stanton RA, Kolb SE, Gonzalez F. A large multicenter outcome study of female genital plastic surgery. *J Sex Med* 2010;**7**:1565–77

2. Ali AH, Thabet SM. Reduction clitoro-labiaplasty versus clitoro-labiectomy in managing adult onset clitoro-labiomegaly. *Gynecol Obstet Invest* 2009;**68**:224–9.

3. Girling VR, Salisbury M, Ersek RA. Vaginal labiaplasty. *Plast Reconstr Surg* 2005;**115**:1792–3.

4. Rubayi S. Aesthetic vaginal labiaplasty. *Plast Reconstr Surg* 1985;**75**:608.

5. Miklos JR, Moore RD. Labiaplasty of the labia minora: Patient's indications for pursuing surgery *J Sex Med* 2008;**5**:1492–5.

6. Pardo J, Sola P, Ricci P, Guilloff E. Laser labiaplasty of the labia minora. *Int J Gynec Obst* 2005;**93**:38–43.

7. Krizko M, Krizko M, Janek L. Plastic adjustment of the labia minora. *Ceska Gynekol* 2005;**70**:446–9.

8. Alter GJ. A new technique for aesthetic labia minora reduction. *Ann Plastic Surg* 1998;**40**:287–90.

9. Munhoz AM, Filassi JR, Ricci MD, Aldrighi C, Correira LD, Aldrighi JM, Ferreira MC. Aesthetic labia minora reduction with inferior wedge resection and superior pedicle flap reconstruction. *Plast Reconstr Surg* 2006;**118**:1237–47.

10. Rouzier R, Louis-Sylvestre C, Paniel BJ, Hadded B. Hypertrophy of the labia minora; Experience with 163 reductions. *Am J Obstet Gynecol* 2000;**182**:35–40.

11. DiGiorgi V, Salvini C, Mannone F, Carelli G, Carli P. Reconstruction of the vulvar labia minora with a wedge resection. *Dermatol Surg* 2004;**30**:1583–6.

12. Choi HY, Kim CT. A new method for aesthetic reduction of labia minora (the deepithelialized reduction labiaplasty). *Plast Reconstr Surg* 2000;**105**:419–22.

13. Giraldo F, Gonzalez C, deHaro F. Central wedge nymphectomy with a 90-degree Z-plasty for aesthetic reduction of the labia minora. *Plast Reconstr Surg* 2004;**113**:1820–5.

14. Goldstein AT, Romanzi LJ. Z-plasty reduction labiaplasty. *J Sex Med* 2007;**4**:550–3.

15. Alter GJ. Management of the mons pubis and labia majora in the massive weight loss patient. *Aesthet Surg J* 2009;**29**:432–42.

16. Bloom JMP, Van Kouwenberg E, Davenport M, et al. Aesthetic and functional satisfaction after monsplasty in the massive weight loss population. *Aesthet Surg J* 2012;**32**(7):877–85.

17. El-Khatib HA. Mons pubis ptosis: Classification and strategy for treatment. *Aesthet Plast Surg* 2011;**35**(1):24–30.

18. Michaels VJ, Friedman T, Coon D, et al. Mons rejuvenation in the massive weight loss patient using superficial fascial system suspension. *Plast Reconstr Surg* 2010;**126**(1):45e–6e.

19. Hughes III CE. Body contouring of the suprapubic region. *Aesthet Surg J* 2000;**20**(5):411–2.

CHAPTER 9

Surgical procedures II: perineoplasty, vaginoplasty, colpoperineoplasty ("vaginal rejuvenation")

Robert D. Moore, John R. Miklos, and Orawee Chinthakanan

International Urogynecology Associates, Atlanta, GA, and Beverly Hills, CA, USA

Experience is a hard teacher. She gives the test first and the lesson after.

Vernon Law

Introduction

Vaginal rejuvenation and cosmetic vaginal surgery have been performed and popularized increasingly in gynecology, urogynecology, and plastic surgery. However, the subject itself is hotly debated rather than the in-depth surgical techniques. The line between cosmetic and medically indicated surgical procedures is a gray area, and procedures are performed for both purposes. This chapter will review the background and history of these procedures and the available data to support them, as well as review techniques and complications. In addition, we will discuss some of the controversy surrounding these procedures. Finally, we will also attempt to shed light on what is myth and what is science in this relatively new field of elective vaginal surgery for sexual function and cosmesis of the female vagina and vulva.

This chapter covers "vaginal rejuvenation" procedures. Many use the term "vaginal rejuvenation" to encompass all elective vaginal/vulvar surgery. However, we feel that it should be used only to refer to functional procedures of the internal vaginal canal and introitus that are designed to enhance sexual function, which includes ensuring adequate support of the pelvic floor, internal vaginal canal repairs, and repair of the introitus.

Vaginal rejuvenation

Vaginal rejuvenation is a relatively new term that refers to repair of the vaginal canal and opening of the vagina for enhancement of sexual function. The concept may be referred to as "vaginal rejuvenation," "aesthetic vaginal surgery," "vaginoplasty," "vaginal tightening," or "cosmetic vaginal surgery." The term of "vaginal rejuvenation" has recently created considerable controversy in the field of gynecology and urogynecology as well as in the public eye. There seems to be misinformation and confusion over what the term actually refers to and what procedures are actually being done and where on the body they are undertaken.

Some of these terms refer to cosmetic external surgery of the vagina and vulva, that is, labiaplasty or hymen restoration procedures. Other terms refer to surgery to enhance sexual function. In this chapter, "vaginal rejuvenation" is used to refer to surgical procedures of the internal vagina and the introitus that are designed to repair vaginal relaxation and to enhance or improve sexual function and sensation of the female vagina, and we reserve the term "cosmetic genital surgery" to refer to the outside of the vagina. Vaginal rejuvenation has also been defined to include perineoplasty and vaginoplasty, which are techniques to "tighten" the vaginal canal and to elevate and strengthen the perineal body [1].

Female Genital Plastic and Cosmetic Surgery, First Edition. Edited by Michael P. Goodman.
© 2016 John Wiley & Sons, Ltd. Published 2016 by John Wiley & Sons, Ltd.

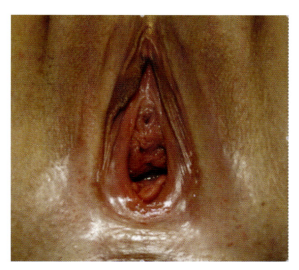

Figure 9.1 Picture of relaxed introitus and vaginal canal.
Source: R. Moore and J. Miklos. Reproduced with permission.

The purpose of these procedures is not to correct pelvic floor defects; they are modifications of traditional colporrhaphy and are frequently performed concomitantly with reconstructive procedures for pelvic organ prolapse. These procedures involve vaginal reconstructive techniques to anatomically modify the vaginal caliber by decreasing the diameter of the vaginal canal while reconstructing the perineal body [2–4].

Utilizing this definition, one realizes that this is not a new field at all, that is, gynecologists have been dealing with sexual dysfunction related to vaginal pathology resulting mostly from vaginal childbirth for hundreds of years. However, the implication of our definition is to listen to women's complaints of altered sexual function secondary to vaginal relaxation/looseness and possibly to do vaginal repairs prior to developing symptoms of vaginal prolapse or presenting with advanced prolapse. As will be discussed later, many women who are candidates for vaginal rejuvenation in fact have symptoms and clinical findings of prolapse. Therefore, a proper repair must involve restoring the foundation of pelvic floor support and encompass some of the newer concepts of vaginal rejuvenation in the repair.

Prolapse and vaginal relaxation (Figure 9.1) occurring after vaginal childbirth is not a new concept. We have clear evidence that vaginal delivery increases risks for vaginal support problems, vaginal relaxation, prolapse, and incontinence. Various pathophysiologic studies have demonstrated marked changes after vaginal delivery to levator

muscles [5,6], nerves [7], and pelvic support [8]. It is obvious that parous women are more likely to have pelvic organ prolapse, fecal incontinence, and urinary incontinence than women who have not borne children [9].

There is ample epidemiological evidence that vaginal delivery appears to be the strongest risk factor for pelvic floor disorders [10]. Utilizing data from the Women's Health Initiative study [11], women who have borne at least one child are twice as likely to have uterine prolapse, rectocele, and cystocele as nulliparas, after adjusting for age, ethnicity, body mass index, and other factors. The amount of damage at the time of vaginal childbirth has also been shown to be strongly correlated with sexual function. At 6 months postpartum, women with an intact perineum or first-degree perineal tear are less likely to experience sexual dysfunction than those with greater perineal trauma [12,13]. Interestingly, 80.4% of urogynecologists stated that they would agree to perform an elective primary cesarean section at time of delivery [14).

Prolapse and sexual function

Female sexual dysfunction is defined as a disorder of sexual desire, sexual arousal, orgasm, and/or sexual pain contributing to personal distress [15]. Sexual dysfunction is a multifactorial disorder; biological, psychosocial, and relational factors can contribute to female sexual dysfunction. Among these factors, the pelvic floor appears to have an important influence. Dysfunction of vaginal support leading to incontinence, prolapse, and sexual dysfunction is highly prevalent [16]. Surprisingly, little research has been undertaken regarding the sexual function part of pelvic floor disorder. One would agree that surgery to correct pelvic organ prolapse or incontinence is justified.

The American Urogynecologic Society has stated that any surgery for pelvic organ support should take into account restoration of the normal anatomy and function of the pelvic floor and vagina, including maintaining support and also maintaining or correcting bowel, bladder, AND sexual function. Despite these goals, very little information regarding sexual function and vaginal relaxation exists in the literature. In the landmark textbooks by leaders in the field of urogynecology, there are no chapters at all regarding sexual function and prolapse [17–19]. Two of these references are nearly 20 years old, and very little or no reference is made to it throughout the texts [20].

Therefore, the questions that need to be answered are [1] does prolapse and/or vaginal relaxation cause sexual dysfunction; and [2] does repair improve sexual function and/or the sensation of the female vagina? We will examine the existing data and make some educated conclusions regarding vaginal relaxation and sexual function. Finally, we will address whether repair of vaginal relaxation, which may not be severe enough to cause symptomatic prolapse, results in an improvement of sexual function.

It is beyond the scope of this chapter to review all of the anatomy and neuroanatomy of pelvic floor support and its relation to sexual function; however, suffice it to say that we do have good evidence that vaginal childbirth, as well as some other environmental and genetic factors, can lead to issues with pelvic floor support that in turn can affect sexual function. Again, repairs of pelvic floor and vaginal support have been performed for many, many years and one would not argue that one of the goals of any of these repairs is to "restore sexual function," therefore we must make the assumption that vaginal relaxation and prolapse affect sexual function in a negative way. The Pelvic Organ Prolapse/Incontinence Sexual Questionnaire (PISQ) and the Female Sexual Function Index (FSFI), among other tools, are validated questionnaires on sexual function and are necessary instruments to measure sexual function [21].

Many studies support this theory as well. Novi et al. compared sexual function in women with and without prolapse using PISQ [22]. They found that prolapse had a significant negative impact on sexual function, when compared to the group without prolapse. The study also reports that the PISQ scores were not significantly different between patients who had pelvic surgery to correct prolapse in the past and patients who never had prolapse. This may indicate that the surgical repair of prolapse improved their sexual function scores.

Botros et al. studied the impact of childbirth on female sexual function using an identical twin study design [23]. The PISQ was administered to 276 identical, sexually active twins to examine their sexual function. The analysis showed that nulliparous women reported superior sexual satisfaction scores compared to parous women. Barber et al. evaluated sexual function in women with urinary incontinence and pelvic organ prolapse and reported that prolapse was more likely than incontinence to affect sexual activity and sexual relations [24]. Rogers et al. also reported that women with urinary incontinence and/or pelvic organ prolapse, when compared to women without these conditions,

had significantly poorer sexual function on the PISQ score and reported less sexual activity [25]. In addition, impairment of sexual relations and duration of abstinence were strongly associated with worsening pelvic organ prolapse [26]. These studies confirm that prolapse, albeit a more severe form of vaginal relaxation, but certainly relaxation, can contribute to sexual dysfunction.

Srikrishna et al. also evaluated whether prolapse may impact sexual function and found that 83.6% of women presenting for prolapse surgery reported improved sexual function as one of their major goals for surgery [27]. This clearly indicated that women with prolapse are stating the prolapse has affected their sexual function and improving sexual function is a goal of their prolapse repair. They also found a significant improvement in sexual function after the prolapse repair was completed.

Azar et al. utilized FSFI to evaluate women before and after surgery for prolapse and also found that sexual function was improved post-operatively after repair of the prolapse [28]. Stoutjesdijk et al. also found a significant improvement in dyspareunia and increased frequency and satisfaction with intercourse after vaginal reconstructive surgery (29). These findings were also recently confirmed by Rogers et al. in a multicenter prospective study evaluating sexual function after surgery for prolapse and/or incontinence with improved sexual function scores after repair [30].

Recent studies also show similar results of improvement in sexual function 6 months after postsurgical treatment of prolapse and incontinence by using PISQ-12 [31,32] and FSFI [32]. Handa et al. assessed sexual function in 224 women, originally enrolled in the CARE trial, with sexual partners before and 1 year after abdominal sacrocolpopexy for prolapse stage II–IV using PISQ score [33]. They found that the proportion of sexually active women increased, the proportion who avoided sex because of prolapse symptoms decreased, and the mean PISQ scores improved at 1 year after surgery.

Salamon et al. compared pre- and 1-year postoperative PISQ-12 in a cohort of patients who underwent laparoscopic sacrocolpopexy utilizing porcine graft or polypropylene mesh. They reported that laparoscopic sacrocolpopexy improved female sexual function regardless of whether a porcine dermis or a polypropylene mesh material was used [34]. According to the medium term outcomes, there were no differences in PISQ score between short-term (6 weeks to 6 months) and medium-term (18–36 months) follow-up after prolapse repair surgery [35,36].

We feel that the posterior vaginal wall anatomically controls most of the vaginal caliber secondary to its relationship to the levator ani and genital hiatus. Repair of this wall is a major portion of most rejuvenation-type procedures. Therefore, studies evaluating rectocele repairs may have more of a direct correlation to vaginal caliber and sexual function.

Brandner et al. reported that posterior repair had a positive impact on sexual function. They examined FSFI scores before and after surgical rectocele repair in sexually active patients who had symptomatic rectoceles. There were significant improvements in FSFI scores in domains of sexual desire, satisfaction, and pain [37]. Komesu et al. investigated the effect of posterior repair on sexual function by using PISQ score [38]. They included a cohort of patients who underwent pelvic floor reconstructive surgery with and without posterior repair and found that both groups significantly improved in sexual function.

Tunuguntla and Gousse found that while posterior repair with levatorplasty leads to sexual dysfunction and pain in many women, posterior colporrhaphy completed alone, with the avoidance of levator ani plication, improves sexual function [39]. Komesu et al. evaluated the effect of posterior repair on sexual function in women who underwent surgical treatment for prolapse and/or incontinence and reported that women with posterior repair had improvements in sexual function on PISQ scores [38]. Paraiso et al. compared three different methods of vaginal rectocele repair including one that utilized a graft and reported that all three approaches resulted in statistically significant improvements in the PISQ score [40].

Prolapse repair not only improves female sexual function but also improves male sexual function. Kuhn et al. evaluated sexual function in female patients and their male partners by using FSFI for female patients and Brief Male Sexual Inventory (BMSI) for their partners. FSFI scores in women improved significantly in the domains desire, arousal, lubrication, overall satisfaction, and pain. For their partners, there were significant improvements in sexual drive and overall satisfaction. However, erection, ejaculatory function, and orgasm remained unchanged [41].

Vaginal relaxation and effect on sexual function and sensation

It is clear from the published literature that prolapse plays a role in creating sexual dysfunction. The difficulty with this is that certainly sexual function is multifactorial and can, because of this, be a very difficult area to study. It is also clear from the above studies that vaginal repair improves sexual function and sexual quality of life, but is it because of the prolapse creating discomfort causing the woman to avoid intercourse, or because of self-image issues regarding the prolapse? Or is it because vaginal relaxation and prolapse may cause decreased sensation leading to sexual dysfunction, that is, feeling less, more difficulty achieving orgasm, or feeling self-conscious about the fact that she feels her vagina is loose, stretched or relaxed? Again, this is a very difficult issue to study and to date the literature is lacking in this regard [42]. We can, however, study basic anatomy and function of the vagina in relation to sensation, orgasm, and sexual function and propose educated conclusions by putting together the available data, anatomy, and function as well as considering the data previously presented showing that repair of vaginal prolapse improves sexual function.

Ozel et al. recently published one of the first reports evaluating libido, sexual excitement, vaginal sensation, and ability to orgasm in a group of women with prolapse compared to women without prolapse. They found that women with prolapse and vaginal relaxation were significantly more likely to report an absence of libido and lack of sexual excitement during intercourse and a much lower frequency of achieving orgasm during intercourse (all statistically significant) compared to women with the same demographics without prolapse (i.e., multiparous, similar age, marital status, etc.) [43]. This is a landmark study as it is one of the first studies evaluating the sensation of the vagina and the changes that may occur following relaxation of the tissues that causes prolapse.

The reasons why vaginal relaxation or prolapse may affect sensation are multifactorial and difficult to ascertain. It has been shown that when voluntarily contracted, the pelvic floor muscles can intensify orgasms for women [44]. Decreased sensation and difficulty achieving orgasm may be secondary to nerve damage from childbirth, muscular changes, or soft tissue changes, and to date we have no way of studying or confirming the exact cause prior to surgery. We can assume, however, that if most women with prolapse have improved sexual function following repair, that even in this more extreme situation causing true symptomatic prolapse, any associated nerve damage that may exist is overcome by the repair of the prolapse and returning the vagina back to its normal anatomic state.

It also makes logical sense that vaginal caliber can affect vaginal sensation. This has been studied and it has been shown that vaginal tone affects vaginal sensation and the ability to orgasm [45]. Tone is comprised of two variables, both levator muscle tone and the elasticity of the vaginal tissues attached to the muscles. The vaginal caliber is directly related to the elasticity of the endopelvic fascia surrounding the vaginal canal and the tone of the levator ani muscles that the tissues are attached to. If the levator muscles are atrophied this affects the overall pressure that the vagina can produce. Similarly, if the vaginal support tissues that are attached to the muscles are stretched, damaged, or disconnected from their connections to the levators (i.e., at the white line or the arcus), this will also affect vaginal tone and size, which ultimately can reduce vaginal sensation and the ability to orgasm.

Kline utilized a perineometer to evaluate vaginal tone and control (woman's ability to create a sustained contraction and improve vaginal tone) and showed that women with decreased tone or levator atrophy found it more difficult to reach coital orgasm, and if reversed the women's ability to achieve coital orgasm improved. It can be clearly seen in a cross-section view of the pelvis that the vaginal canal is attached laterally to the levators and when the levators contract, the vaginal caliber is reduced and pressure increased. Some argue that Kegel exercises alone can achieve this in a patient with decreased vaginal tone, and this certainly can be true in patients with true levator atrophy. However in women in whom the endopelvic fascia is stretched beyond its elastic capability to recover or not attached to the levators at all, the levators, no matter how strong, cannot overcome this and create a taught vaginal canal, and this will affect vaginal sensation.

We have shown so far in this chapter that vaginal prolapse can definitely affect sexual function and its repair can improve sexual function and ability to orgasm. The question, though, is how much vaginal relaxation does a women need to have to have decreased sensation or sexual dysfunction? And if women do have a sense of a relaxed or loose vagina that is causing them to have sexual dysfunction prior to having any of the traditionally described symptoms of prolapse (i.e., feeling or seeing a bulge, incontinence, voiding dysfunction, or bowel dysfunction), will a repair of the caliber of the vagina reverse these changes and improve sexual function? Clearly on examination, we see women present with a damaged perineal body from episiotomy or laceration during childbirth and a relaxed vaginal canal that do not have a true cystocele or rectocele (Figure 9.1). The patient states that the opening of her vagina feels wide open, her vagina feels very loose and relaxed, she has less sensation during intercourse, doesn't achieve coital orgasm as she did before, and would like a repair to return her vagina to its normal anatomic size and state. In the past, we turned these patients away because their only symptom was sexual dysfunction and they did not have true prolapse and therefore did not have an indication for surgical repair. We were ignoring one of the major aspects of quality of life in a couple's relationship, which is sexual function. This is what vaginal rejuvenation is all about: completing a vaginal repair of a relaxed vaginal opening and vaginal canal for sexual function and the woman's subjective symptoms of feeling as if her vagina is loose and/or wide open.

Data to support vaginal rejuvenation techniques

The theory that vaginal size is related to sexual sensation has been studied by Pardo *et al.* in a group of women who presented with symptoms of a wide or relaxed vagina and were interested in vaginal repair for sexual function alone. The women had no symptoms of prolapse or incontinence. Inclusion criteria included a sensation of a wide or loose vagina alone in combination with a decrease or lack of ability to reach orgasm. Exclusion critera included symptomatic prolapse (cystocele, rectocele, or vault/uterine prolapse), dyspareunia, primary anorgasmia or psychologic impairment (all patients had psychological evaluation pre-operatively), or partner sexual dysfunction. Fifty-three patients were included in the study, and 96% of the patients experienced decreased vaginal sensation, 73% described difficulty achieving orgasm, and 27% could not reach orgasm prior to surgery. All but two patients had previous vaginal deliveries. Following surgical repair of the vaginal caliber and tightening of the vagina (colpoperineoplasty using YAG laser for dissection), 90% of women reported their sexual satisfaction was much or sufficiently improved and 94% of women were able to reach orgasm. No patient reported worsened sexual function; however, 4% of patients reported regretting undergoing the procedure [2]. In a follow-up study, Pardo *et al.* confirmed their findings in a second group of patients as well [46]. This confirmed that vaginal size has a direct impact on sensation and ability to orgasm and when repaired sexual function improves.

Matlock and Simopoulos conducted a study to evaluate sexual function in women presenting with subjective symptoms of vaginal relaxation with or without stress urinary incontinence following laser vaginal rejuvenation using PISQ score. Ninety-six patients underwent the procedure and completed PISQ before and 6 months after surgery. All patients presented with the chief complaint of relaxed vagina. Of those 65% had stage II POP-Q. This finding suggests that early pelvic organ prolapse may manifest as vaginal relaxation. The overall sexual function improved after surgery. There were only 13% of women who had decreased PISQ scores post-operatively. In addition, 53% reported increased intensity of orgasm during sexual intercourse [47].

Goodman *et al.* led a recent multicenter U.S. study on women undergoing female genital plastic surgery including vaginoplasty/perineoplasty for vaginal relaxation affecting sexual function. This study gathered data from diverse practices and surgical specialties and surgeons who utilized more than a single technique to achieve a common goal, is a strength of this study. The authors of this chapter were one of the centers involved in the study. Pre-operatively 70% of women reported their sexual function was fair/poor. Post-operatively it was found that 86% of 81 women following vaginoplasty/perineoplasty for sexual function reported enhanced sexual function following repair with only 1% reporting a negative effect on sexual function, confirming repair of the vaginal caliber may lead to improved sexual function in women presenting with relaxation. Eighty-three percent of women were satisfied with the outcome of vaginal rejuvenation. The predominant reasons for surgery from the perspective of both physicians and patients were feelings of looseness and lack of coital friction and sexual pleasure [48].

A literature review by Goodman indicated that female genital plastic surgery procedures including vaginal rejuvenation appear to fulfill the majority of patients' desires for cosmetic and functional improvement, as well as enhancement of the sexual experience. The majority of patients reported improvement of overall satisfaction and subjective enhancement of sexual function and body image [49].

Vaginal rejuvenation—surgical techniques

Importance of proper evaluation and diagnosis

Proper pre-operative evaluation is a vital process for a patient who presents with an interest in surgery to repair what she conceives is a loose or relaxed vagina and would like it tightened for sexual enhancement or to correct the feeling of having a "wide-open" vagina, that is, vaginal rejuvenation surgery. This includes proper medical history, psychosocial evaluation for sexual dysfunction, and/or sexual satisfaction prior to any of the anatomical changes she may have noted since childbirth. Marital or relationship issues or concerns and an evaluation of her expectations of surgery and the reason why she is interested in the procedure should be discussed as well. It is true that most women that present to our clinic had a very satisfactory sexual life and then experienced a major change following their pregnancies and deliveries or gradually by aging. However, sexual dysfunction is very complex and multifactorial and of course a surgical procedure to repair vaginal support and reduce the vaginal caliber will not reverse or change psychological or psychosocial sexual dysfunction arising from previous abuse, primary anorgasmia, relationship issues, depression, or other more complex psychological dysfunction.

In addition to a medical and psychosocial history, an adequate urogynecological history and physical examination must be completed. Since sexual dysfunction related to a sense of a relaxed or loose vagina may be the first sign of the beginning stages of pelvic floor dysfunction and prolapse, an adequate history must be taken. We have actually found that as many as 50–75% of patients who present for vaginal rejuvenation, when asked, have symptoms including urinary incontinence, overactive bladder or voiding dysfunction such as difficult emptying, feelings of pressure or the sense that their organs are falling, defecatory dysfunction, or dyspareunia related to the uterus being impacted during intercourse because of prolapse. It is vitally important to have an adequate understanding of the symptoms that prolapse can cause, and we use validated questionnaires such as the UDI-6, IIQ-7, and the PISQ-IR [50] to evaluate patients for these symptoms as well as a general urogynecologic history form. If significant symptoms of urogynecologic pathology are present, these must be evaluated pre-operatively so that they can be addressed properly during surgery. Any prolapse that is present must be repaired properly at time of surgery including uterine/vault prolapse, enterocele, cystocele, or rectocele as vaginal rejuvenation procedures do NOT adequately treat these defects. The foundation of the pelvic floor support must be intact prior to any technique that will tighten the caliber of the vagina or introitus.

Surgical procedures

The surgical procedure required is determined by the patient's physical examination and her personal goals for surgery. Many women who present interested in vaginal rejuvenation–type surgery, or surgery to correct a feeling of a loose or wide vagina, are found to have prolapse in the form of cystocele, rectocele, or uterine/vault prolapse. In most instances it is POP-Q stage II or less; however, it is present and should be repaired. This is what determines what surgery will need to be undertaken as *the prolapse must be corrected first*, prior to any rejuvenation procedures being completed, and is really the first step in an overall repair or "rejuvenation" of the vagina and pelvic floor. If significant uterine/vault prolapse and/or anterior compartment (cystocele) defects are encountered, these typically should be repaired abdominally/laparoscopically/robotically or vaginally prior to addressing the posterior compartment and the caliber of the vagina.

Rejuvenation of the vaginal canal and introitus

Repair of the posterior vaginal wall and the introitus are the key aspects to any vaginal rejuvenation procedure. Vaginal rejuvenation surgeries are alterations and modifications of vaginal repairs for prolapse that focus on the final diameter and caliber of the vagina and attempt to restore it back to its pre-childbirth state. They do, however, go far beyond the simple traditional posterior repairs and perineoplasty of old. The focus of these older procedures was simply to restore and reduce the bulge, whereas the focus of vaginal rejuvenation is to restore the caliber of the vagina and genital hiatus back to the

pre-childbirth state from the introitus all the way up to the apex. They are much more extensive and meticulous procedures.

No "drop-offs," "dips," "ridges," or depressions should be felt, and there should be no tension placed on the levators, which causes lateral banding of the vagina. Additionally, the cosmetic appearance of the introitus and perineal body should also be taken into account and requires an intricate dissection and repair to not only restore function of the introitus but also obtain an appearance that the woman wants. That look is of the vaginal opening being closed, not gaping or wide open with a normal length perineal body that does not bulge out following the repair. This look is sometimes difficult to obtain without making the introitus too tight, which will cause pain with intercourse.

Posterior wall, introitus, and rejuvenation

The posterior vaginal wall is the focus of any vaginal rejuvenation procedure. In a woman with a mild cystocele or mild relaxation of the anterior vaginal wall, a small anterior colporrhaphy can be completed to take care of this prior to repair of the posterior wall. However, one needs to be very careful with this, as if the repair of the anterior wall is too aggressive, it will lead to lateral banding and constriction of the vagina, before reconstruction of the posterior wall is even started.

An incision is made at the introitus, typically in a trapezoid pattern, which will also be used in the perineoplasty portion of the procedure [Figure 9.2(a)]. A small incision is then made in a vertical fashion on the posterior wall and the vaginal epithelium is dissected off the underlying rectovaginal fascia all the way laterally out to the levators [Figure 9.2(b) and (c)]. The dissection must be taken all the way up to the apex of the vagina, as the repair needs to incorporate the entire posterior wall to restore the caliber of the full length of the vagina [Figure 9.2(d) and (e)]. The dissection of the vaginal epithelium may be completed using laser, as championed by Dr. David Matlock, or radiofrequency (RF) energy (Drs. Red Alinsod and Michael Goodman) or completed utilizing more standard techniques with sharp scissors or electrocautery. Care needs to be taken with any electrical energy source near the rectum.

If a rectocele is present, the fascia is repaired in a site-specific fashion with delayed absorbable suture for the first layer of the repair. This may be a lateral repair of

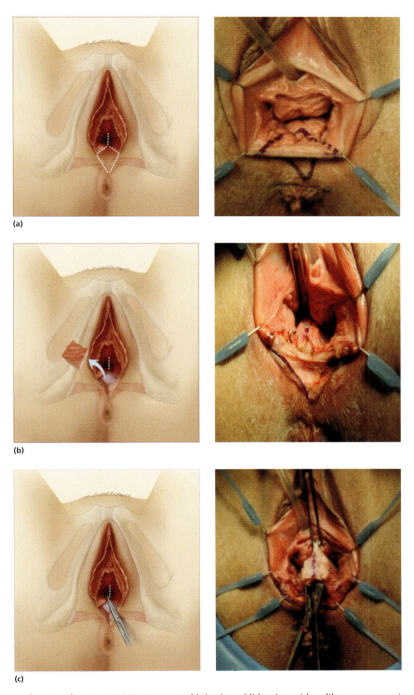

Figure 9.2 Surgical procedure step by step. (a) We recommend injection of lidocaine with a dilute vasoconstrictor below the vaginal epithelium to aid with dissection and hemostasis. (b) Next, a diamond-shaped incision is made using sharp or electrocautery dissection. (c) The vaginal wall is dissected over this undermined area and, with the help of sharp and blunt dissection, the mucosa is dissected laterally from its underlying fascia.

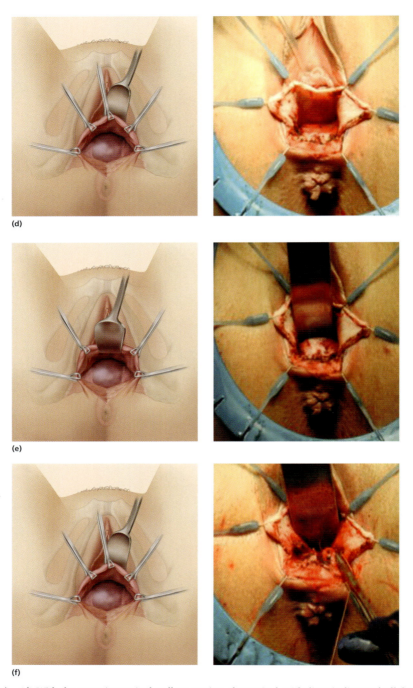

Figure 9.2 (*Continued*)   (d) With the posterior vaginal wall on tension, the vaginal epithelium is dissected off the rectovaginal septum out laterally to the levators bilaterally all the way up to the ischial spines/vaginal apex with either laser or sharp dissection. (e) Dissection reveals relaxed or stretched out rectovaginal fascia leading to relaxed vaginal caliber. (f) Defects in fascia corrected and/or first layer of plication of the fascia completed (i.e., repair of any rectocele).

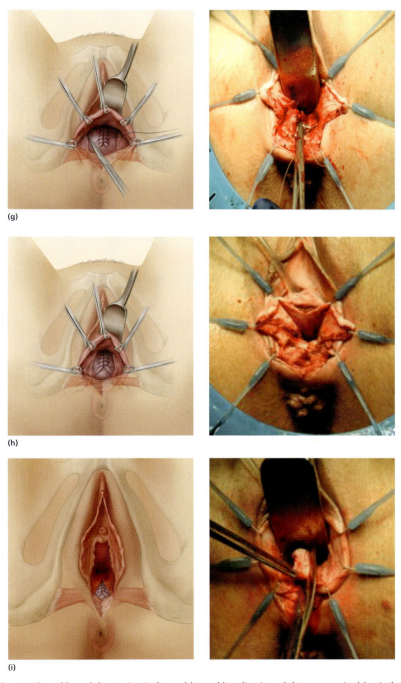

(g)

(h)

(i)

Figure 9.2 (*Continued*)   (g) The caliber of the vagina is then addressed by plication of the rectovaginal fascia/levator junction in the midline with delayed absorbable sutures. (h) Levator plication is avoided; however, the diameter of the vagina is constantly measured and several layers of plication may be needed to reduce the genital hiatus and reduce the caliber of the vagina to an appropriate level. The superficial transverse perineal muscles are brought together in the midline. (i) A small amount of vaginal epithelium is then excised and the incision closed in a running fashion.

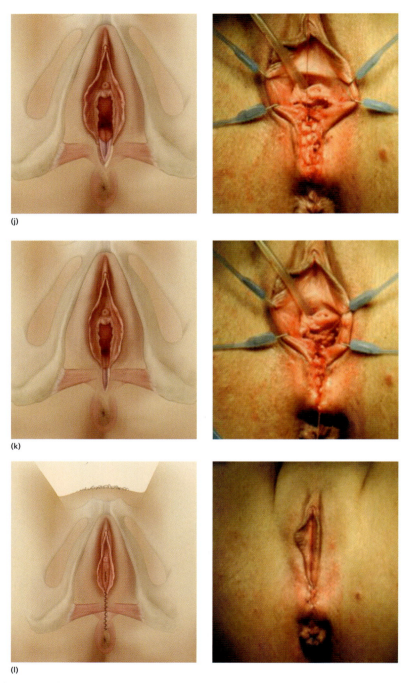

(j)

(k)

(l)

Figure 9.2 (*Continued*)   (j) A multilayer repair (typically this may involve 4 or 5 layers) is completed at the perineum and introitus with 2–0 delayed absorbable suture used throughout the repair and 4–0 Vicryl on the superficial skin of the perineum. (k) A perineoplasty is then completed. (l) After vaginal rejuvenation. Source: R. Moore and J. Miklos. Reproduced with permission.

the defects, a midline plication, or a combination [Figure 9.2(f)]. The caliber of the vagina is then addressed by plication of the rectovaginal fascia in the midline with delayed absorbable sutures. Levator plication is avoided, and the diameter of the vagina is constantly measured with the surgeon's fingers. Several layers of plication may be needed to reduce the genital hiatus and reduce the caliber of the vagina to an appropriate level [Figure 9.2(g) and (h)]. A small amount of vaginal epithelium is then excised [Figure 9.2(i)] and the incision closed in a running fashion [Figure 9.2(j)].

A perineoplasty is then completed, involving a meticulous and detailed dissection out laterally to obtain the lacerated edges of the deep and superficial transverse perineal muscles and bring them back together in the midline to achieve uniformity at the same level of the posterior wall repair. The inferior edges of the labia majora that will make up the posterior fourchette of the vaginal opening must be marked at the beginning of the procedure so that these edges match up during the closure to form the vaginal introitus. An appropriate amount of skin must also be excised from the perineum and introitus to result in a cosmetically pleasing appearance of the opening of the vagina for the patient. A multilayer repair (typically this may involve 4 or 5 layers) is completed at the perineum and introitus [Figure 9.2(k) and (l)].

When a repair is primarily because of vaginal relaxation for sexual function it becomes a much more meticulous dissection and repair as the surgeon has to constantly judge and measure vaginal caliber to try to restore the entire vaginal length to its pre-childbirth state. If this is not done, the results will be poor and the patient's sexual function may not change or may worsen secondary to pain, vaginal shortening, scar tissue formation, and/or constrictions.

(Editor's note: While the procedure may be performed under general, conduction, or local infiltration anesthesia, an advantage of "local" is the ability of the conscious patient, upon demand, to contract her levator muscles for guidance during suture placement in reconstruction of the pelvic floor.)

Post-operative care

Routine post-operative care is given to patients undergoing vaginal surgery. Many of the procedures are completed on an outpatient basis and the surgery is completed under local, spinal, or general anesthesia.

A pudendal block may also be given prior to or during the procedure to help decrease post-operative pain. Vaginal packing is left in post-operatively and removed prior to the patient being discharged. Routine instructions for vaginal surgery are given to the patient and she is seen for follow-up at 4 weeks post-operatively or sooner as indicated. The vaginal introitus and caliber are assessed and if felt necessary the patient will begin perineal massage in a warm water bath for 1 to 2 weeks prior to resuming penetrative sexual intercourse.

Risks/complications

The potential complications of vaginal rejuvenation are infection, bleeding, wound dehiscence, dyspareunia, inadequate tightening, introital narrowing, and recto-perineal/rectovaginal fistula (48,51). These are discussed in detail in Chapter 16. According to the study by Goodman *et al.*, 4% of women had temporary stricture of the vaginal apex, 2% wound dehiscence, 2% excessive post-operative pain, 2% inadequate tightening, 2% microtear at 1 year follow-up, 2% introital tightening, and 2% bleeding after first sexual intercourse.

Conclusion

Vaginal rejuvenation surgery is one of the latest trends in elective vaginal surgery for women. It is a restoration of the vaginal caliber in women who suffer from decreased vaginal sensation or feelings of a loose or wide vagina that affects their sexual life. In many instances, women who present with these symptoms are found to have other urogynecologic pathology such as prolapse that must also be addressed in any repair contemplated. Sexual dysfunction or decreased sexual sensation may be one of the first symptoms that women suffer from in the progression of prolapse and therefore a proper examination is vital prior to any repair. We have ample evidence, as presented in this chapter, that prolapse and vaginal relaxation can create sexual dysfunction and that repair may reverse these changes in many women. However, when dealing with sexual dysfunction alone and the caliber or width of the vagina, the surgical repair must be meticulous and precise in order to enhance sensation and function and not impair it. This sums up the statement "The Art of Surgery"!

References

1. Goodman MP. Female cosmetic genital surgery. *Obstet Gynecol* 2009;**113**(1):154–9.

2. Pardo JS, Solà VD, Ricci PA, Guiloff EF, Freundlich OK. Colpoperineoplasty in women with a sensation of a wide vagina. *Acta Obstet Gynecol Scand* 2006;**85**(9):1125–7.

3. Moore RD, Miklos JR. Vaginal reconstruction and rejuvenation Surgery: Is there data to support improved sexual function? *Am J Cosmet Surg* 2012;**29**(2):97–113.

4. Dobbeleir JM, Van Landuyt K, Monstrey SJ. *Aesthetic surgery of the female genitalia*. Paper presented at Seminars in Plastic Surgery, 2011.

5. DeLancey JOL, Kearney R, Chou Q, Speights S, Binno S. The appearance of levator ani muscle abnormalities in magnetic resonance images after vaginal delivery. *Obstet Gynecol* 2003;**101**(1):46–53.

6. Lien KC, Mooney B, DeLancey JOL, Ashton-Miller JA. Levator ani muscle stretch induced by simulated vaginal birth. *Obstet Gynecol* 2004;**103**(1):31–40.

7. Allen RE, Hosker GL, Smith ARB, Warrell DW. Pelvic floor damage and childbirth: A neurophysiological study. *BJOG* 1990;**97**(9):770–9.

8. Dietz HP. Pelvic floor trauma following vaginal delivery. *Curr Opin Obstet Gynecol* 2006;**18**(5):528–37.

9. DeLancey JOL. The hidden epidemic of pelvic floor dysfunction: Achievable goals for improved prevention and treatment. *Am J Obstet Gynecol* 2005;**192**(5):1488–95.

10. Mant J, Painter R, Vessey M. Epidemiology of genital prolapse: Observations from the Oxford Family Planning Association Study. *BJOG* 1997;**104**(5):579–85.

11. Hendrix SL, Clark A, Nygaard I, Aragaki A, Barnabei V, McTiernan A. Pelvic organ prolapse in the women's health initiative: Gravity and gravidity. *Am J Obstet Gynecol* 2002;**186**(6):1160–6.

12. Brubaker L, Handa VL, Bradley CS, et al. Sexual function 6 months after first delivery. *Obstet Gynecol* 2008;**111**(5):1040.

13. Signorello LB, Harlow BL, Chekos AK, Repke JT. Postpartum sexual functioning and its relationship to perineal trauma: A retrospective cohort study of primiparous women. *Am J Obstet Gynecol* 2001;**184**(5):881–90.

14. Wu JM, Hundley AF, Visco AG. Elective primary cesarean delivery: Attitudes of urogynecology and maternal-fetal medicine specialists. *Obstet Gynecol* 2005;**105**(2):301–6.

15. Basson R, Berman J, Burnett A, et al. Report of the International Consensus Development Conference on female sexual dysfunction: Definitions and classifications. *J Urol* 2000;**163**(3):888–93.

16. Pauls RN, Segal JL, Silva WA, Kleeman SD, Karram MM. Sexual function in patients presenting to a urogynecology practice. *Int Urogynecol J* 2006;**17**(6):576–80.

17. Brubaker LT, Saclarides TJ. *The Female pelvic Floor: Disorders of Function and Support*. Philadelphia: FA Davis Co., 1996.

18. Walters MD, Karram MM. *Urogynecology and Reconstructive Pelvic Surgery*. Amsterdam: Elsevier Health Sciences, 2006.

19. Nichols DH, Randall CL, Diedrick MD. *Vaginal surgery*. Baltimore: Williams & Wilkins, 1996.

20. Lowenstein L, Pierce K, Pauls R. Urogynecology and sexual function research. How are we doing? *J Sex Med* 2009;**6**(1):199–204.

21. Barber MD, Maher C. Epidemiology and outcome assessment of pelvic organ prolapse. *Int Urogynecol J* 2013;**24**(11):1783–90.

22. Novi JM, Jeronis S, Morgan MA, Arya LA. Sexual function in women with pelvic organ prolapse compared to women without pelvic organ prolapse. *J Urol* 2005;**173**(5):1669–72.

23. Botros SM, Abramov Y, Miller J-JR, et al. Effect of parity on sexual function: An identical twin study. *Obstet Gynecol* 2006;**107**(4):765–70.

24. Barber MD, Visco AG, Wyman JF, Fantl JA, Bump RC. Sexual function in women with urinary incontinence and pelvic organ prolapse. *Obstet Gynecol* 2002;**99**(2):281–9.

25. Rogers RG, Kammerer-Doak D, Villarreal A, Coates K, Qualls C. A new instrument to measure sexual function in women with urinary incontinence or pelvic organ prolapse. *Am J Obstet Gynecol* 2001;**184**(4):552–8.

26. Ellerkmann RM, Cundiff GW, Melick CF, Nihira MA, Leffler K, Bent AE. Correlation of symptoms with location and severity of pelvic organ prolapse. *Am J Obstet Gynecol* 2001;**185**(6):1332–8.

27. Srikrishna S, Robinson D, Cardozo L, Cartwright R. Experiences and expectations of women with urogenital prolapse: A quantitative and qualitative exploration. *BJOG* 2008;**115**(11):1362–8.

28. Azar M, Noohi S, Radfar S, Radfar MH. Sexual function in women after surgery for pelvic organ prolapse. *Int Urogynecol J* 2008;**19**(1):53–7.

29. Stoutjesdijk JA, Vierhout ME, Spruijt JW, Massolt ET. Does vaginal reconstructive surgery with or without vaginal hysterectomy or trachelectomy improve sexual well being? A prospective follow-up study. *Int Urogynecol J* 2006;**17**(2):131–5.

30. Rogers RG, Kammerer-Doak D, Darrow A, et al. Does sexual function change after surgery for stress urinary incontinence and/or pelvic organ prolapse? A multicenter prospective study. *Am J Obstet Gynecol* 2006;**195**(5):e1–4.

31. Celik DB, Kizilkaya Beji N, Yalcin O. Sexual function in women after urinary incontinence and/or pelvic organ prolapse surgery. *J Clin Nurs* 2014;**23**(17–18):2637–48.

32. Kim SR, Moon YJ, Kim SK, Bai SW. Changes in sexual function and comparison of questionnaires following surgery for pelvic organ prolapse. *Yonsei Med J* 2014;**55**(1):170–7.

33. Handa VL, Zyczynski HM, Brubaker L, et al. Sexual function before and after sacrocolpopexy for pelvic organ prolapse. *Am J Obstet Gynecol* 2007;**197**(6):e621–9.

34. Salamon CG, Lewis CM, Priestley J, Culligan PJ. Sexual function before and 1 year after laparoscopic sacrocolpopexy. *Female Pelvic Med Reconstructive Surg* 2014;**20**(1): 44–7.

35. Kim-Fine S, Smith CY, Gebhart JB, Occhino JA. Medium-term changes in vaginal accommodation and sexual function after vaginal reconstructive surgery. *Female Pelvic Med Reconstructive Surg* 2014;**20**(1):27–32.

36. Thibault F, Costa P, Thanigasalam R, et al. Impact of laparoscopic sacrocolpopexy on symptoms, health-related quality of life and sexuality: A medium-term analysis. *BJU Int* 2013;**112**(8):1143–9.

37. Brandner S, Monga A, Mueller MD, Herrmann G, Kuhn A. Sexual function after rectocele repair. *J Sex Med* 2011;**8**(2): 583–8.

38. Komesu YM, Rogers RG, Kammerer-Doak DN, Barber MD, Olsen AL. Posterior repair and sexual function. *Am J Obstet Gynecol* 2007;**197**(1):e101–6.

39. Tunuguntla HS, Gousse AE. Female sexual dysfunction following vaginal surgery: A review. *J Urol* 2006;**175**(2): 439–46.

40. Paraiso MFR, Barber MD, Muir TW, Walters MD. Rectocele repair: A randomized trial of three surgical techniques including graft augmentation. *Am J Obstet Gynecol* 2006;**195**(6): 1762–71.

41. Kuhn A, Brunnmayr G, Stadlmayr W, Kuhn P, Mueller MD. Male and female sexual function after surgical repair of female organ prolapse. *J Sex Med* 2009;**6**(5):1324–34.

42. Shaw D, Lefebvre G, Bouchard C, et al. Female genital cosmetic surgery. *J Obstet Gynaecol Canada* 2013;**35**(12):1108–12.

43. Ozel B, White T, Urwitz-Lane R, Minaglia S. The impact of pelvic organ prolapse on sexual function in women with urinary incontinence. *Int Urogynecol J* 2006;**17**(1): 14–17.

44. Baytur Y, Deveci A, Uyar Y, Ozcakir H, Kizilkaya S, Caglar H. Mode of delivery and pelvic floor muscle strength and sexual function after childbirth. *Int J Gynecol Obstet* 2005;**88**(3):276–80.

45. Kline G, Graber B. Case studies of perineometer resistive exercises of orgasmic dysfunction. In: *Circumvaginal Musculature and Sexual Function*, pp. 25–42. Basil, Switzerland: S. Karger, 1982.

46. Pardo J, Sola V, Ricci P. Colpoperineoplasty for vaginal relaxation: A follow-up study. *Int Urogynecol J Pelvic Floor Dysfunct* 2007;**18**:S147.

47. Matlock DL, Simopoulos AF. The application of the Pelvic Organ Prolapse/Urinary Incontinence Sexual Questionnaire (PISQ-12) to laser assisted anterior and posterior colporrhaphy with perineorraphy: A pilot study. *World Congress on Female and Male Cosmetic Genital Surgery*, 2011, Las Vegas, Nevada.

48. Goodman MP, Placik OJ, Benson III RH, et al. A large multicenter outcome study of female genital plastic surgery. *J Sex Med* 2010;**7**(4 pt 1):1565–77.

49. Goodman MP. Female genital cosmetic and plastic surgery: A review. *J Sex Med* 2011;**8**(6):1813–25.

50. Rogers R, Rockwood T, Constantine M, et al. A new measure of sexual function in women with pelvic floor disorders (PFD): The Pelvic Organ Prolapse/Incontinence Sexual Questionnaire, IUGA-Revised (PISQ-IR). *Int Urogynecol J* 2013;**24**(7):1091–103.

51. Iglesia CB, Yurteri-Kaplan L, Alinsod R. Female genital cosmetic surgery: A review of techniques and outcomes. *Int Urogynecol J* 2013;**24**(12):1997–2009.

CHAPTER 10

The biomechanics and physiology of clitoral and vaginally activated orgasm: impact of vaginal tightening operations

Michael P. Goodman

Caring for Women Wellness Center, Davis, CA, USA

I have a simple philosophy: Fill what's empty; empty what's full; scratch where it itches.

Alice Roosevelt Longworth

It is well documented that pelvic relaxation adversely affects sexual function and that, when repaired, function improves [1]. Treatment should be tailored toward improvement of sexual function. Cardozo's group in the UK found that 83.6% of women presenting for prolapse surgery list "improved sexual function" as part of their goal for surgery [2].

In order to understand the physiology and biomechanics involved in so-called "vaginal tightening operations" ("vaginal rejuvenation," VRJ; perineoplasty, PP; vaginoplasty, VP; colpoperineoplasty, CP), one must first understand two fundamental points: [1] exactly what these operations are, how they are performed, and what they accomplish anatomically, and [2] the biomechanics, psychology, and physiology involved in the two proposed types of orgasmic function in women: "clitoral orgasm" (CO) and "vaginally activated orgasm" (VAO).

The effect of childbirth on pelvic floor musculature and levator hiatal dimensions now has some evidence base [3]. In a previous chapter (Chapter 9), Moore, Miklos, and Chinthakanan reported that vaginal wall tightening operations are variations on classic pelvic floor perineorrhaphy + site-specific repair procedures modified specifically for improvement of sexual function by including a multilayered pelvic floor repair, reconstructing and elevating the perineal body, minimizing vaginal caliber, better approximating levator and transverse perineal musculature, and effecting an improved cosmetic introital, vestibular, and perineal appearance.

Vaginal tone (thought to be due to a combination of anatomic proximity and muscular strength) affects vaginal sensation and ability to orgasm [4,5]. Increases in vaginal tone may be produced in several ways. Pelvic floor muscular strength may become more robust by regular and repeated pelvic floor strengthening exercises (aka "Kegel's") with or without the aid of a pelvic floor physical therapist and with or without the aid of various vaginal floor stimulation and biofeedback exercise units such In-Tone™, Apex™, and various vaginally held spherical devices (Luna Beads™, modifications of "Ben Wah balls," etc.), cones, rods, and so forth. Investigators have shown that supervised pelvic floor muscle training can increase muscle volume, close the levator hiatus, shorten muscle length, and elevate the resting position of the bladder and rectum [6,7]. Additionally, the circumferential "tightening" produced by CP/VRJ surgical procedures increases vaginal pressure as measured by a perineometer (8, and personal measurements conducted by the author, J. Miklos and R. Moore, and M. Pelosi II and M. Pelosi III).

Anatomic relationships

Understanding the biomechanics necessitates an understanding of the anatomic positioning of the vaginal canal and relationships of the clitoral complex and the nerve-rich anterior vaginal wall, which also contains the erectile tissue of the bulbs and crurae of the clitoris as it "roots" around the urethra in the anterior vaginal wall (Figure 10.1). Understanding the physiology involved requires knowledge of the neurophysiology and probable differences in orgasmic potential of women.

The nulliparous vagina, in addition to possessing muscular vigor and certainly a narrower caliber than the multiparous vaginal canal, follows a distinctly downward angle as it proceeds from introitus to fornix (Figure 10.2) This angulation pushes the inserted object against the anterior vaginal wall, including the anterior distal vaginal area known as the "G-spot" or "G-area" (see Chapter 11), resulting in stretching and friction in this area as well as other (posterior vaginal wall and

cervix) areas of the vaginal canal (Figure 10.3) [9]. In many instances, the multiparous vagina loses this angle via pressure necrosis of muscle fibers from fetal head pressure and shearing/separating forces from the fetal presenting part as it slowly descends against and through the pelvic floor. The levator musculature becomes attenuated, the introitus gapes, the perineal body becomes lax and its size diminished, and the vaginal canal assumes a more horizontal angle. This has sexual consequences for many women, who complain of a "sensation of wide vagina" [a term coined by J. Pardo et al. from Chile [10], and A. Ostrzenski from the United States [11]], loss of friction, and less pressure from an inserted object against the anterior vaginal wall (AVW) and clitoral complex. This results in loss of sensation and difficulty achieving orgasm (Figure 10.4). The perineum may also gape because a tear or episiotomy has been poorly repaired.

With its proximity to periurethral tissue, including Skene's glands, clitoral bulbs, and crurae, and its rich skeletal (via the dorsal nerve of clitoris, a branch of the pudendal nerve) and autonomic (via hypogastric) nerve supply, the AVW is an important anatomic area intimately involved, along with the external clitoris, labia, and other parts of the vulva and distal vagina, in sexual pleasure [12]. A "relaxed" vagina engenders less pressure in this area, while a toned vagina (or, conversely, a large penis) engenders greater sexual satisfaction. The vagina, especially in its distal (AVW) portion, contains enough nerves to participate in sexual response, as well as the whole biochemical machinery known to mediate penile excitation [13–16].

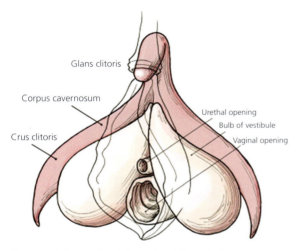

Figure 10.1 Anatomic relationships of the clitoris.

Glans clitoris

Corpus cavernosum

Crus clitoris

Urethal opening
Bulb of vestibule
Vaginal opening

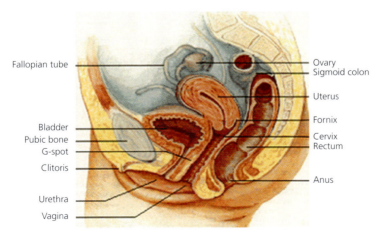

Fallopian tube

Ovary
Sigmoid colon

Uterus

Bladder
Pubic bone
G-spot
Clitoris

Fornix

Cervix
Rectum

Anus

Urethra

Vagina

Figure 10.2 Anatomic relationship of the vaginal canal and adjacent organs, portraying vaginal angulation.

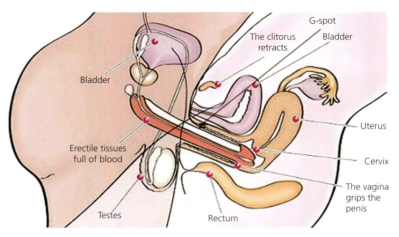

Figure 10.3 Angle of penile penetration, showing pressure against "G-spot" and clitoral body/glans.

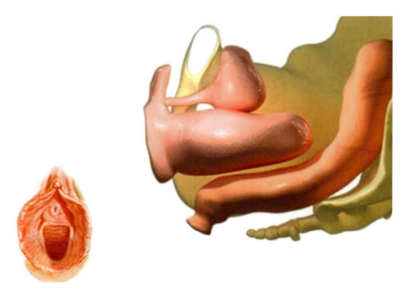

Figure 10.4 Relaxed introitus and vaginal canal.

Orgasm physiology

The existence of different types of female orgasms (CO and VAO) has been successfully argued [16]. Sexual arousal may lead to orgasm/multiple orgasms. Orgasm (from the Greek *lagnos- lustful*) is a cerebral event with local effects, including activation of sympathetic fibers via the hypogastric nerves and inferior hypogastric plexus to the uterovaginal plexus, accompanied by reflex waves of contraction of skeletal muscles of the vagina, urethra, and anus mediated by pudendal nerve, plus uterine smooth muscle contractions mediated by autonomic nerves [13].

Clitoral orgasm, from local/digital stimulation, and mediated through the clitoral nerve, a branch of the pudendal n., is described as "warm" or "electrical," whereas VAO is described as more intense, more internal, throbbing, deep, and is triggered more by internal stimulation and distension of the vaginal walls and manipulation of the cervix and is more under the control of autonomic nerves [17]. In contrast to CO, VAO refers to a woman's orgasm triggered by penile-vaginal (or surrogate) intercourse. Awareness of vaginal and cervical stimulation is uniquely different from awareness of clitoral stimulation. Vaginal and cervical stimulation generate their own unique sensory input to the brain separate and distinct from clitoral sensory input and are adequate on their own to generate orgasm, a fact noted by Komisurak, Whipple, *et al.* [18] in their landmark work investigating orgasm in spinal cord–severed women who indeed were orgasmic with vaginal stimulation, proving that the hypogastric plexus, via the vagus nerve, conveys vaginal and cervical stimulation directly to the brain, bypassing the spinal cord.

There is an intimate relationship between the distal portion of the vagina, including the AVW, the urethra, introitus, and vulva. These separate organs appear to act as an inter-related unit, with a shared blood supply and innervation, and respond as a unit during stimulation [12]. Additionally, there is a close relationship between the "internal" portions of the clitoral unit and the AVW, which exhibits a special sensitivity secondary to pressure and movement of the clitoral unit, as well as the autonomic receptors. A penis, or other inserted object, exerts a force on the AVW against the pubic symphysis, stretching the clitoris. One might assume, then, that the tighter the vaginal barrel, the greater the force and greater the resultant stretch.

What do vaginal tightening operations accomplish?

There is a rich body of evidence, much of it from Stuart Brody and his group at the University of West Scotland in Paisley and well reported in the popular media [19,20], asserting that women who have a greater VAO constancy have a slight tendency to prefer men with a longer, thicker penis [21], although the veracity of these statements may certainly be challenged; bigger may indeed be better, but only up to a point [22]! Brody asserts that 1. Sexual desire is greater for women who have vaginal orgasm, and more frequent vaginal orgasm is associated with experiencing greater excitement from deep vaginal stimulation [5,23,24]. 2. Intimate relationship quality is better for women who experience vaginal orgasm [23,25–27]. 3. A history of vaginal orgasm is a protective factor against female arousal disorder [27].

4. A history of vaginal orgasm is a protective factor against global orgasmic dysfunction [28]. 5. Women with greater intercourse orgasm constancy have better concordance of vaginal and subjective responses to erotica [29,30]. 6. Women who have greater vaginal orgasm constancy have better attention to vaginal sensations during intercourse [21]. 7. Women with a history of vaginal orgasm manifest less pelvic and vertebral functional muscular disturbance [31]. 8. Frequency of penile-vaginal intercourse orgasm (but not frequency of other orgasm sources) and specifically having a vaginal orgasm is associated with greater sexual satisfaction [10,21,22,32–34]. 9. In women, stimulation of the clitoris, vagina, and cervix activated different regions of the brain, indicating that different genital regions produce different brain responses [18]. 10. Women who have vaginal orgasm are more satisfied with their own sexual health [21,23].

It certainly can be postulated that the increased AVW and cervical pressure engendered by vaginal tightening and strengthening and elevating the pelvic floor produces a similar biomechanical milieu as exists with increasing penile length and girth. Multiparous women, as they age, frequently experience vaginal laxity. Men, as they age, frequently experience less robust erectile quality. Understanding Brody, Weiss *et al.*'s data, it is small wonder that reports from the literature [10,35,36] confirm the enhancement of sexual pleasure noted in women undergoing vaginal tightening operations.

Vaginal tightening procedures, by re-establishing the downward angle of the vagina and increasing pressure against the AVW, cervix, and clitoral complex with insertion of a toy or penis, help correct the parturition-induced relaxation of the perineum and vaginal canal. When the vaginal caliber is repaired in a group of women presenting with decreased vaginal sensation or decreased friction, sexual function improves [37]. Postsurgical pelvic floor exercises compound this improvement. There is clear evidence in the medical literature that, in addition to the psychological improvement generated by what women feel is a cosmetic improvement to the appearance of the introitus, the biomechanical changes attendant with vaginal tightening procedures improve sexual pleasure and sexual health, are reproducible, and are secondary to the biomechanical tightening of the vaginal barrel produced by this surgery.

References

1. Webbe SA, Kellogg S, Whitmore K. Urogenital complaints and female sexual dysfunction. Part 2. *J Sex Med* 2010;**7**: 2305–17.

2. Srikrishna S, Robinson D, Cardozo L, Cartwright R. Experiences and expectations of women with urogenital prolapse: A quantitative and qualitative explanation. *BJOG* 2008;**11**:1362–8.

3. Shek KL, Dietz HP. The effect of childbirth on hiatal dimensions. *Obstet Gynecol* 2009;**113**:1272–8.

4. Kline G, Graber B. Case studies of perineometer resistive exercises of orgasmic dysfunction. In: *Circumvaginal Musculature and Sexual Function*, pp. 25–42. Basil, Switzerland: S. Karger, 1982.

5. Brody S, Klapilova K, Krejcova M. More frequent vaginal orgasm is associated with experiencing greater excitement from deep vaginal stimulation. *J Sex Med* 2013;**10**:1730–6.

6. Rosenbaum TY. Pelvic floor involvement in male and female sexual dysfunction and the role of pelvic floor rehabilitation in treatment: A literature review *J Sex Med* 2007; **4**:4–14.

7. Broekken IH, Majida M, Engh ME, Bo K. Morphological changes after pelvic floor muscle training measured by 3-dimensional ultrasonography. *Obstet Gynecol* 2010;**115**: 317–24.

8. Kline G, Graber B. Case studies of perineometer resistive exercises of orgasmic dysfunction. In: *Circumvaginal Musculature and Sexual Function*, pp. 25–42. Basil, Switzerland: S. Karger, 1982.

9. Kilchevsky A, Vardi Y, Lowenstein L, Gruenwald I. Is the female G-spot truly a distinct anatomic entity? *J Sex Med* 2012;**9**:719–26.

10. Pardo J, Sola V, Ricci P, Guiloff E, Freundlich D. Colpoperineoplasty in women with a sensation of a wide vagina. *Acta Obstet Gynecol Scand* 2006;**85**:1125–8.

11. Ostrzenski A. An acquired sensation of wide/smooth vagina: A new classification. *Eur J Obst Gynec Reprod Biol* 2011;**158**:97–100.

12. O'Connell HE, Eizenberg N, Rahman M, Cleeve J. The anatomy of the distal vagina: Towards unity. *J Sex Med* 2008;**5**:1883–91.

13. D'Amati G, di Gioia CR, Bologna M, et al. Type 5 phosphodiesterase expression in the human vagina. *Urology* 2002;**60**:191–5.

14. D'Amati G, di Gioia CR, Proietti L, et al. Functional anatomy of the human vagina. *J Endocrinol Invest* 2003;**26**:92–6.

15. Janini EA, D'Amati G, Lenzi A. Histology and immunohistological studies of female genital tissue. In: *Women's Sexual Function and Dysfunction: Study, Diagnosis and Treatment*, pp. 126–33. London: Taylor and Francis, 2006.

16. Jannini EA, Rubio-Casillas, Whipple B, Buisson O, Komisaruk BR, Brody S. Female orgasm(s): One, two, several. *J Sex Med* 2012;**9**:956–65.

17. Brody S, Kruger TH. The post-orgasmic prolactin increase following intercourse is greater than following masturbation and suggests greater satiety. *Biol Psychol* 2006;**71**: 312–5.

18. Komisaruk BR, Whipple B, Crawford A, Liu WC, Kalnin A, Mosier K. Brain activation during vaginocervical self-stimulation and orgasm in women with complete spinal cord injury: fMRI evidence of mediation by the vagus nerves. *Brain Res* 2004;**1024**:77–88.

19. http://www.dailymail.co.uk/sciencetech/article-2127901/ Put-away-road-map-lads-Scientists-present-new-proof-women-climax-intercourse-alone.html?ito=feeds-newsxml.

20. http://onlinelibrary.wiley.com/doi/10.1111/j.1743-6109. 2012s.02694.x/abstract/.

21. Brody S, Weiss P. Vaginal orgasm is associated with vaginal (not clitoral) sex education, focusing mental attention on vaginal sensations, intercourse duration, and a preference for a longer penis. *J Sex Med* 2010;**7**:2774–81.

22. Veale D, Eshkevari E, Read J, Miles S, Troglia A, Phillips R, Carmona L, Fiorito C, Wylie K, Muir G. Beliefs about penis size: Validation of a scale for men ashamed about their penis size. *J Sex Med* 2014;**11**:84–92.

23. Brody S. Vaginal orgasm is associated with better psychological function. *Sex Relat Ther* 2007;**22**:173–91.

24. Nutter DE, Condron MK. Sexual fantasy and activity patterns of females with inhibited sexual desire versus normal controls. *J Sex Marital Ther* 1983;**9**:276–82.

25. Weiss P, Brody S. International Index of Erectile Function (HEF) scores generated by men or female partners correlate equally well with own satisfaction (sexual, partnership, life and mental health). *J Sex Med* 2011;**8**:1404–10.

26. Costa RM, Brody S. Women's relationship quality is associated with specifically penile-vaginal intercourse orgasm and frequency. *J Sex Marital Ther* 2007;**33**:319–27.

27. Weiss P, Brody S. Female sexual arousal disorder with and without a distress criterion: Prevalence and correlates in a representative Czech sample. *J Sex Med* 2009;**6**: 3385–94.

28. Fugl-Meyer KS, Oberg K, Lundberg PO, Lewin B, Fugl-Meyer A. On orgasm, sexual techniques, and erotic perceptions in 18- to 74-year-old Swedish women. *J Sex Med* 2006;**3**:56–68.

29. Brody S, Laan E, van Lunsen RH. Concordance between women's physiologic and subjective sexual arousal is associated with consistency of orgasm during intercourse, but not other sexual behavior. *J Sex Marital Ther* 2003;**29**: 15–23.

30. Brody S. Intercourse orgasm consistency, concordance of women's genital and subjective sexual arousal, and erotic stimulus presentation sequence. *J Sex Marital Ther* 2007;**33**: 31–9.

31. Nicholas A, Brody S, de Sutter P, de Carufel F. A woman's history of vaginal orgasm is discernible from her walk. *J Sex Med* 2008;**5**:2119–24.

32. Tao P, Brody S. Sexual behavior predictors of satisfaction in Chinese sample. *J Sex Med* 2011;**8**:455–60.

33. Brody S, Costa RM. Satisfaction (sexual, life, relationship, health) is associated directly with penile-vaginal intercourse, but inversely with other sexual behavior frequencies. *J Sex Med* 2009;**6**:1947–54.

34. Phillipsohn S, Hartmann U. Determination of sexual satisfaction in a sample of German women. *J Sex Med* 2009;**8**:1001–10.

35. Brody S. The relative health benefits of different sexual activities. *J Sex Med* 2010;**7**:1336–61.

36. Goodman MP, Placik OJ, Benson RH III, Miklos JR, Moore RD, Jason RA, Matlock DL, Simopoulos AF, Stern BH, Stanton RA, Kolb SE, Gonzalez F. A large multicenter outcome study of female genital plastic surgery. *J Sex Med* 2010;**7**:165–77.

37. Moore RD, Miklos JR, Chinthakanan D. Evaluation of sexual function outcomes in women undergoing vaginal rejuvenation/vaginolasty procedures for symptoms of vaginal laxity/decreased vaginal sensation utilizing validated sexual function questionnaire PISQ-12. *Surg Tech Int* 2014;**24**:253–60.

CHAPTER 11

The G-spot

Dudley Robinson and Linda Cardozo

Department of Urogynaecology, King's College Hospital, London, UK

I know the answer! The answer lies within the heart of all mankind! The answer is twelve? I think I'm in the wrong building.

Charles Schulz

Introduction

Ernst Grafenberg, a German obstetrician and gynecologist working in Berlin, first described a distinct erogenous zone in the anterior vaginal wall along the course of the urethra in 1950. He noted that during orgasm this area was pressed downward, seemed to be surrounded by erectile tissue, and that the most stimulating area was located in the upper posterior urethra where it arises from the bladder neck. In addition he also noted that stimulation of this area lead to the production of fluid from the urethra, possibly from the intraurethral glands [1]. Although this concept was first proposed in 1950, it was not until 30 years later that the term "G-spot" was first coined by Addiego and colleagues, referring to an "erotically sensitive spot" located in the pelvic urethra and palpable through the anterior vaginal wall [2].

The concept of the G-spot, however, remains controversial, and the scientific evidence supporting the concept is poor and very limited. This is perhaps best summed up by Terence Hines, an American neuroscientist: "Until a thorough and careful histological investigation of the relevant tissue is undertaken, the G-spot will remain a sort of gynaecological UFO (Unidentified Foreign Object): much searched for, much discussed, but unverified by objective means" [3]. A more recent review of all the published evidence has also concluded that the G-spot does not exist [4] although other authors continue to debate the anatomical and scientific evidence [5].

Evaluating the evidence: genetic studies

The genetic and environmental influences on the presence of the G-spot have recently been evaluated in a large study of 1,804 twins aged 22–83 years. All were asked to complete questionnaires regarding female sexual function and asked about the presence of the G-spot. Overall 56% of women reported having a G-spot and the prevalence decreased with age. Variance component analyses revealed that variation in G-spot reported frequency was almost entirely as a result of individual experiences and random measurement error (>89%) with no genetic influence. In addition, correlations with general sexual behaviour, relationship satisfaction, and attitudes toward sexuality suggested that the G-spot is most likely a secondary pseudophenomenon with no physiological or physical basis [6].

Female Genital Plastic and Cosmetic Surgery, First Edition. Edited by Michael P. Goodman.
© 2016 John Wiley & Sons, Ltd. Published 2016 by John Wiley & Sons, Ltd.

Evaluating the evidence: anatomical studies

The evidence suggesting that the G-spot is a distinct anatomical entity also remains controversial [7]. A study of seven fresh Korean cadavers has been reported investigating the innervation of the vagina using microdissection and immunohistochemistry. Overall the distal anterior vaginal wall was found to have significantly denser nerve innervation than the surrounding structures, prompting the authors to suggest that this may be related to the G-spot [8]. However, this would seem to contradict the findings previously observed and reported by Grafenberg.

A more recent case study has also reported on the anatomical findings of the G-spot based on the dissection of a fresh 83-year-old cadaver [9]. The author reported that the G-spot had a distinguishable anatomic structure that was located on the dorsal aspect of the perineal membrane, 16.5 mm from the upper part of the urethral meatus, and it created a 35° angle with the lateral border of the urethra. It was described as a well-delineated sac (8.1 mm × 1.5 mm–3.6 mm × 0.4 mm) with walls resembling fibroconnective and erectile tissue that had three distinct areas and contained blue grapelike structures. A distal tail was also identified, which disappeared into the surrounding tissues. These findings from a single dissection have been highly contentious, in part secondary to the absence of histological verification in the data presented [10].

More recently a literature review (1950–2011) has been reported to assess any valid objective data that evaluated the existence of an anatomically distinct G-spot [11]. While there were many papers reported in the literature investigating the existence of the G-spot, attempts to characterise vaginal innervation have not been reproducible. Furthermore, while the majority of women were found to believe a G-spot actually exists, not all women were able to locate it for themselves. In addition, imaging studies have been unable to demonstrate a unique entity, other than the clitoris, whose direct stimulation leads to a vaginal orgasm. The authors conclude that while objective measures have failed to provide consistent evidence, reliable anecdotal reports of a highly sensitive area in the distal anterior vaginal wall continue to support the existence of the G-spot.

Evaluating the evidence: imaging studies

Despite the lack of evidence supporting the existence of the G-spot as a distinct anatomical area, a small study in five volunteers has been reported investigating the use of ultrasound to detect the movement of the clitoris and its anatomical relationship with the anterior vaginal wall during perineal contraction and penetration without orgasm. Imaging in the coronal plane demonstrated a close relationship between the root of the clitoris and the anterior vaginal wall, suggesting that the increased sensitivity of the lower anterior vaginal wall may be explained by pressure and movement of the hood of the clitoris during penetration and perineal contraction [12]. These findings would suggest that the area of increased sensitivity may be related to the clitoris rather than the G-spot.

This work has also been repeated during penetrative sexual intercourse with a volunteer couple [13]. Coronal ultrasound performed over the upper aspect of the vulva demonstrated that the penis inflated the vagina and stretched the root of the clitoris and that this had a very close relationship with the anterior vaginal wall. Consequently this anatomical functional unit may explain the findings attributable to the G-spot, although it suggests that the clitoris may be the source of increased stimulation.

Evaluating the evidence: clinical studies

While evidence to support the existence of the G-spot from anatomical dissection and imaging studies remains contradictory, there is a little more clinical evidence regarding the concept of the G- spot.

A prospective cohort study of 50 uncircumcised and 125 circumcised women with mild anterior vaginal wall prolapse has been reported from Egypt [14]. Pre-operative sexual examination was performed in order to map the site of the G-spot in addition to other anatomical landmarks. Women were then followed up with sexual function questionnaires and a histological examination of the excised vaginal tissue was performed. Overall the G-spot was functionally proven in 82.3% of women and anatomically proven in 65.9%. Histological assessment confirmed that the two small flaccid balloonlike masses located on either side of the lower urethra and the G-spot were composed of epithelial, glandular, and erectile tissue; these were identified in 47.4% of women. In addition sexual function scores were significantly higher in the women with histologically identified G-spot tissue, and these scores dropped significantly after anterior vaginal wall surgery. Conversely female circumcision was not found to have a significant effect.

A further descriptive randomised prospective study, also from Egypt, has been reported in 1,500 women, of whom 500 underwent vaginal and/or vulvar surgery [15]. According to information from the study, the G-spot was "found to be present in all women; in 58% as a localised spot and in 42% as a diffuse area." Associated female ejaculation was reported in all localised cases and in 24.5% of the diffuse cases. In addition the G-spot was found to be "connected to the hymen in all cases, the urethra in 52.7%, the vulva in 82.2% and the cervix in 10.8% of cases." This data is confusing; it appears that the tissue located maintained anatomic connections, although exact information is vague. Furthermore sexual function scores were found to be reduced in those women having surgery involving the G-spot area (e.g., anterior colporrhaphy that intruded upon the approximate anatomic location ascribed to the G-spot).

The evidence from these two studies from one Egyptian institution would appear to give some support to the G-spot being an anatomical structure, although these findings have not been reproduced by other studies.

G-spot amplification

If the G-spot does exist, then, theoretically, augmenting the size of the G-spot may lead to more friction during intercourse and this may possibly lead to increased sexual satisfaction. This has lead to the development of G-spot amplification procedures, of which perhaps the best known is the G-Shot.

The G-Shot is a technique first described by Dr. David Matlock, a cosmetic gynecologist in Los Angeles (www.drmatlock.com). It is described as an office-based procedure where a bioengineered human high molecular weight hyaluraonic acid is injected in the area of the G-spot as localized by the patient in order to augment sensation during intercourse. The procedure is performed under local anesthetic and takes 15 minutes.

The injection lasts approximately 4–6 months and then needs to be repeated periodically.

To date there are no publications supporting the efficacy of the procedure, although in a small pilot study of 20 women 87% claimed enhanced sexual gratification and arousal (www.drmatlock.com). These results have never been reported in a peer review journal and there are no data to support the safety of the procedure.

Concerns regarding the efficacy and safety of these procedures have been addressed by the American Congress of Obstetricians and Gynecologists (ACOG) [16]. The guidelines state that G-spot amplification is a procedure offered by some practitioners although not medically indicated, and the safety and effectiveness have not been documented. The guidelines also state that women should be informed regarding the lack of data and also the potential complications including infection, altered sensation, dyspareunia, adhesions, and scarring.

More recently the Society of Obstetricians and Gynaecologists of Canada have also issued guidelines regarding genital cosmetic surgery [17]. Having performed systematic review of the literature, they concluded that there was little evidence to support any female genital cosmetic surgery in terms of improvement to sexual satisfaction or self-image and, furthermore, terms such as "G-spot enhancement" should be recognised as marketing terms only, have no medical origin, and therefore cannot be scientifically evaluated.

Conclusion

The published evidence regarding the existence of the G-spot remains highly divisive and controversial. While twin studies have shown no evidence of a genetic influence some anatomical studies have reported the presence of structures within the anterior wall that consist of contractile tissue and have dense innervation. There is also some clinical evidence, although limited, to support these findings. Conversely, however, imaging studies have suggested that it is perhaps the proximity of the clitoris to the anterior vaginal wall and urethra that is responsible for this localised area of increased sensitivity.

While the concept of the G-spot remains an intellectual enigma it also has significant commercial significance attached to it, and augmentation of sexual response by using G-spot amplification techniques is becoming more common despite a lack of evidence regarding safety and efficacy. Consequently there is currently a pressing need to validate anatomical and physiological studies so the controversy regarding the existence of the G-spot may be finally settled without exposing more women to unproven and potentially harmful treatments.

References

1. Grafenberg E. The role of urethra in female orgasm. *Int J Sexol* 1950;**3**:145–8.
2. Addiego F, Belzer EG, Comolli J, Moger W, Perry JD, Whipple B. Female ejaculation: A case study. *J Sex Res* 1981;**17**:13–21.
3. Hines T. The G spot: A modern gynaecologic myth. *Am J Obstet Gynecol* 2001;**185**:359–62.
4. Puppo V, Gruenwald I. Does the G spot exist? A review of the current literature. *Int Urogynecol J* 2012;**23**:1665–9.
5. Jannini EA, Whipple B, Kingsberg SA, Buisson O, Foldes P, Vardi Y. Who's afraid of the G spot? *J Sex Med* 2010;**7**:25–34.
6. Burri AV, Cherkas L, Spector TD. Genetic and environmental influences on self reported G spots in women; a twin study. *J Sex Med* 2010;**7**:1842–52.
7. Puppo V. Embryology and anatomy of the vulva: The female orgasm and women's sexual health. *Eur J Obstet Gynaecol Reprod Biol* 2011;**154**:3–8.
8. Song YB, Hwang K, Kim DJ, Han SH. Innervation of vagina: Microdissection and immunohistochemical study. *J Sex Marital Ther* 2009;**35**:144–53.
9. Ostrzenski A. G spot anatomy: A new discovery. *J Sex Med* 2012;**9**:1355–9.
10. Hines T, Kilchevsky A. The G spot discovered? Comments on Ostrezenski's article. *J Sex Med* 2013;**10**:887–8.
11. Kilchevsky A, Vardi Y, Lowenstein L, Gruenwald I. Is the female G spot truly a distinct anatomic entity? *J Sex Med* 2012;**9**:719–26.
12. Foldes P, Buisson O. The clitoral complex: A dynamic sonographic study. *J Sex Med* 2009;**6**:1223–31.
13. Buisson O, Foldes P, Jannini E, Mimoun S. Coitus as revealed by ultrasound in one volunteer couple. *J Sex Med* 2010;**7**:2750–4.
14. Thabet SM. Reality of the G spot and its relation to female circumcision and vaginal surgery. *J Obstet Gyanecol Res* 2009;**35**:967–73.
15. Thabet SM. New findings and concepts about the G spot in normal and absent vagina: Precautions possibly needed for preservation of the G spot and sexuality during surgery. *J Obstet Gyanaecol Res* 2013;**39**:1339–46.
16. American College of Obstetrics and Gynecology. Committee Opinion #378. Vaginal "rejuvenation" and cosmetic vaginal procedures. *Obstet Gynecol* 2007;**110**:737–8.
17. Shaw D, Lefebvre G, Bouchard C, et al. Society of Obstetricians and Gyanecologists of Canada. Female genital cosmetic surgery. *J Obstet Gynaecol Can* 2013;**35**:1108–14.

CHAPTER 12

Post-operative care

Michael P. Goodman

Caring for Women Wellness Center, Davis, CA, USA

> I went to a bookstore and asked the saleswoman, "Where's the self- help section?" She said if she told me, it would defeat the purpose.
>
> *George Carlin*

Several steps are involved in achieving a successful outcome in FGPS. Pre-operative patient choice and preparation, choice of specific procedure, suture material, choice of anesthesia, and meticulous surgical technique are important, but all is for naught if the surgeon is not aware of/does not instruct his/her patient in appropriate post-operative care or if the patient fails to follow instructions or is not a good candidate for elective vulvovaginal aesthetic surgery.

This cannot be stressed enough: careful, clear post-op instructions from the physician and/or patient care coordinator and re-emphasis to be certain your patient fully understands the instructions and the importance of following them are imperative. *Outcome is proportional to cautious post-op care on the part of your properly chosen patient.*

A common misconception is that these are "simple" operations. It is the surgeon's responsibility to clearly inform the patient that outcome is dependent equally upon her ability to follow instructions as on the surgeon's technique.

Pre-operative preparation for post-operative care

Post-operative care must be discussed with your patient at a visit well prior to her surgical date. Has she arranged for a ride home if it is your impression that, because of the complexity of surgery or the length or difficulty of the journey, she should not drive herself home? If her journey is significant—especially if it involves air transit, passenger terminals, long walks/transfers—have local lodging arrangements been made, if appropriate, until such time (1–3 days) as when she will be able to travel, especially if she is "on her own"? What arrangements have been made for her children? Her family? For time off from work? Has she been instructed to refrain from ingesting aspirin and NSAIDS for 10–14 days prior to surgery, to refrain from tobacco for at least 3–4 weeks prior to and 3–4 weeks after her procedure? If she has a history of recurrent herpes genitalis, have you prescribed peri-operative prophylaxis? She should refrain from self-tanning for a minimum of 3 weeks post-operatively.

Both general post-operative protocol and "tailoring" for her individual situation and procedure should be discussed on at least two occasions, the first well prior to the date of surgery, and again in-office prior to her procedure, and clear written instructions should be given at these times.

Specific instructions

Labiaplasty, minora (LP-m), majora (LP-M); reduction, clitoral hood (RCH)

(**NB: *Instructions described herein are for the average curvilinear resection LP-m, RCH, and LP-M. Patients with more involved incisions and for V-wedge modifications should be*

Female Genital Plastic and Cosmetic Surgery, First Edition. Edited by Michael P. Goodman.
© 2016 John Wiley & Sons, Ltd. Published 2016 by John Wiley & Sons, Ltd.

instructed to extend these typical recovery times, precautions, and proscriptions by ~25%.)

- *Day 0 to day 5*: If *arnica* is to be given, it should begin from a day prior to or immediately following her procedure. *Icing* should begin within a couple of hours of surgery with a small, flexible, re-freezable soft pack, or bags of frozen peas or corn, or a form-fitting moistened and frozen sanitary napkin and should be effected for 15–20 minutes 6–8 times/day for the first 3–5 days after surgery. *Hygiene*: We advise periodic rinses with a peri-bottle and daily showers preferably

with a hand-held shower device. Full immersion should be avoided for 2 weeks. A witch hazel impregnated wipe such as Tucks is soothing for personal hygiene. *Observation by the patient*: We encourage observation, *but not manipulation*, of the surgical area for the first 36 hours to observe for signs of excessive bleeding, hematoma, or wound separation. We strongly discourage "handling" at any time and discourage close observation after the first 36 hours. Patients are counseled and re-counseled that the area may become significantly ecchymotic and edematous,

POST-OPERATIVE INSTRUCTIONS FOR LABIAL/VULVAR PLASTIC SURGERY

The ultimate success of your surgery is partially dependent on your self-care in the weeks after your procedure. Instructions are as follows:

1. **Bathing:** Starting the evening of surgery you may begin once–twice daily rinses of the surgical area with a hand-held shower device, or direct the shower stream toward the surgical area. You may utilize a hand-held "peri-bottle" to rinse at any time. Pat (DO NOT RUB) dry with a soft cloth/towel or dry with a hair dryer (low heat; high blow), then apply a clean maxi pad with a non-stick surface.

2. **Keeping clean:** Rinse yourself with your "peri-bottle" and dab the area with the "Tucks™" or generic witch-hazel pads after each urination and bowel movement, then apply a clean non-stick sanitary pad.

3. **Icing:** You will be given two re-usable ice packs from the office. Cover with a hand towel and place one against the labia for 15–20 minutes, 5–6 times per day for the first 4–5 days after surgery to help with swelling and discomfort. (You may also do this by filling a surgical glove or plastic "zip-lock" bag with crushed ice or utilize frozen peas or corn.)

4. **Medications & creams:** Remember to continue your Arnica, which you began in the office prior to surgery, on an empty stomach 5–6 times daily. Take your pain medication along with 2 OTC ibuprofen or 1 OTC naprosyn every 3–6 hours if needed, but with food in your stomach. If you were given Cu-3 intensive hydrating gel by the office, gently apply it to your incisions twice daily following your rinses for the first week. Alternatively, you may use an OTC antibiotic ointment such as poly/neosporin. (*If you purchased the Arnica cream instead of tablets, you may use this along with your Cu-3 gel.) You may utilize Dermaplast™ spray as needed for minor surface stinging or itching. If itching becomes problematic, call Dr. _____ and (s)he will prescribe an anti-itch oral medication.

5. **Shaving/waxing:** You should NOT shave or wax in the vaginal area until cleared by Dr. _____ at your 1-month post-op appointment.

6. **Significant swelling:** If you feel your swelling is significant, you may get relief from taking OTC ibuprofen, 600 mg, with food every 6–8 hours round-the-clock for 3–4 days as needed.

Figure 12.1 Post-operative instruction sheet for labiaplasty.

7. For **2 FULL WEEKS** after surgery it is <u>extremely</u> important **NOT** to do any heavy lifting, vigorous activities or exercising, including but not limited to: fast walking, stair climbing, dancing, swimming, etc. Sexual intercourse, horseback riding, biking, and running should be withheld for a minimum of **1 MONTH**. Do not have intercourse or insert anything into the vagina until cleared by Dr. _____. (*Please use <u>pads only</u> with your first period after surgery.)

8. "Looking/touching/rubbing…" Your vulva will become VERY discolored and swollen from ~day 1 to day 7 after your surgery. Please evaluate yourself (without tugging on or near the incision lines) for signs of excessive bleeding, wound separation, or "goose-egg" formation in the 36 hours after surgery. After that, it is best to not visualize the area frequently, nor handle it excessively, as the appearance will change day-by-day, and the changes and irregularities noted initially will "…*drive you crazy*…" Put your Cu-3 on only 2 times/day, after cleansing. Use your Dermaplast spray only for surface stinging. Don't "handle" it excessively!!

You will have your first post-op visit 5–10 days after surgery for evaluation.

*It is normal to have: a small to sometimes significant amount of bloody <u>spotting</u>, swelling, and bruising or discoloration in the area.

*Danger signs include: evidence of infection (redness, swelling and perhaps a yellowish discharge, and/or fever), increasing day-by-day pain, and bleeding that is more than light–moderate spotting. If you notice that one area/side is <u>significantly</u> more swollen than others, please apply 5 minutes of firm pressure to the area with a pad or washcloth, using the heel of your hand. Look at the area; if it is still bleeding or if the "egg" has reappeared, call your doctor and apply additional pressure.

**If you have any questions or concerns at any time, please call Dr._____ at the office or through his/her urgent number, (   )_____

Figure 12.1 (*Continued*)

will lose its natural appearance and contour, and will swell irregularly, there may be a disparity in size bilaterally, and that, in short, it may look positively awful! The author personally shows patients post-operative day 1–7 vulvar photographs to emphasize these points. Patients must be made aware that initial postoperative appearance will not necessarily (see Figures 12.3–12.7) parallel long-term outcome. *Activities*: Patients are counseled to avoid up/down/ "swish-swish-swish" walking activities and squatting, to avoid any activity that produces rubbing/chafing of their incisional area. They may climb stairs, but slowly, one at a time, and limit trips. Similarly with driving: trips are to be limited, automatic transmission only, and great care to be taken with transfers in and out of the vehicle. Patients are also instructed to elevate their hips and legs when possible. *Analgesia*:

Ibuprofen 600–800 mg or naprosyn 220–440 mg may be utilized for mild pain; hydrocodone 5–10 mg + acetaminophen 325 mg with or without the addition of ibuprofen 400 mg q 4–6 hours is suggested for more significant discomfort, and the author personally encourages q.4 hr. ingestion of pain medications starting 1 hour prior to anticipated end of local anesthesia and continuing for the initial 12–18 hours postoperatively. All pain medication must be ingested with food. *Significant edema*: Patients may be counseled to ingest ibuprofen 600 mg q 6–8 hours round-the-clock for 3–4 days to reduce symptomatic edema. *Dressings*: Patients may utilize copper-containing topical ointments ("Cu-3") or antibiotic ointment gently applied to the incision or to a telfa or gauze pad applied to the wound after cleansings to prevent adhesion of dressing or undergarments.

POST-OPERATIVE INSTRUCTIONS FOR PERINEAL AND INTRA-VAGINAL PROCEDURES

The ultimate success of your surgery is partially dependent on your self-care in the weeks after your procedure/s. Instructions are as follows:

1. Starting the evening of your surgery, take warm sitz baths (soak the perineal area in clean warm water) for about 15–20 minutes and/or rinse with a "peri-bottle" 2–3 times daily for a week. Wipe yourself with witch hazel pads (Tucks™) after each urination and bowel movement. (** If you have had labial reduction surgery along with your vaginal tightening procedure, ask your surgeon whether you should use sitz baths or not…)

2. It is extremely important to minimize vigorous activities including fast walking, stair climbing, "ups & downs," heavy lifting, etc. for the first week or two after your surgery or until you've been instructed at your first post-op visit. You may resume modest activities in 1 week, but wait until a minimum of 3 WEEKS before resuming full physical activities.

3. Do not resume intercourse or insert anything into the vagina until you have been cleared by Dr. _____ (usually 6-9 weeks after surgery.

4. If given medication by Dr. _____ (antibiotics, pain meds, etc.), please take as directed.

5. It is normal to have a modest amount of thin blood or bloody discharge for up to 2-3 weeks,

6. If you experience painful urination, inability to urinate, or urinary frequency, drink plenty of fluids and try emptying your bladder while taking a long warm shower or bath. If symptoms persist, please call Dr. _____. Make sure you drink lots of water, eat 10–12 prunes daily, be up and around, take a stool softener ("DSS") and a mild laxative (Miralax™, Smooth Move™ tea, senna, etc.)

7. Danger signs include: Fever of 100 degrees or higher, foul-smelling vaginal discharge, increasing vaginal/rectal pressure (although a moderate amount of rectal pressure is normal because of all the sutures in the pelvic floor), and increasing pain and/or swelling of the incisional area.

You will have your first post-op appointment 5–10 days after surgery for evaluation. If you have any questions or concerns prior to or after that, please call Dr. _____ at the office; outside of office hours you can reach him by calling ( ) _____.

Figure 12.2 Post-operative instruction sheet for VRJ/CP/PP/VP.

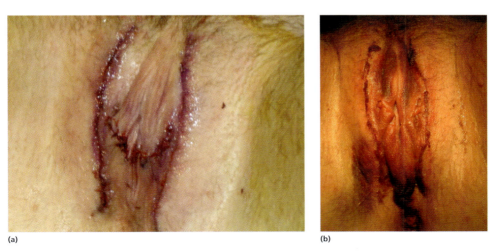

(a)   (b)

Figure 12.3 (a) Immediately post-op V-wedge LP-m and LP-M. (b) Same patient, 1 week post-op. Source: M. Goodman. Reproduced with permission.

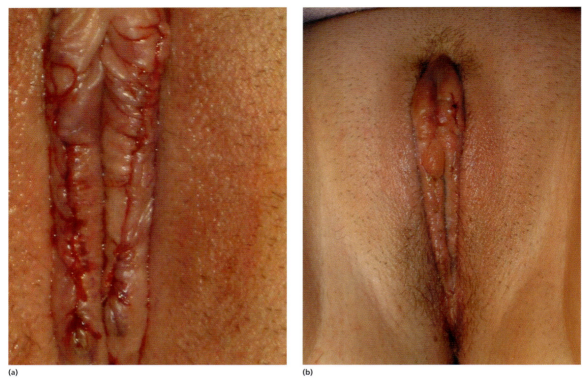

Figure 12.4 (a) Immediately post-op straightforward LP-m. (b) One week post-op. Source: M. Goodman. Reproduced with permission.

- Beware of patients who have a cavalier attitude. Their rest and limitation of activities during this time period is crucial to the outcome and their satisfaction.
- *Day 6 to day 10*: Icing may discontinue. Hygiene continues the same. The patient may begin assuming more normal ambulation and may return to *sedentary* work activities such as school, office work, and so forth. Still no active walking, running, sexual activities involving the genital area, or other similar activities. The first post-operative visit, either in person or, if she lives at a distance precluding an in-person exam, "virtually" with a file of in-focus photos ("selfies") is scheduled for ~5–10 days after surgery.
- *Day 11 to day 21*: Hygiene continues the same. Menstrual hygiene during the first month post-op should be with pads rather than tampons. Still nothing per vagina. More active work and home responsibilities may be resumed depending on specific procedure and appearance at first post-operative evaluation. The patient may resume normal but not vigorous ambulation and may return to upper body work at her gym. No squats!

- *Day 22 to day 42*: Swimming and running may usually resume at 3 weeks, pending individual recovery and stability of the suture line. Cycling and coital activities may proceed at ~4–6 weeks, pending results of your (hopefully in-person) ~4–6 week evaluation. This is a good time to remind your patient that she cannot fully evaluate her individual long-term outcome for at least another 3+ months, and counsel her that, should she be unhappy with an aspect of her outcome, that the wound is still healing, and that you do not advise any possible revisions until a minimum of 3 months post-op, when the incision has "softened" and re-vascularized. Some surgeons advocate gentle massage for desensitization of resolving dysesthesias, if present.

PP/VP/CP/"VRJ"

General instructions are similar to the above, with the following caveats.

1 Sitz baths are encouraged, once or twice daily, unless patient has had a concomitant LP.
2 Icing is utilized only for perineal swelling or comfort.

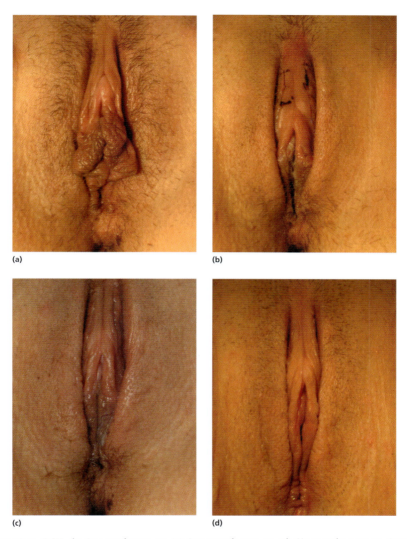

Figure 12.5 (a) Pre-op LP-m, RCH. (b) One week post-op. (c) One month post-op. (d) Six months post-op. Source: M. Goodman. Reproduced with permission.

3 Stool softeners, prunes, and pushing fluids are encouraged.

4 Physical activities/lifting are geared to the extent of the repair, and whether anterior and/or posterior colporrhaphy have been performed. Lifting items >20 pounds is discouraged for 2–3 weeks for perineoplasty, and up to 4–5 weeks if an anterior colporrhaphy was performed.

5 Intra- or peri-operative antibiotic use is universal; some surgeons utilize pre-operative parenteral antibiotic therapy while others utilize oral therapy for 48–72 hours pre-op and 24–48 hours post-operatively for office-based procedures. A second- or third-generation cephalosporin or equivalent may be used parenterally; cephalexin or amoxicillin/clavulanic acid are good oral choices.

6 Patients are evaluated at 6 weeks post-op for ongoing post-operative pelvic floor physical therapy and/or the need for vaginal dilatation if over-tightening has occurred. If stenosis is present, after ensuring that the vagina is adequately estrogenized, dilatation with

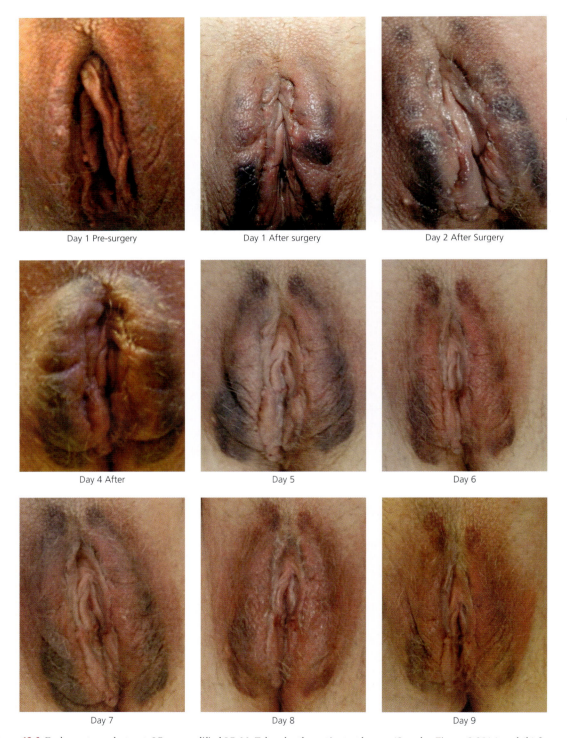

Figure 12.6 Early post-op photoset, LP-m, modified LP-M. Taken by the patient at home. (See also Figure 8.28(a) and (b) for pre- and 1-month post-op photos.) Source: M. Goodman. Reproduced with permission.

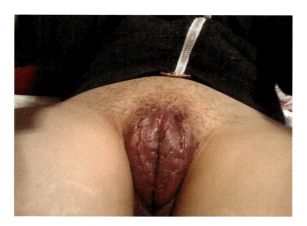

Figure 12.7 One week post-op, LP-m and LP-M. Marked edema, ecchymoses. (See also Figure 17.4 for additional photos of this patient.) Source: M. Goodman. Reproduced with permission.

progressively sized coned or beveled dilators is affected. Pelvic floor physical therapy with the use of biofeedback and/or TENS- type units such as APEX™

or In-Tone™ and/or intra-vaginal inserts (weights, "balls") are utilized by many surgeons.

Typical post-operative instruction sheets are reproduced in Figures 12.1 and 12.2.

For your patients residing at a distance, it is imperative that you ascertain that they have a personal physician or facility they can visit and you can communicate with should a post-operative concern mandate evaluation not possible by you personally at your center.

Availability and the ability to anticipate, empathize, and frequently "hand-hold" are requisites for the women's genital plastic/cosmetic surgeon. A telephone call to the patient from the physician or office surgical coordinator the day after surgery is a welcome touch.

Several representative photos taken immediately following surgery and during the first post-operative weeks follow in Figures 12.3–12.7. It is instructive to visualize the changes probable in the recovery period and to share these with our patients during pre-operative consultation. This will save much angst on the part of both patients and their physicians.

CHAPTER 13

Aesthetic male-to-female transsexual surgery

Marci Bowers

Mills-Peninsula Hospital, Burlingame, CA, USA

Cosmetic one-stage vaginoplasty: introduction

As evidenced by instances of castration throughout history, the concept of transsexualism has likely always been a part of the human experience. The Bible, for example, includes some 63 references to eunuchs [1]. These early castrated males might be considered transsexuals of their era. Examples of intersex masculinized females are also dotted throughout history, including the suspected installation of Pope John/Joan in the 10th century.

Body modification—hormones and surgery for the treatment of transsexualism—first found traction in the early 20th century. Much of the early research began in pre–World War II Berlin. There, psychologist Magnus Hirschfeld and his colleague Eugene Steinach advanced sexuality and the concept of gender identity from a scientific perspective [2]. Once known as the "Einstein of Sexuality," Dr. Hirschfeld described cross-dressing ("transvestit"), worked to elucidate the chemical nature of hormones, experimented with gonadal transplantation, and began rudimentary treatment of transsexual individuals. This progress ultimately resulted in what is considered the first surgical change of sex in 1930. The patient, in fact, was Ms. Lili Elbe who, after a series of ill-fated operations, ultimately succumbed to complications as a result of this endeavor. Berlin gradually came to be known as the most tolerant lesbian/gay/bisexual/transgender (LGBT) haven of European cities. Tolerant, that is, until the rise of the Third Reich. In 1933, just 3 months after Hitler's installation as German chancellor, storm troopers sacked and incinerated the laboratories of Drs. Hirschfeld/Steinach. However, from that inferno fled a young psychiatry student by the name of Harry Benjamin to the United States. While practicing in New York until the age of 104, Dr. Benjamin continued and greatly expanded the work of his predecessors, eventually becoming the international face of transsexualism when his name was immortalized as the Harry Benjamin International Gender Dysphoria Association (HBIGDA), now the World Association for Transgender Health (WPATH). WPATH sets current standards of care and advances health, education, and science for those in the transsexual/transgender community. (Note: Although often used synonymously, the term "transgender" is considered more inclusive and embracing than the term "transsexual." Transgender can include broad categories of gender variance including cross-dressing, drag, non-op transsexualism, etc. Transsexual, on the other hand, is specific to those whose discomfort with their own secondary sex characteristics is such that only a surgical solution allows for resolution of the discomfort.)

The *modern* surgical history of transsexualism improved significantly with Dr. George Burou's description of the so-called penile inversion technique of male-to-female (MTF) vaginoplasty in the late 1950s. Dr. Burou, a French-born gynecologist, performed these surgeries for transsexual women in Casablanca, Morocco [3]. His penile inversion surgical template became the de facto model for the most prevalent and preferred modern methods of male-to-female genital confirmation surgery (GCS) [4]. Many followed Dr. Burou, including the late Dr. Stanley Biber, as well as Drs. Meltzer, Brassard, Monstrey, and

Female Genital Plastic and Cosmetic Surgery, First Edition. Edited by Michael P. Goodman.

many others. With subsequent innovations and modifications, the technique is still highly individual but has shown gradual refinement. This chapter's author, who joined Dr. Biber in Trinidad, Colorado, at one time nicknamed the "Sex Change Capital of the World," has performed more than 1,200 MTF vaginoplasties. It is this work that will now be detailed and shared. Dr. Bowers is additionally acknowledged as the world's first transsexual woman and only current gynecologist to herself perform genital reassignment surgery (GRS).

Management

It is now generally accepted that hormonal and surgical treatment of gender dysphoria has conclusive social and psychological benefit for transsexual individuals [4,5]. Early dissenters who had argued against "surgical treatment for a psychological problem" have largely relented under the crush of medical and psychosocial evidence in support of treatment. Supportive evidence has also come from the recognition that gender identity is generally established at an early age and that psychological treatment to dissuade gender nonconforming behavior is largely futile [6].

The author is a member of WPATH and follows its established standards of care (SOC) [7]. Patients are required to undergo psychological evaluation by mental health specialists well versed in the management of gender dysphoria in accordance with WPATH SOC. Specifically, patients are required to live in their desired gender role for a period of at least *one year* and to have been on cross-sex hormone therapy for a period of *one year* prior to engaging in GRS. Other forms of gender confirming surgeries such as facial feminization or breast augmentation may be utilized during the evaluation period but are not held to as rigidly defined standards as genital surgery. Patients must provide, in general, *two letters* of psychological assessment prior to proceeding with vaginoplasty.

Preparation for surgery

Patients are asked to provide a full medical history, psychological summary letters, medical clearance (if indicated), and a recent EKG and HIV test—at least 6 weeks prior to surgery. HIV positive patients are not excluded if health is otherwise excellent, HIV is under active treatment, viral load is zero, and CD4 count exceeds 400/hpf. Patients are seen at least 1 day prior to surgery for pre-operative evaluation where review of letters, adherence to WPATH SOC, and general medical health are evaluated. The author ultimately decides whether or not patients have met the criteria for surgery. Patients are then examined, consented, and given a bowel prep regimen consisting of 2 tabs of Dulcolax and Go-lytely. The patient is shaved.

Demographics

Demographics are summarized in Figures 13.1 through 13.5. It is important to note that wrongly gendered feelings began in 94% of surgical clients prior to the age of puberty. This may partially explain the low rate of regret found in this population.

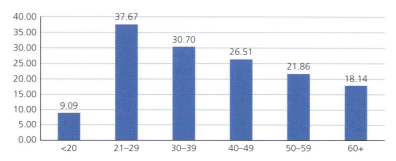

Figure 13.1 Age at time of GRS by %, all years combined. Although this series shows the majority of surgeries older than age 40, the median age at time of GRS is declining. This is due to more insurance coverage and earlier recognition, treatment, and acceptance.

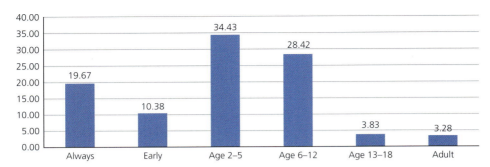

Figure 13.2 Earliest memories of gender dysphoria by %.

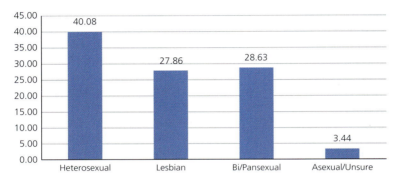

Figure 13.3 Sexual orientation at time of GRS by % (n = 262). Very even distribution of sexual attraction despite predominant pre-operative affection for females. Heterosexual defined as "attracted to males," etc.

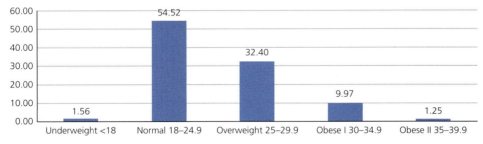

Figure 13.4 Distribution of body habitus at time of GRS by %, based on BMI, all years combined.

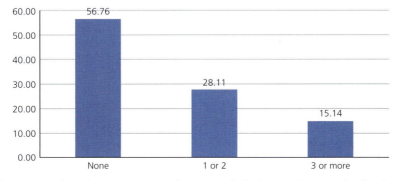

Figure 13.5 Had children at time of GRS by % (n = 185). Reflects generally heterosexual (attracted to females) pre-operative status.

Surgery

The keys to our surgical approach are through an understanding of hypospadias in biological males. In the embryology of the male fetus, each male anatomically passes from female to male. Through the various degrees of hypospadias, we gain knowledge of how such a reversal process ought to work in order to gain both functional and cosmetic ideals [8] for those seeking to revert from male to female.

Following induction of anesthesia, the patient is positioned in high lithotomy, prepped, and draped. The patient is marked (Figure 13.6). The tip of the penis is grasped with a penetrating towel clamp. The penis is extended with the non-dominant hand. Transverse horizontal lines are drawn from the superior aspect of the

base of the penis outward bilaterally. A similar vertical line is drawn from the mid-shaft toward the umbilicus. These serve as reference points for the initial incisions and for defining the position of midline structures such as the urethra, clitoral hood, and so forth later in the procedure.

The *deconstructive phase* of the operation begins as incisions are made. The scrotal/perineal skin is excised. The excised scrotal skin is then stretched with hemostats on a Koban-wrapped cutting board (Figure 13.7).

Metzenbaum scissors are used to de-fat and thin the tissue, removing as much Camper's fascia and connective tissue as possible until a suitable full thickness epithelial graft is achieved. The graft is left stretched but covered with saline-moistened towel or sponge and set aside for later stent coverage. This graft will become the future deep vagina (Figure 13.8).

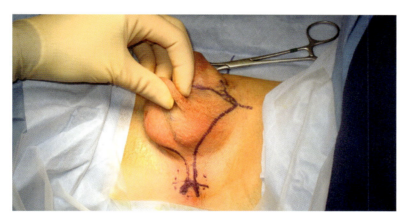

Figure 13.6 Initial surgical site markings. Source: M. Bowers. Reproduced with permission.

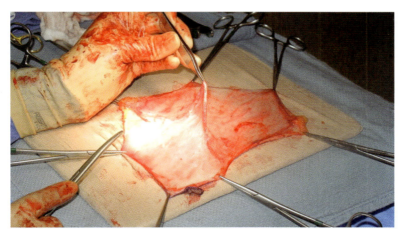

Figure 13.7 Preparation of scrotal skin as full thickness skin graft. Source: M. Bowers. Reproduced with permission.

Each testicle is then grasped with penetrating towel clamps. The testicles are then serially elevated as electrocautery is used to dissect free excess adipose as the inguinal ring and base of the spermatic cord are gradually exposed (Figure 13.9). Dissection proceeds to the inguinal ring as a medium Richardson retractor is used to expose but also sweep tissue cephalad toward the ring assuring protection of the genitofemoral nerve, which can be injured as it passes inferiorly. The base of the spermatic cord is doubly ligated. Additionally, the ring is closed to prevent potential hernia.

Cautery is used to separate the spongiosum from the underlying paired penile cavernosa along the intercavernous septum. A Foley is inserted near the distal end of the spongiosum by entering the urethra 4 cm below the tip.

The neoclitoris is created by extending the penile shaft downward. The bases of the paired bulbocavernosa are injected with 5 cc of 1:100 dilution of 1% lidocaine-epinephrine mixture. An elliptical incision is made from the prepuce inferiorly into the corona of the dorsal aspect of the penis (Figure 13.10). Mayo scissors are used to free the tip from the ventral portions of the cavernosa and circumferentially around each incision, thus freeing the cavernous bodies from the overlying penile skin circumferentially. The penis is then "inverted," allowing the surgeon to place two non-dominant fingers up from below within the subcutaneous

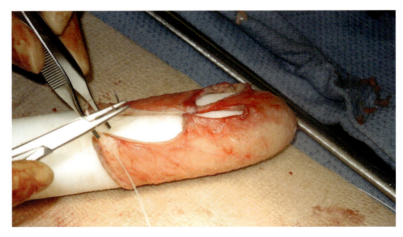

Figure 13.8 Sewing of scrotal skin to become neovagina. Source: M. Bowers. Reproduced with permission.

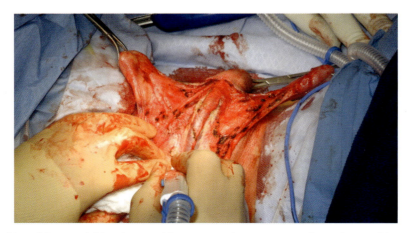

Figure 13.9 After excision of the scrotal skin prior to orchiectomy exposing cavernosa and spongiosum with spermatic cords/testicles on traction. Source: M. Bowers. Reproduced with permission.

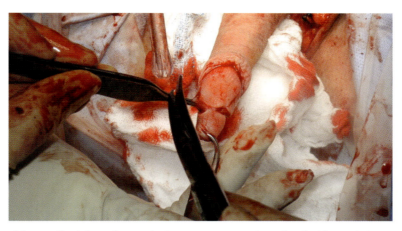

Figure 13.10 Creation of the neoclitoris from glans penis. Source: M. Bowers. Reproduced with permission.

space. Mayo scissors cut to complete the separation of the skin and cavernous structures. The tip is unclamped and clamped again as the skin and cavernous structures should now be completely separated.

Electrocautery is used to cut deeply along the cavernosa bilaterally at 3 and 9 o'clock from the symphysis pubis distally out along the shaft to along and beneath the neoclitoral incisions.

Mayo scissors complete this dissection, progressing from the remaining coronal tip incisions and midline septum to horizontally bi-valve the cavernosa. The ventral portions of the bi-valved cavernosa are excised at the level of the crus/pubic symphysis and discarded. Bleeding can be vigorous, particularly if there is residual tumescence. Caution, cautery, and suction are particularly useful during these portions of the procedure. The excised ventral base of each cavernosa is then ligated with single figure-of-eight ligatures of 3-0 Vicryl. The dorsal neurovascular sheath contains the elliptical portion of corona/prepuce or neoclitoris. Mayo scissors are used to thin the neurovascular sheath by removing excess spongi tissue. The neurovascular pedicle should be 2–3 cm at its widest, the narrower the better while preserving vascular flow to the clitoral tip.

The neoclitoris is completed by taking 4 bites of suture along the cut ventral surfaces beneath the clitoris to purse string the tissue beneath the corona and effectively cone the clitoral tip. The neurovascular sheath is then folded upon itself and sewn to the anterior symphisis and longitudinal connective tissue along each side. The clitoris is later drawn through a slit created in the spongiosum, thus allowing the clitoris and hood to

be completely lined by urethral mucosa (see below, Figure 13.13).

The *dissection phase* of the operation is intended to create the space for the future neovagina. The bladder is first drained. A folded sponge is placed between the perineum and catheterized spongiosum, which is tractioned up and against the patient. A lighted right angle retractor (Ferreira Style Breast Retractor with fiber-optic light and 4-inch blade 110-675 CC5 custom) allows the assistant to protect the urinary structures anteriorly while lifting upon the central tendon of the perineum. This has the effect of allowing the rectum to drop as the central tendon is serially released by electrocautery or sharp dissection. Care is taken to always keep the central tendon and a small amount of spongiosum muscle posteriorly until the prostate is reached. It is of critical importance to avoid entering the rectum, as this constitutes the greatest risk for rectovaginal fistula. The central tendon is the aponeurosis of the bulbospongiosum and is the key landmark throughout this dissection. The Foley should be palpable anteriorly along the dissection plane. Upon passing through the inferior pole of the prostate, orientation of the fibers changes slightly to less spongi. The tissue should also release slightly, allowing the superior aspect of the dissection to proceed with a combination of blunt finger dissection and electrocautery. If bleeding is encountered, ligatures of 2-0 chromic are placed. Finger dissection should push from the center bilaterally. Upon completion, depth should approach 6 inches typically and often greater, aided often with the use of a stick sponge, which can be directed from anterior to posterior, sweeping open the tissue with reasonable ease. A rolled

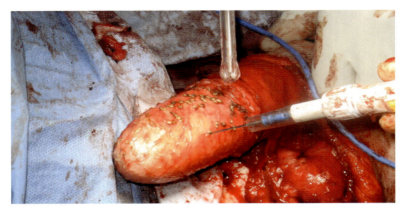

Figure 13.11 Cauterization of hair follicles of scrotal sewn to inverted penile skin over stent. Source: M. Bowers. Reproduced with permission.

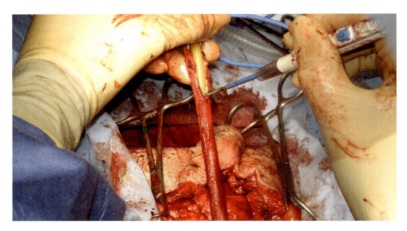

Figure 13.12 Division of spongiosum to create labial lining and neourethra. Source: M. Bowers. Reproduced with permission.

cigar consisting of four tightly rolled 4 x 4 sponges is placed within the neovaginal cavity as a placeholder and to tamponade and absorb blood as the case proceeds, thus completing the second stage of the procedure.

The *reconstructive phase* begins by fitting the de-fatted and thinned full-thickness scrotal graft over a large stent (Figure 13.11). The edges are trimmed to fit the stent and sewn to cover as much stent as possible. Edges are cleaned. Hair follicles are then serially obliterated with needle-tip cautery. Small holes serve as drainage portals, much as Swiss-cheesing is done to split thickness grafts. The dermal/squamous side of the graft faces the stent to line the future vagina.

The catheterized spongiosum is lifted anteriorly and divided vertically from the distal end to the base of the spongiosum muscle (Figure 13.12). The edges are trimmed of excess spongi tissue. A small vertical defect is created mid-shaft to allow passage of the neoclitoris. This will serve as the clitoris's new and final resting position. The clitoris is drawn through the defect, then sewn into location with 3-0-Vicryl circumferentially (Figure 13.13). The distal excess spongiosum is trimmed.

The scrotal skin-covered stent is passed through the inverted patient penile skin and sewn in place circumferentially with 2-0 Vicryl. The midline of the penile/neovaginal graft is divided so as to allow a comfortable placement as the neovagina. No internal fixation of the neovagina is necessary. The neovagina assimilates within 6 days, attributable to fibrosis and eventual neovascularization of the graft. Expulsion, rejection, or prolapse

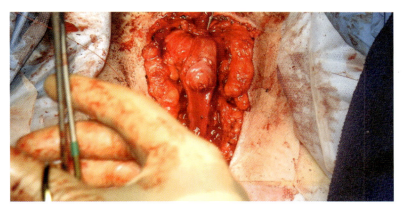

Figure 13.13 Neoclitoris through slit in spongiosum. Source: M. Bowers. Reproduced with permission.

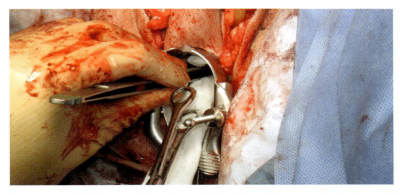

Figure 13.14 Packing of neovagina with 2-inch vaginal packing soaked with vaginal metronidazole. Source: M. Bowers. Reproduced with permission.

of these grafts is rare. A speculum is placed in the neovagina that is packed with vaginal packing soaked in vaginal .05% metronidazole (Figure 13.14). The packing is left for 6 nights until its removal in the office. The speculum is removed and the posterior attachment and introital flap are secured with 2-0 Vicryl interrupted ligatures. The neourethra and labia minora are defined next by dividing the midline from inferior to anterior. Pre-operative midline markings allow the surgeon to maintain symmetry with critical incisions. The midline perineal tissue is grasped and tented with Adson forceps, allowing vertical incision for labia placement. The splayed open spongiosum containing the neoclitoris is brought through the midline defect and then anchored posteriorly and anteriorly with a single ligature of 2-0 Vicryl. The raw edges of the spongiosum are sewn bilaterally to the midline perineal incision. A second imbricating is used to define the labia minora and clitoral hood (Figure 13.15).

Hemostasis is confirmed beneath each flap. Excess fat is trimmed and/or repositioned. A Pratt drain is placed though the left buttock via trocar. The drain is snaked up along each labial bed up to and around the neoclitoris and down to the other side, trimmed to fit. The proximal end is sewn in and the end placed on bulb suction.

The labia majora are closed in three layers, the first with a 3-0 Vicryl subcutaneous running stitch followed by a 3-0 Vicryl subdermal closure followed by a running 3-0 Monocryl subcuticular closure of the skin (Figure 13.16).

Pressure dressings are then carefully applied. This includes a 1-inch diameter "cigar" of rolled 4 × 4 sponges placed centrally followed by 4 × 4s followed by an ABD pad followed by foam tape stretched to create as much pressure as possible. Dressings are removed in 36–48 hours when the patient is ambulated for the first time.

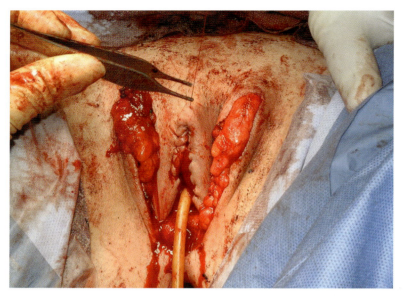

Figure 13.15 Clitoral hood labia minora formation. Source: M. Bowers. Reproduced with permission.

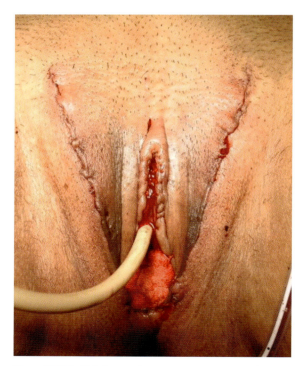

Figure 13.16 Labial closure. Source: M. Bowers. Reproduced with permission

Recovery

Recovery is rapid and surprisingly low in pain relative to other cosmetic procedures; most patients are off narcotics within 72–96 hours. Patients are ambulated within 48 hours. Diet is advanced overnight. The dressing is removed on the morning of the second post-operative day. Topical Neosporin is applied to incisions twice daily. Pressure dressings remain until the morning of the second post-operative day. The Blake drain is removed and patients are discharged the morning of the third post-operative day. Discharge medications include oral antibiotics and analgesics only. Patients are given detailed wound care and post-op instructions as well as emergency contact phone numbers. A Foley is left in place until the morning of the sixth post-operative day, at which time the vaginal packing is removed. Dilation instruction is then initiated with a series of three acrylic vaginal dilators given to each patient. A regular dilation sequence is established and dilation continued indefinitely. Patients are instructed to dilate for 15 minutes 3 times daily for 3 months, then twice daily for nine months, then once daily. Generous lubrication is encouraged. See Figure 13.17 for the final result.

Outcomes

Evidence suggests that the *quality of the surgical treatment* afforded to transsexual individuals has a significant correlation with satisfaction and lack of regret following sex reassignment [9]. This implies that the choice of a surgeon and surgical technique are equally important factors in determining outcome. Accessibility issues remain with few properly trained or willing surgeons in many regions of the United States and around the world. Cost remains a significant barrier as well when health plans or national insurance coverage is lacking. There is also no one definitive technique for MTF vaginoplasty although there is growing consensus that a single stage vaginoplasty is ideal in terms of quality and economy.

Blood loss averages 250 cc. The surgical procedure takes approximately 3 hours to perform. Patients are typically able to orgasm, often within 12 weeks of surgery. Long-term rates of orgasm approach 90% [4]. Receptive intercourse is possible with vaginal depths typically in excess of 20 cm (6 inches) (Figure 13.18). Retention of glands including Cowper's, the prostate, and seminal vesicle allow patients to release pre- and post-ejaculatory fluid similar in quality to that of homologous female structures [9]. Vaginal lubrication per se is not possible and supplemental lubrication is normally required. The vaginal flora that gradually establishes itself differs bacteriologically but not qualitatively from that of natal females. The absence of glycogen in the vaginal epithelium accounts for the majority of this difference. Glycogen in the natal vaginal epithelium facilitates culture of the vagina with lactobacilli, whereas, in transsexual women, this predominant bacterial composition is lacking. Post-op, vaginal pH is alkaline.

Complications

While relatively rare, potential complications can be significant (Table 13.1). *Rectovaginal (RV) fistula* remains the single most feared complication of MTF vaginoplasty.

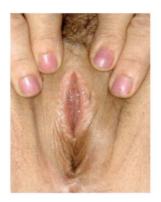 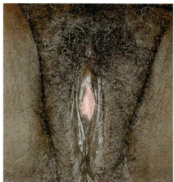

Figure 13.17 Final result. Typical recovery to this point is at least 3 months. Source: M. Bowers. Reproduced with permission.

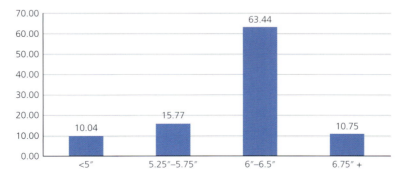

Figure 13.18 Vaginal depth at initial GRS by %. Average = 6.02″.

Table 13.1 Complications.

Complications (GRS) # = 577	Number
Enterotomy	3(2 with RV fistula)
Urethrotomy	1
Clitoral necrosis	9(?)
Skin separation	22
Chronic pain	2
Loss of depth	6(?)
Transfusion	1
Infection	0(?)

Its occurrence can result in multiple additional surgeries, loss of the neovagina, and colostomy. The single greatest risk factor for RV fistula is intraoperative enterotomy. For this reason, bowel prep is mandatory for all patients undergoing vaginoplasty. In our experience, primary enterotomy repair failed in 2/3 patients although one resulted in passage of gas only. *Urinary complications*, while possible, are rare. Others have reported urethral stenosis and lower urinary tract symptoms (LUTS) [10], although urinary complications were not seen in our series, likely due to the splaying effect of the spongiosum and lining of the labia minora with urethral mucosa. Incontinence was also not seen. Infection also is unusual. Relatively common complications include *wound breakdown* and *poor healing*. *Granulation tissue* is also somewhat common (5%) and easily treated in most cases. For *cosmetic shortcomings*, an interval labiaplasty can be useful after at least 3 months of convalescence. Follow-up was difficult in this clientele due to relocation and to simply "moving on" following surgical completion. This may falsely diminish the reported relatively low number of wound-related complications.

Summary

The cosmetic surgical management of MTF transsexualism is best approached as a one-stage, modified penile inversion technique with scrotal grafting. Retention of neurovascular structures of the natal penis allows the new vulva to attain a highly functional and visually aesthetic state. The procedure can be accomplished with relatively low risk and a short hospital stay. Patient satisfaction is high. Critics of MTF gender reassignment point to persistent incidence of suicide and other examples

supposedly suggesting maladaptation following surgery [11]. In fact, the road for transgender persons is not easy—before, after, or during transition. Violence, discrimination, and challenges in acceptance persist for the transgender community, despite advancing civil rights and legal protection. What should be most striking is that, despite these hardships and the financial and emotional toll and pain, transgender persons only very rarely regret their decisions to seek sex reassignment [9].

Thanks to Drs. Julie Nicole and Simon Cebers.

References

1. Cheney V. *Castration: The Advantages and the Disadvantages*. Bloomington, IN: 1st Books, 2003, pp. 69–70, 130, 148–9.
2. Meyerowitz J. *How Sex Changed: A History of Transsexuality in the United States*. Cambridge, MA: Harvard University Press, 2004, pp. 18–21, 29–30.
3. Wesser DR. A single stage operative technique for castration, vaginal construction and perineoplasty in transsexuals. *Arch Sex Behav* 1978;**7**:309–23.
4. Selvaggi G, Monstrey S, Ceulemans P, T'Sjoen G, De Cuypere G, Hoebeke P. Satisfaction after sex reassignment surgery in transsexual patients. *Ann Plast Surg* 2007;**4**:427–33.
5. Jokić-Begić N, Korajlija AL, Jurin T. Psychosocial adjustment to sex reassignment surgery: A qualitative examination and personal experiences of six transsexual persons in Croatia. *Scientific World Journal* 2014, http://dx.doi.org/10.1155/2014/960745.
6. American Psychological Association. Just the Facts about Sexual Orientation and Youth: A Primer for Principals, Educators, and School Personnel 2008, 1–24. www.apa.org/pi/lgbc/publications/justthefacts.html.
7. World Professional Association for Transgender Health. Global Applicability of the Standards of Care and Surgery, WPATH Standards of Care Version 7 2012, 1–4, 54–64. www.wpath.org.
8. Salm D. Psychological and Emotional Aspects of Hypospadias: General Aspects of Hypospadias 2012, 1(1). http://www.hypospadias-emotions.com.
9. Lawrence AA. Factors associated with satisfaction or regret among male-to-female transsexuals undergoing sex reassignment surgery. *Arch Sex Behav* 2003;**32**:299–315.
10. Goddard JC, Vickery RM, Qureshi A. Feminizing genitoplasty in adult transsexuals: Early and long-term results. *Brit J Urol* 2007;607–13.
11. Dhejne C, Lichtenstein P, Boman M, Johansson ALV, Långström N, Landén M. Long-term follow-up of transsexual persons undergoing sex reassignment surgery: Cohort study in Sweden. *PLoS One* 2011;**6**(2):e16885. Published online February 22, 2011. doi:10.1371/journal.pone.0016885.

CHAPTER 14

Anesthetic choices and office-based surgery

Michael P. Goodman

Caring for Women Wellness Center, Davis, CA, USA

I've had so much plastic surgery, when I die they will donate my body to Tupperware.

Joan Rivers

Choices are available for you and your patients in both anesthetic method and surgical venue.

Anesthesia

Although novice surgeons may do well to begin their genital plastic work in a hospital or surgical center operating room under general or conduction anesthesia, certainly vulvar procedures, and in experienced hands even intra-vaginal procedures, lend themselves to an outpatient venue and local and local tumescent anesthesia.

Of course both general and sub-arachnoid block will supply adequate anesthesia for vulvar and vaginal genital plastic procedures. However, for a well-prepared patient and physician, local infiltrative anesthesia or a regional block works well, with or without pre-operative sedation.

If the procedure is to be performed in a surgical center or hospital environment, choices of anesthesia are legion and include general endo-tracheal, sub-arachnoid block, regional block, or local tumescent with or without conscious sedation. Certainly local with conscious sedation or spinal anesthesia are safe and elegant anesthetics and usually have the additional benefit of expedited recovery.

Sedation

Sedation may be helpful for alleviating anxiety especially at the outset of a procedure where the patient is awake. An anxiolytic and/or a narcotic analgesic may be suitable. Personally, in his "awake" cases in an office setting, the author uses 1 mg lorazepam p.o. 30–45 minutes prior to surgery. Another 1 mg lorazepam may be given sub-lingually, as decided by the patient and her office circulating RN, several minutes prior to prep. Both other benzodiazepines and types and doses of analgesics may be substituted, and the route may be either oral or parenteral.

For office procedures, patients are instructed to pre-hydrate and eat a light meal prior to coming to the office, but in any case all patients are given a fiber/protein bar and a large (22 oz.) bottle of Gatorade (tm) or equivalent upon arrival to the office, in an effort to further hydrate and prevent post-procedure hypotension.

Regional block

A pudendal block is an elegant anesthetic for work on the vulva and distal vagina and may be an anesthetic of choice in an outpatient setting for those women amenable to this choice and physicians facile in utilizing this modality. The author prefers a total of ~5–10 ml 0.25–0. % bupivacaine with epinephrine per side for

Female Genital Plastic and Cosmetic Surgery, First Edition. Edited by Michael P. Goodman.
© 2016 John Wiley & Sons, Ltd. Published 2016 by John Wiley & Sons, Ltd.

long-lasting (3–5 hour) anesthesia. However, technical difficulties with administration and risk of vascular injection, nerve or vascular injury, and failure of achieving anesthesia of ~10–20% are risks of regional pudendal nerve block.

Local infiltrative

The author prefers local incisional injection as his agent of choice for office-based vulvo-vaginal aesthetic surgery, as it is reproducible, extremely safe, and, depending upon the agent, confers relatively long-acting anesthesia.

Any local injectable anesthetic agent singly or in combination, with or without epinephrine, may be utilized. The author prefers 0.5% bupivacaine with

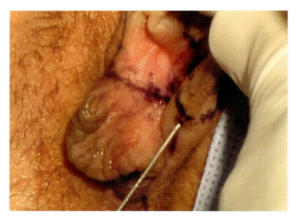

Figure 14.1 Initial injection of local at the base of the incision line. Source: M. Goodman. Reproduced with permission.

epinephrine, if the patient has no known sensitivity to either agent. Care must be taken with any of the local anesthetics, both to avoid intravascular injection and to not exceed toxicity dosages. A conservative limit per patient for 0.5% bupivacaine is 30 ml; 60 ml for 0.25% bupivacaine. Local anesthetic agents are acidic, causing discomfort upon injection. This may be diminished by buffering the solution with ~0.15 ml sodium bicarbonate/10 ml anesthetic.

Local anesthetic volume makes a difference. The greater the volume, the greater the difficulty in precise control of bleeders. The greater the anesthetic volume and the greater the use of electrocautery, the greater the amount of tissue necrosis, and the greater the risk of excessive post-operative edema, discomfort, and distortion of epithelium, adversely affecting final results.

Technique for labia minora/clitoral hood local injection

The mixture of local anesthetic and sodium bicarbonate is drawn from a medicine cup into a 3–5 ml syringe. A 25 or 27 ga. 1.5-inch needle is utilized for injection. A small bleb of anesthetic is injected at the base of the labum or initiation of the surgical line (Figure 14.1). The needle is advanced superficially sub-cutaneously laterally to the drawn incision lines on the lateral labial surfaces, medially on the mucosal surfaces, and a thin ribbon of anesthesia is slowly laid down as the needle is withdrawn (Figure 14.2). As one advances along the incision line care is taken to utilize already injected areas as needle entry sites. If operating on a conscious patient, "verbal analgesia" via

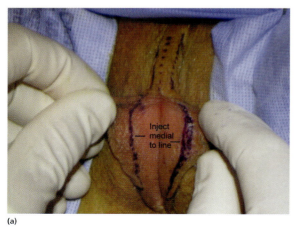

(a)

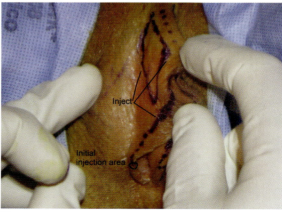

(b)

Figure 14.2 (a) Injection diagram 1. (b) Injection diagram 2. Source: M. Goodman. Reproduced with permission.

communication with the patient by the surgeon, and "hand-holding" via the surgical suite nurse or surgical assistant is helpful. The patient should have been informed pre-operatively by her surgeon about the discomfort inherent in the injection, but that the time necessary is very short (usually well <30–60 seconds per side). The surgeon may limit individual injections to 20-second intervals, which may be counted out with the patient by the physician or nurse assistant. Incision lines are tested with a forceps prior to skin incision. At least 5 minutes should be allowed to elapse for the epinephrine to take effect and induce vasoconstriction.

Several different methods have been proposed to aid in skin analgesia prior to injection, including applying 4% Emla cream or 5% lidocaine gel to the area and occluding with plastic film an hour or so prior to procedure, or applying ethyl chloride spray or a local anesthetic spray just prior to local injection. This author has given fair trial to them all and has found all wanting. The time and effort do not appear to offer any advantage. By the time the patient is evaluated, readied, prepped, and lines drawn, the cream/gel analgesia wears off, ethyl chloride spray application is almost as uncomfortable as the needle stick, and, even if the momentary skin penetration pain is mitigated, the sub-cutaneous infiltration is still painful. The author has found that buffering the anesthetic with sodium bicarbonate as described appears to offer the best reduction of injection pain.

On average, no more than a total of 6–10 ml total is necessary for labiaplasty, depending on the complexity of the incision lines and whether hood reduction is part of the procedure.

Technique for labia majora local injection

Anesthetic preparation is similar as for labia minoraplasty, but injection with needles <25 gauge is difficult secondary to resistance of the labia majora epithelium. A total volume of ~8–10 ml usually suffices for both sides. Injection is made just outside of the incision lines (Figure 14.3).

Technique for PP and HP local injection (office cases, local tumescent anesthesia)

Anesthetic mixture is the same, but close attention must be paid to total volume utilized. In my hands, I rarely use more than 20–30 ml, averaging 15–25 ml for PP, and approximately one-quarter of that for hymenoplasty. When PP alone is performed, 0.5% bupivacaine solution may be used, but if combining procedures (e.g., LP+ PP),

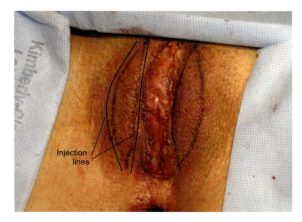

Figure 14.3 Injection lines for LP-M. Source: M. Goodman. Reproduced with permission.

I will estimate the size and complexity and will frequently either mix 0.5% with 0.25% bupivacaine 50/50, giving a 0.375% solution, with a maximal allowed volume of 45 ml, or utilize 0.25% bupivacaine. No side-by-side studies exist, but the amount of anesthesia produced with the more concentrated solution is impressive, with less volume necessary for anesthesia, resulting in better hemostasis.

Performing PP or HP under a local anesthetic with mild sedation is a technique reserved for only the occasional surgeon well experienced in both PP/VRJ type procedures, and in working on other vulvar aesthetic procedures in-office under local anesthetics.

Perineoplasty/vaginoplasty or hymenoplasty procedures, whether performed in a surgical center/hospital or office setting, are greatly facilitated by the usage of the Lone Star Retractor System (Cooper Surgical, Inc., 75 Corporate Dr., Turnbull, CT 06611), especially the self-affixing horseshoe-shaped model designed by Dr. Red Alinsod, of Laguna Beach, California. Dr. Alinsod is the pioneering surgeon who first began performing perineoplasty in an office-based,setting under local anesthesia. This retractor system is imperative for procedures performed in an office setting. Prior to placing the retractor system the vulvar vestibule and perineum are manually separated and a small mark made with a sterile marking pen at ~2:30, 4:00, 8:00, and 9:30 o'clock just inside or just outside of the hymenal ring as placement sites for a minimum of 4 rubber stays that provide retraction and visualization, as well as marks at the apex in the mid-pelvic floor, the nadir of the incision line above the anal verge, and the lateral-most points of dissection at both the hymenal ring and vulvar vestibule, and an initial "dotted line" drawing is produced, linking these areas. (See also Chapter 9.) This drawing will be formalized after the retractor system is placed. Small blebs of anesthetic agent are injected sub-mucosally at the retractor hook sites, and the stays are attached to the previously placed retractor horseshoe.

After placement, the lines are formalized, and local anesthetic is injected sub-cutaneously and sub-mucosally along the lines and deeper into the levator, transversalis, and anal sphincter muscle sheaths and rectovaginal fascial sheath in several different locations (Figures 14.4 and 14.5).

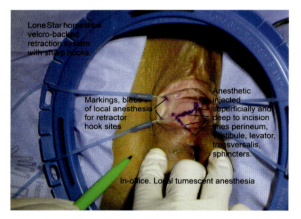

Figure 14.4 Office perineoplasty. Source: M. Goodman. Reproduced with permission.

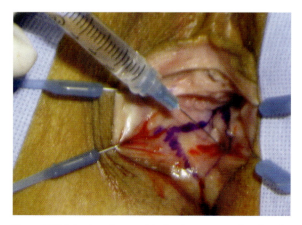

Figure 14.5 Injection. Source: M. Goodman. Reproduced with permission.

Candidates

Anesthetic choice depends on physician comfort with the procedure, patient choices, and finances, as both facility and anesthesia fees are significantly more costly in a surgical center/hospital environment. It is advisable for the surgeon to have a requisite number of cases under her or his belt under general or conduction anesthesia to feel confident and at ease prior to operating on an awake patient.

Novice genital plastic surgeons may attempt placing a pudendal block or local tumescent anesthesia in patients scheduled for general, converting to conscious sedation if the block is successful, while utilizing the block for initial post-operative analgesia. Additionally, novice surgeons may become facile with local tumescent anesthesia by injecting after induction of general anesthesia, additionally utilizing the local anesthetic for initial post-operative analgesia.

For a physician to utilize awake anesthesia, the patient must not be overly anxious, the physician must be trained in the technique, and the patient should have an attendant to comfort her during the injection.

Office-based surgery

Surgical venues may include hospital OR, a freestanding surgical center, or an office-based facility. If office-based, minimal medical, mechanical, and IV supplies sufficient for resuscitation must be available. That said, what—besides expertise, a comfortable patient, and a savvy surgeon—is requisite for successful office-based surgery?

Room setup

A space of adequate size is needed to hold an exam/operative table, back table, generator and cautery unit (Figure 14.6), supply cabinets, space to move around, and space at the head of the table for a friend or partner if the patient so desires. There must be space at the foot of the table for either a slide-out table-mount unit or Mayo stand of sufficient size to both hold instruments and for the surgeon to lean his or her elbows to both steady hands and minimize fatigue. One or two spotlights either ceiling mounted overhead or wall or stand mounted behind the surgeon is recommended.

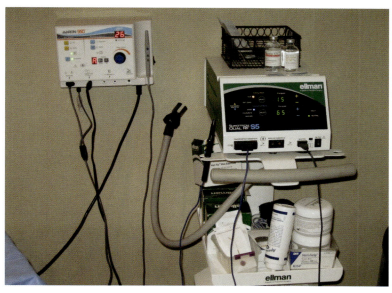

Figure 14.6 RF generator and cautery units.

Equipment and supplies

1 *Gynecological exam/surgical table.* Can be power or fixed, but must have drawers and ability to change out stirrups for either padded knee crutches or Allen-type leg rests. Knee crutches should be padded with foam, towels, and so forth and must have multi-positioning capability. A slide-out end is preferable for instruments and as a surgeon's arm rest; a mayo stand or the "cut-out Mayo" designed by Dr. Alinsod is elegant.

2 *Cutting and cautery capability.* Many choices are available for cutting and hemostasis, including scalpel, scissors, electrosurgical units for needle-point cutting, as well as cautery capability. Alternative power generators may be utilized if desired and are elegant and helpful for the precise scrolling work frequently required for cosmetic genital procedures. The author utilizes an RF generator for cutting and minor hemostasis and a separate Bovie™ or Valleylab™-type unit for hemostasis. Several manufacturers make RF generators. Requisites are bipolar pure cutting current, as well as fulguration or hemostatic capabilities. Many surgeons utilize laser equipment (see Chapter 8), which also is an excellent tool for these procedures. Both RF and laser are wonderfully precise cutting tools and, although both supply hemostatic options, neither has the capability for the cauterization requisite for safe genital plastic/cosmetic procedures.

3 *Smoke evacuator.* If utilizing RF, laser, or electrosurgical equipment, a small canister-type smoke evacuation system is mandated. The evacuation tip may be placed under the drapes just above the surgical field.

4 *Surgical lighting.* Many incandescent or halogen surgical lighting systems are available. These may either be ceiling mount, wall mount, or freestanding. The author uses an incandescent freestanding and a halogen wall-mount unit projecting light onto the surgical field from different angles.

5 *Draping.* One of several commercially available surgical drape kits with table covers, under-buttocks drape, leggings, and abdominal drape may be utilized. Most come with sterile surgical gowns, or these may be purchased separately.

6 *Surgical prep equipment.* Several different prep kits with iodine or other antiseptic soap and prep solutions are available. Prep must cover entire surgical field, buttocks, and distal one-third of vagina (vulvar surgery) and entire vagina for intra-vaginal tightening operations.

Surgical setup, instruments, and suture material (Figure 14.7)

1 *Back table* (e.g. Lakeside cart or equivalent). *Instruments/supplies*: 4 × 4 gauze sponges, draping supplies, sterile paper hand-drying wipes, gloves are

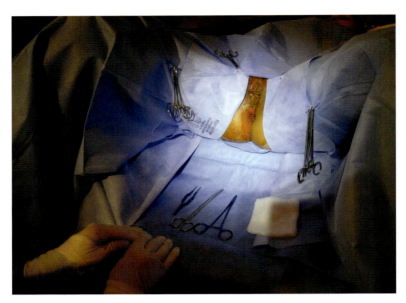

Figure 14.7 Op table setup. Source: M. Goodman. Reproduced with permission.

available on the "back table." The author's instrument set consists of (1) ~5" needle driver; (2) delicate (Addson- type) forceps; (3) baby Metzenbaum or Kaye scissors; (4) suture scissors; (5) two mosquito clamps; (6) two Allis clamps; (7) one Kelly or Mayo-type clamp to hold ancillary equipment (RF unit, cautery, etc.) to drape; (8) two towel clips or clamps to secure draping; (9) sterile fine-tipped marking pen; (10) ~50 ml medicine cup for drawing up anesthetic agent. Short-handled equipment (~5") is preferable.

For vaginal tightening procedures (PP; VRJ), *add*: 2–4 Allis-Adair or T-type clamps and heavier Metzenbaum or Mayo-type dissecting scissors. Heany-type curved jaw needle holder is preferable.

2 *Anesthesia supplies*: 0.25, 0.5% bupivacaine with and without epinephrine (multi-dose vial); sodium bicarbonate (multi-dose vial); 3–5 cc syringe with 18 or 20 ga. needle for drawing solution and 25 or 27 ga. needle for injecting; small (~50 ml) stainless steel medicine cup for mixing solution and drawing into syringe.

3 *Suture material*:

a *For labiaplasty, minora (LP-m); clitoral hood reduction (RCH)*: 5-0 Monocryl on PC-5 needle; 5-0 or 4-0 Vicryl on a SH-1 needle for sub-cutaneous closure; 5-0 Vicryl Rapide or 5-0 Vicryl on a PC-3 needle for skin (sub-cuticular or interrupted/mattress skin closure).

b *For labiaplasty, majora (LP-M)*: the author uses 4-0 Vicryl, 4-0 Monocryl, or 4-0 PDS on SH or SH-1 needle for the cubcutaneous layer, and 5-0 Monocryl on a PC-5 needle for sub-cuticular closure, or 5-0 nylon on a PS-3 needle for skin closure. (Sutures removed in 7–8 days.)

c *For PP, VRJ*: the author uses 2-0 Monocryl on a CT-2 needle for deep layers (levators; perineal body); 3-0 or 4-0 Monocryl on an SH or CT-2 needle for second (rectovaginal fascia) layer; and 3-0 or 4-0 Vicryl on an SH-I needle for vaginal mucosa and perineal closure.

Medications, ancillary supplies

Pre-op sedation/analgesia and anesthesia supplies have been reviewed earlier. Extra instruments, singly packaged, should be available.

"Goodie Bag"

Our office supplies our patients with a supply bag containing many items they will need for their recovery, including:

a Medium-sized latex gloves

b Disposable panties

c 4 × 4s

d Telfa pads

e Arnica tablets

f 30 gm container of Cu-3 Hydrating Gel, a copper-based hydrating gel to be gently placed on the surface of the incision lines b.i.d.

g Canister of Dermaplast analgesic spray.

h Inflatable "doughnut" cushion.

i Two reusable small-sized soft ice packs.

j Angled sprayer squeezable peri-bottle for hygiene.

k Package of witch-hazel wipes for hygiene.

Personnel

Procedure room personnel may certainly vary with personal preference. The author prefers a surgical assistant (two office employees who have learned under his tutelage alternate) and an RN who acts as a "hand-holder" and circulating nurse, monitors the patient, manages emergency supplies, keeps the surgical record, helps position the patient, monitors any friend/family members present, recovers the patient, and cleans up/sterilizes equipment.

Estimated operative, post-op, and recovery time

Operative times of course vary with surgeon and patient, and there certainly is a learning curve, but a properly performed LP-m varies between 45 minutes–1.75 hours, depending on complexity and amount of hood and/or posterior commisure to be included; LP-M approximately 1–1.25 hours; simple PP approximately 1–1.25 hours, and PP/VP 1.25–2 hrs surgical time.

CHAPTER 15

Non-surgical cosmetic vulvovaginal procedures

Gustavo Leibaschoff[1] and Pablo Gonzalez Isaza[2]

[1] World Society of Cosmetic Gynecology; International Union of Lipoplasty, Dallas, TX, USA
[2] Department of Obstetrics and Gynecology Hospital, Universitario San Jorge, Pereira, Colombia

(Editor's note: Radiofrequency [RF] and laser energy, fat transfer, and other methods of non-surgical tissue shrinkage and bulking techniques have been applied to the vulva and vagina. This chapter will briefly review these non-surgical modalities.)

Autologous fat grafting (AFG) and platelet-rich plasma (PRP)

Gustavo Leibaschoff

The transplantation of fat from one area of the body to another is a safe and effective procedure when performed by the hands of a qualified surgeon. Fat transfer requires more than just the action of filling an area with fat tissue and is additionally dependent on the regenerative action from adult stem-stromal cells for survival.

For AFG to emerge as a mainstream technique, it must be safe, yield reproducible results, and be based on stringent surgical principles. What began as an apparently simple technique of suctioning fat with implantation into areas for cosmetic and reconstructive purposes has now evolved into a complex menu of clinical choices.

The four variables commonly considered important to the overall success of fat grafting include harvesting, handling, transplantation or placement, and preparation of the recipient site. These four steps have developed and matured, leading to a multitude of techniques, technologies, and various opinions about each area. Additionally, quality of the fat can be enhanced with a variety of additives including adipocyte-derived stem cells and PRP. Autologous fat will vascularize without reinjection if delivered in small aliquots. There is no cost for the fat and it is available in sufficient quantities from almost any patient.

AFG meets all of the fundamental criteria for the "ideal" augmentation material: availability, minimal donor morbidity, and reproducible and predictable results, while avoiding non-autograft disease transmission or incompatibility. Considering these facts, autologous fat transfer provides a very appealing resource for soft tissue volume augmentation with both small and large volumes, made possible by the regenerative action from the autologous fat stem cells, preadipocyte, endothelial cells, and stromal vascular fraction.

It is important to consider and follow these guidelines for fat grafting as detailed by Shiffman [1] and listed below.

Guidelines for AFG
Guideline 1: Selection of appropriate recipient sites

This technique is for use in healthy individuals. Remember the following phrase: THE FAT LIVES IN THE FAT! This was our first concept but today following the new studies of Yosimura *et al.* [2] we know about the presence of adipocyte and stem cells in the fat tissue, so we can use the fat tissue in areas without fat.

Primary recipient sites are locations where fat normally resides but has been lost, including facial and body depressions due to loss of subdermal fat deposits, malar and sub-malar areas, glabella, chin, pre- and retroglandular breast areas, post-liposuction deformities, labia majora, and buttocks.

Secondary recipient sites: Locations with adequate vascularity and limited tissue density such as labial aspect of the nasolabial folds, submucosal (lingual) aspect of the lips, mucocutaneous area of the lips; and various depressions associated with scarring or trauma.

Female Genital Plastic and Cosmetic Surgery, First Edition. Edited by Michael P. Goodman.
© 2016 John Wiley & Sons, Ltd. Published 2016 by John Wiley & Sons, Ltd.

Recipient site considerations: Sites should be gently pre-tunneled prior to injection of fat into the recipient bed [3]. Pre-tunneling may be utilized in the donor and recipient areas, with different indications. In the donor area, pre-tunneling without aspiration allows better distribution of the local solution, thus improving the effectiveness of the tumescent fluid. In the recipient area, pre-tunneling will enhance mobilization of the fat tissue without compromising graft quality, while liberation of growth factors allows better contact of the graft with normal fat tissue.

Recipient sites should not be infiltrated with fluids prior to fat introduction (lidocaine and vasoconstriction) [4]. Fat transplantation should be avoided into areas of pre-existing inflammation or compromised circulation. Avoid attempts to place grafted tissue directly into the dermal plane or dense intra-lesional scar sites (this guideline is in revision today following the new studies with autologous adipose stem cells). Selection of access opening for introduction of autologous fat grafts should be made to ensure maximal cosmetic result.

Guideline 2: Selection of appropriate donor sites [3]

The donor site fat has "memory." Fat from the lower abdomen placed in the face behaves like fat in the lower abdomen.

Screening for potential candidates and donor areas is important. Clearly identify the individual patient's areas of long-term difficulties with fat deposition and maintained storage locations (i.e., diet and exercise-resistant sites and sites with more LPL and alpha 2 receptors). Ideal donor areas are locations where cells are genetically designated as active in storage and are metabolically resistant, thus allowing better long-term survival. Sites should be easily accessible for ease of harvesting and be located to achieve the best aesthetic result.

The *most common donor sites* are the lower abdomen, pubis, flanks, thigh, buttocks, and knees; less commonly, calves, upper arms, and the lateral thoracic area.

Guideline 3: Harvesting

Low-pressure harvesting of autologous fat [5] with a small syringe is ideal for small fat grafting, or a large syringe for breast or buttocks. A low-pressure pump may also be used for larger areas of fat grafting. Always utilize appropriate sterile surgical technique. Pre-operative broad-spectrum systemic antibiotics may be appropriate prior to initiation of any harvest (24 hours before the procedure and continuing for 5 days). Selected donor and recipient sites should be marked with the patient in the upright position. Remember, all procedures in lipoplasty should begin with accurate and adequate marking. Photos should document both donor and recipient sites and should be taken without marking.

Graft harvesting: Fat harvesting seems to have high cell viability and good predictability of results when grafts are removed with low-pressure using a closed-syringe technique [5]. Today, new techniques allow pumps utilizing lower pressure to be connected to special devices for collection of the fat tissue. Isotonic sterile saline is utilized within the harvesting syringe; the use of hypertonic or hypotonic solutions will damage the fat cell to be grafted.

Extraction should be performed with the correct type of cannula, such as a polished edge Cobra, size 2.1 to 3.7 mm in diameter. Smaller cannulas are utilized for face or hands; larger for buttocks or breast augmentation.

Guideline 4: Donor sites

Donor sites are gently injected with tumescent anesthesia pre-tunneling. 2.1–3.0 mm Cobra cannulas or 16G needles are utilized for harvesting. Wait 20 minutes after placing the tumescent anesthesia prior to gently pre-tunneling in all areas.

Minimal repetitions provide for minimal trauma through the areas being harvested, resulting in cleaner fat cell removal.

Following aspiration of a small volume of normal saline into the harvesting syringe, the plunger should be moved back approximately one-fourth to one-third the volume of the syringe barrel (NS [normal saline]). For a 10 ml syringe use 2 ml NS; draw plunger to 3 ml, when this 3 ml is full of fat move the plunger another 3 ml and repeat the maneuver until the syringe is full of fat tissue with tumescent solution. For a 35 ml syringe use 5 ml NS; draw plunger to 5 ml, continue as with the 10 ml syringe. For a 60 ml syringe use 10 ml NS; draw plunger in 10 ml, continue as with the 10 ml syringe.

In *patients seeking lipocontouring* at the same time, it is recommended that all fat harvesting for transfer be obtained prior to fat reduction and contouring procedures.

Guideline 5: Handling and preparation of harvested fat [5]

Harvested fat should be allowed to decant thoroughly in order to separate the fat to be transferred from the infranatant layer containing saline and blood elements (see Figures 15.1 and 15.2).

Decanting: Placement of the syringe should be in the vertical position, plunger up. Extraction of the infranatant layer is performed with subsequent addition of equal volumes of normal saline to facilitate cleansing. It is important to repeat decanting until the infranatant layer is clear (average 4–5 times).

Centrifugation [6] is performed at 3,000 rpm for 3 minutes. Infranatant fluid levels should be clearly identified and carefully expressed from the syringe used to transfer the fat cells. Today there are new devices for harvesting and cleaning fat tissue. However, rinsing should be done at least four times to remove the lidocaine contained in the tumescent anesthetic solution.

Clean sterile normal saline should be used to provide complete washing of the potential graft material. Depending on the purity of the harvest, this may require multiple [4,5] rinsing efforts to accomplish the cleansing.

The supranatant layer is comprised of fatty oils and debris. This material should not be included in the actual grafting procedure. Failure to avoid injection of this material may lead to a greater tissue inflammatory response and thereby lessen the viability of grafted cells.

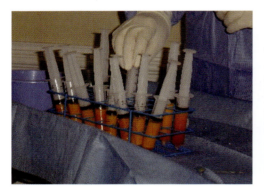
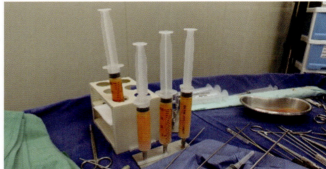

Figure 15.1 Harvested fat awaiting preparation. © G. Leibaschoff. Used with permission.

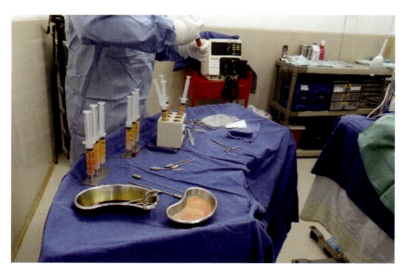

Figure 15.2 "Good" fat tissue awaiting transplantation. © G. Leibaschoff. Used with permission.

Guideline 6: Transfer

Transfer techniques into recipient sites [5]: Use large blunt cannulas (2.1–3.7 mm) for fat injection into limited, pre-tunneled channels. Using cannulas less than 2.1 mm in diameter may result in exposure of graft cells to high pressures with increased potential for cellular damage and less successful augmentation. Use a small syringe for placement of the fat tissue, 1 ml for the face and hands, 5–10 ml per labum, 10–20 ml for breast and buttocks.

Pre-tunneling with small, blunt-edged cannulas is recommended with the intent of creating appropriate spaces to receive the graft cells with minimal resistance and in close approximation to normal fat tissue in that area.

The pre-tunneled areas afford maximal contact of grafted fat cells with the recipient bed cells, providing better vascularity, nutrition, and oxygenation. Ideally, placement of the fat graft into the tunnels should be in the areas normally occupied by fat cells.

Placement of the grafts should be made [7] in small aliquots (0.5–2.0 cc), into the tunnels and into different levels of the fat tissue, using minimal amounts of pressure and small syringes for placement, overfilling 20–30% to compensate for the volume of normal saline fluid used to suspend the fat cells during their transfer (remember the fluid is absorbed in the first 7 days).

Guideline 7: Storage of fat for delayed transfer

Tissue culture evidence has demonstrated the viability of adipocytes following freezing and storage. Fat placed in the injection syringe to be used for transfer should be capped, sealed, and accurately labeled. These isolated syringes are placed in individual ziplock bags, are gradually reduced to a temperature of -4° C, and are held at that temperature throughout the storage period. There is histological evidence that rapid freezing protocols (e.g., liquid nitrogen) may lead to cellular crystallization.

Storage and survival: The volume of stored fat should be limited to small volume transfer syringes (1, 3, 5, or 10 cc). Specimens to be prepared for transfer are removed 2–3 hours prior to actual procedure time. Specimens are placed in a sterile saline solution at room temperature and are gradually allowed to thaw and return to ambient temperature. Storage has been effective at 1 year from the time of harvest.

The survival of free fat used as autograft is *operator dependent*. This requires delicate handling of the graft tissue, careful washing of the fat to minimize extraneous blood cells, and installation into a site with adequate vascularity.

Complications of fat augmentation

Complications of fat transfer include loss of fat volume, need for repeat injection, bruising, hematoma, swelling, prolonged erythema, tenderness/pain, fibrous capsule formation, infection (rare), protrusions secondary to excessive volume, microcalcifications, and CNS damage secondary to misadventures in the glabellar area.

Controversy concerning the efficacy of AFG seems to be related to the amount of graft retained and the long-term retention of volume increase. Many claim relatively high reabsorption rates (30–60%), which does not account for the fluid volume used to transport graft cells from donor to recipient sites. During the first week there is reabsorption of the liquid including that used for tumescent anesthesia.

Loss of fat volume is the most common problem in fat transfer. Prior to fat transplantation the patient should be informed of this possibility and the need for reinjection.

Factors that have substantial influence on the success of autologous fat transplantation [8]

Some of these include:
1 The patient's systemic health;
2 genetic predisposition for cellular fat storage from the preferred donor sites (so-called "primary" fat deposit locations);
3 pre- and post-grafting patient nutrition;
4 use of minimally traumatic harvest and handling techniques;
5 proper preparation of the recipient bed.

Best donor areas for fat transfer

As we know today, fat tissue containing more alpha 2 receptors (antilipolytic receptors) and large amounts of LPL (lipoprotein lipase) is the best fat for transfer [9]. The sub-cutaneous fat tissue in the lower abdomen and pubis are the areas with more alpha 2 receptors and larger amounts of LPL (like the gluteus femoral area).

LPL is the most important enzyme for lipogenesis. It can increase the size of the fat cells, which will also contain larger numbers of alpha 2 receptors [9]. Women produce more LPL in the sub-cutaneous fat tissue of the lower abdomen and gluteal femoral area. This is the physiologic explanation of why these areas offer the best fat tissue for AFG.

When we utilize fat for lipografting, we typically select areas with a large amount of fat tissue or a zone with localized obesity. These areas may cause problems at the recipient site. In the regions with localized obesity the physiology of the fat tissue may vary. According to the studies of Danielle Lacasa and her group [10], there is an alteration in the viability of the fat cells in these areas. There is more fibrosis, less expression of adipo-nectin and leptin, and an increase the proinflammatory cytokines. There is also an alteration in the normal lipolysis, with decreased beta adrenergic action in fat tissue with fibrosis. It is easy to understand that the quality of the fat tissue varies and that some fat used for grafting may give different results.

How we can improve the quality of the fat tissue: autologous PRP

In addition to pre- and post-grafting patient nutrition, one of the most important influences of grafting adult lipocytes (plus stimulation of rich mesenchymal stem cell components within the fat tissues) is the addition of platelet-derived factors added to the harvested graft materials prior to graft placement [11].

PRP is a volume of autologous plasma that has a concentration of platelets greater than baseline.

The autologous concentration of human platelets in a small volume of plasma is shown in the Figure 15.3, and the pre- and post-centrifugation results in Figure 15.4.

Because there is a high concentration of platelets, there is also an increased concentration of the 7 fundamental protein growth factors proven to be actively secreted by platelets to initiate all wound healing [12]. These growth factors include the 3 isomers of platelet-derived growth factor (PDGF-AA, PDGF-AB, and PDGF-BB) of the numerous transforming growth factors (TGF1 and TGF2), vascular endothelial growth factor, (VEGF) and epithelial growth factor (EGF). All of these growth factors have been documented to exist in platelets.

Growth factors are the biologically active signal peptides released from local tissue or blood products (particularly the platelet fraction) that play a critical role in inducing the initiation and progression of the normal wound-healing process. Such factors synchronize the processes of epithelialization, angiogenesis, and collagen-matrix formation, which are key steps in the wound-healing sequence. These peptides work in a coordinated fashion to orchestrate the normal wound-healing processes.

After rinsing the harvested graft material to effec-tively reduce the intracellular lidocaine concentration and permit the removal of extracellular lipid materials and debris, the PRP is added to the autologous graft materials in an approximate ratio of 5–10% in small volume cases and 10–20% of the total graft prepared for large volume transplantation [13] (Figure 15.5).

Degranulation

Besides the initiation of coagulation processes, the platelets undergo a degranulation process that releases a complex group of growth factors and cytokines (peptides) essential for wound-healing mechanisms.

On the basis of those clinical observations, it is reported that addition of PRP (and the attendant addition of high concentrations of growth factors and

		Physiological clot	Regen PRP clot
	Red blood cells	35–50% hematocrit	<1% hematocrit
	Platelets	Native level	2–4 times native level
	Growth factors	Native level	2–4 times native level
	Fibrin	Native level	Native level

Figure 15.3 Composition of PRP. © G. Leibaschoff. Used with permission.

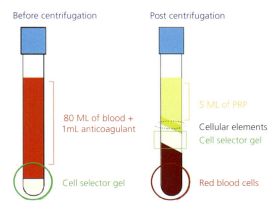

Before centrifugation   **Post centrifugation**

80 ML of blood +
1mL anticoagulant

Cell selector gel

5 ML of PRP

Cellular elements
Cell selector gel

Red blood cells

Figure 15.4 Pre- and post-centrifugation. © G. Leibaschoff. Used with permission.

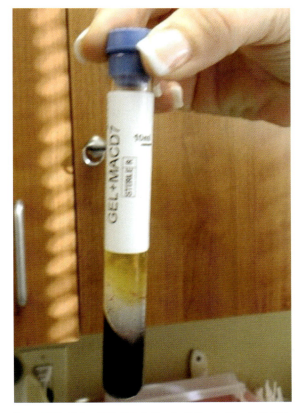

Figure 15.5 Adding PRP. © G. Leibaschoff. Used with permission.

cytokines) [14] increases the retention of the transplanted fat cells, augments the rate of re-vascularization of the grafts, and aids the differentiation of preadipocyte precursor cells into mature adipocytes to further enhance the retained graft volumes.

Introduction of such concentrated growth factors during the preparation and transfer phase seems to potentiate wound healing via normal physiologic mechanisms that control cellular recruitment, migration, and differentiation within the recipient sites. In addition, such additives contribute to the induction and conduction aspects of both the donor and recipient mesenchyme stem cell (undifferentiated) population and in that way significantly contribute to overall fat graft success

AFG + PRP

Our experience suggests that the use of PRP increases the long-term retention of the transplanted fat cells and increases the rate of re-vascularization and survival of the transplanted cells. In addition, clinical experience indicates the addition of PRP is associated with other advantages, including acceleration of the healing processes and, in large volume transfers, reduction of spherical calcifications and lipid cyst formation. This observation has been confirmed by radiographic and ultrasonic visualization [15].

This improvement of the healing rate and graft acceptance is thought to decrease the potential for liponecrosis and lipid cyst formation and the incidence of spherical microcalcifications, particularly within larger volume augmentation (breast and buttock) areas.

The potential of enhanced viability and clinical success of using transplanted fat in both small and large volume applications explains the importance of such combination to promote natural wound-healing mechanisms.

Fat transfer is poised to play a major part in the future of aesthetic medicine, cosmetic surgery, and regenerative surgery. It is not just about the fat cells but the fat tissue, improving the recipient bed, and identifying which processes to minimize and/or optimize.

Important as well is understanding the stromal vascular elements and adult stem cells in the fat tissue, looking at specific reactions and promoting best practices. It is an understanding that we can achieve excellent results without external manipulations of the fat tissue. Still unclear is what happens with external manipulation (removing the stem cells from fat tissue, e.g.) and the changes in these cells.

Use of minimally traumatic harvesting and handling techniques

Fat transplant survival depends on the instrumentation used for harvesting and placement of the fat graft. Damage to the fat graft is inversely related to the diameter of the

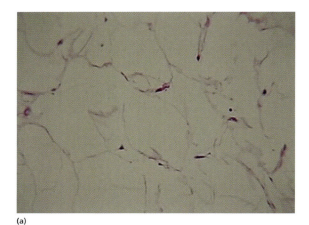

(a)

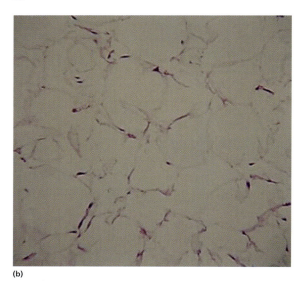

(b)

Figure 15.6 Quality of fat as a function of cannula diameter.
© G. Leibaschoff. Used with permission.

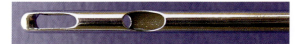

Figure 15.7 Cobra cannula. Courtesy G. Leibaschoff.

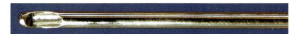

Figure 15.8 Blunt one hole cannula. Courtesy G. Leibaschoff.

instruments used to extract and inject. Large diameter for harvesting and small diameter for placement can destroy the fat graft; therefore it is important to use the same diameter for both procedures [16].

The pressure generated when injecting fat increases as a function of decreasing needle diameter, hence more pressure equals more destruction of the grafted tissue. When using cannulas less than 2 mm in diameter, there is a decrease in the metabolic activity of the fragments and alteration in the anatomy of the graft (Figure 15.6).

With the use of low vacuum pressure, closed syringe technique for harvest, utilizing the correct cannulas for harvest (Cobra) and transfer (blunt, one hole), fat

grafting (large and small volumes) has become more effective and better understood (Figures 15.7 and 15.8).

When discussing fat transplant survival, the presence of blood in the injected fat stimulates macrophage activity, which can decrease the number of fat cells. Thus it is mandatory to thoroughly clean the harvested fat to remove all of the blood. Never use fat containing blood for grafting.

Today we use Coleman's technique with centrifugation at 3,000 rpm for 3 minutes; or decantation (washing the cells in a physiological solution) prior to injection until the infranatant solution is clear (transparent). We can also use the newer devices for harvesting fat tissue that claim to clean the fat tissue for immediate use (see Figure 15.9).

These systems, however, overlook the importance of the presence of lidocaine in the tumescent anesthetic solution. It is well known that solutions containing lidocaine are very lipophilic. The presence of high concentrations of intracellular anesthetic [17] solutions in grafted adipocytes is among the potential negative influential factors in the global success of the graft. Therefore, reasonable reduction of intracellular lidocaine levels is considered advantageous. Lidocaine still exists within the adipocyte, even after three separate rinses using a normal saline solution [18].

In smaller and larger volume transfers such as breast and buttock areas, rinsing and addition of PRP is now favored (see Figures 15.10–15.12).

Proper preparation of the recipient bed is important, and early graft immobilization in the recipient sites during the initial graft acceptance and initiation of the healing cascade is advised.

A technique for improving the PO2 in the recipient bed involves the use of a technique known as carboxitherapy ~3 weeks prior to grafting. The effects of carboxitherapy are purported to be an increase in tissue oxygenation, an increased flow rate and vasodilatation,

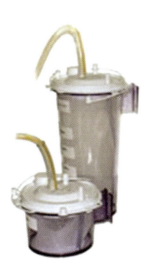
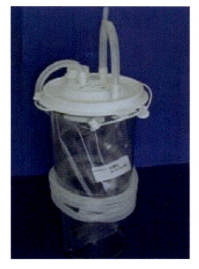
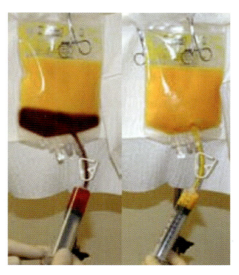

Figure 15.9 Devices for centrifuging fat tissue. © G. Leibaschoff. Used with permission.

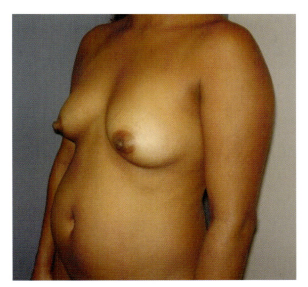
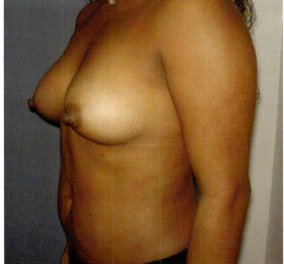

Figure 15.10 Breast augmentation with fat tissue. © G. Rojas and G. Leibaschoff. Used with permission.

and an increase in collagen in the connective tissue [19]. It is felt that the recipient site provides the needed circulation and cellular access for structural cells, so-called "healing cells," and capillary formation [20]. This may explain why small aliquots of graft placed in prepared tunnels surrounded by native fat cells and stroma contributes to and enhances graft survival. In the presence of normal oxygen tensions, the number of fibroblasts and amount of collagen deposits, as well as the number of capillaries, may be increased by increasing the number of macrophages present via liberation of growth factor from the macrophages [21].

Labia majora lipografting

Autologous fat transplant to the labia majora [22] may be utilized to provide an aesthetically enhanced look and a bioregenerative action over the skin and connective tissue of the dermis. Fat is harvested from

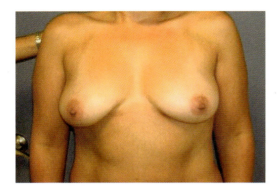

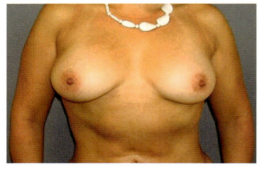

Figure 15.11 Breast augmentation and asymetry correction with fat tissue. © G. Rojas and G. Leibaschoff. Used with permission.

the pubis and the lower abdomen with a 10 cc syringe and 2 mm cobra cannula, taking at least 60 cc of fat tissue (6 syringes). The fat is decanted with normal saline solution and rinsed four times until the solution below the fat is clear (no blood).

Before the placement of the fat tissue, 2 cc of PRP (20%) is added to each syringe and introduced via a 2 mm one hole blunt cannula from the top or bottom of the labia majora, with placement of the fat tissue in small aliquots (micrografts) into three levels: deep, medium, and superficial in the sub-cutaneous tissue of the recipient area. The placement of the fat is via withdrawal of the cannula, increasing the amount of fat tissue in the middle of the labia majora (see Figures 15.13–15.15).

PRP alone is then injected into the dermis 1–2 mm depth with a 1 cc syringe and 30G1/2 needle for the biostimulation of the skin. (Total is 2 cc of PRP.)

Vaginal recalibration by lipograft technique

This procedure consists of reducing vaginal caliber by thickening the vaginal walls with adipose tissue transplant. Although not presently evidence-based, a study by M. Abecassis from France is in press. Practitioners beginning to utilize this technique feel it may be an

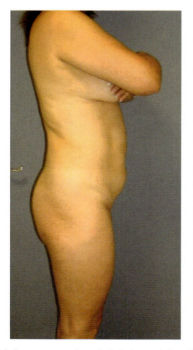

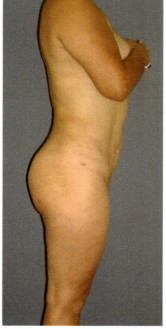

Figure 15.12 Buttocks with fat augmentation. © G. Rojas and G. Leibaschoff. Used with permission.

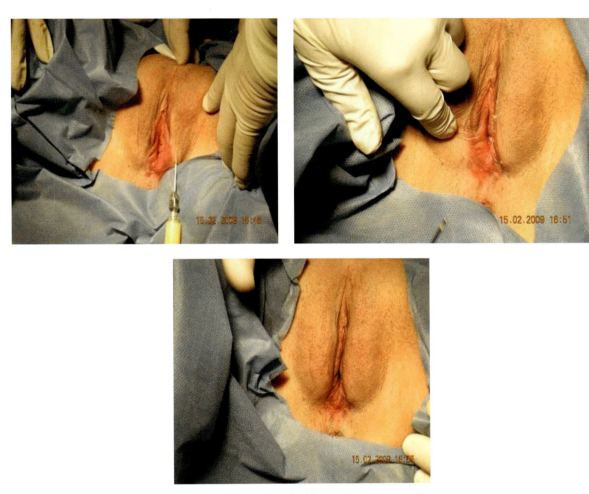

Figure 15.13 Fat grafting in labia majora. © G. Leibaschoff. Used with permission.

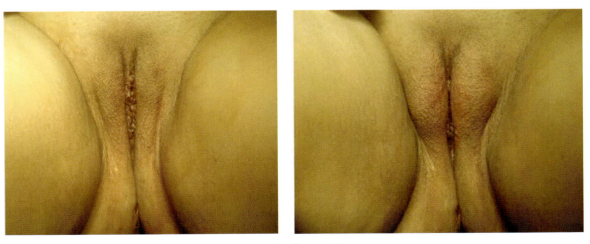

Figure 15.14 Fat grafting, labia majora. © G. Leibaschoff. Used with permission.

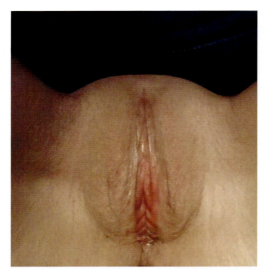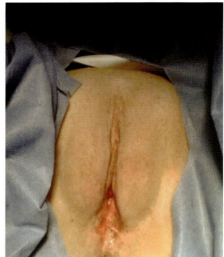

Figure 15.15 Lipografting labia majoria and pubis liposculpture. © G. Leibaschoff. Used with permission.

alternative to surgical correction in those patients with a "sensation of wide vagina" wishing to avoid surgical correction.

The implantation technique avoids the rectovaginal lamina and the anterior wall with its intimate connections with the urethra and the bladder. Entrance points are located at 3:00 and 9:00 hours at the introitus on both sides, but only one entrance is utilized, by which the cannula will deposit the graft in a 5 cm length and a 3 cm height and in "criss-cross" directions in a fan mode.

Placement of the adipose tissue is achieved in two plains; a deep one is necessary to achieve a platform that will sustain the fat that is deposited in a more superficial layer. In Dr. Abecassis's study (in press), 80% of patients questioned declared they were satisfied post-treatment, although follow-up was only 6 months.

The fat's ASCs (adipose stem cells), and "reconstructing cells" [23], along with the "trophicity" of the fat tissue lead to a subjective augmentation of sensation during intercourse, according to patients (personal data).

Conclusion

Many controversies still remain regarding the use of fat grafting, especially in the female breast. There appears no doubt, however, that using PRP will improve the result. Important techniques available to increase the success of AFG include preparation of the recipient area using carboxitherapy, mesotherapy with PRP, adding

PRP to the AFG, using fat containing more alpha 2 receptors, choosing the correct cannula for harvesting and placement, and of course, good technique and operator cognition.

In fat grafting, as other genital plastic/cosmetic procedures. the words of Dr. Pierre Fournier resonate: "No tool can replace talent and experience." "It is not what is in your hand but what is in your head."

References

1. Shiffman MA, ed. *Autologous Fat Grafting*. Berlin: Springer, 2010.
2. Yosimura K, Eto H, Suga H, Aoi N. The fate of adipocytes after non vascularized fat grafting *Plast Reconstr Surg* 2012;**129**: 1081–92.
3. Alexander RW. Liposculpture in the superficial plane: Closed syringe system for improvement in fat removal and free fat transfer. *Am J Cosmet Surg* 1994;**11**:127–34.
4. Shiffman M, Mirrafati S. Fat transfer techniques: The effect of harvest and transfer methods on adipocyte viability and review of the literature. *Dermatol Surg* 2001;**27**:819–26.
5. *Autologous Fat Transplantation*. New York: Marcel Dekker, 2001.
6. Coleman SR. Structural fat grafting. *Plast Reconstr Surg* 2005;**115**:1777–8.
7. Shiffman MA. Fat embolism following liposuction. *Am J Cosmet Surg* 2011;**28**:212–8.
8. Bircoll M. Autologous fat transplantation. *Plast Reconstr Surg* 1987;**79**:492–3.

9. Lafontan M, Langin D. Lipolysis and lipid mobilization in human adipose tissue. *Prog Lipid Res* 2009;**48**:275–97.

10. Divoux A, Tordjman, J, Lacasa D, Veyrie N, Hugol D, Aissat A, Basdevant A, et al. INSERM, Paris. Fibrosis in human adipose tissue: Composition, distribution, and link with lipid metabolism and fat mass loss. *Diabetes* 2010;**59**:2817–25.

11. Alexander RW, Abuzeni PZ. Enhancement of autologous fat transplantation with platelet rich plasma. *Am J Cosmet Surg* 2001;**18**:59–70

12. Ross R, Raines EW, Bowen-Pope DF. The biology of platelet-derived growth factor. *Cell* 1986;**46**(2):155–69.

13. Cervelli V, Palla L, Pascali M, De Angelis B, Curcio BC, Gentile P. Autologous platelet-rich plasma mixed with purified fat graft in aesthetic plastic surgery. *Aesthetic Plast Surg* 2009;**33**:716–21.

14. Bennett NT, Schultz GS. Growth factors and wound healing: Biochemical properties of growth factors and their receptors. *Am J Surg* 1993;**165**(6):728–37.

15. Alexander RW, Sadati K, Corrado A. Platelet rich plasma (PRP) utilized to promote greater graft volume retention in AFG. *Am J Cosmet Surg* 2006;**23**:203–21.

16. Cervelli V, Bocchini T, DiPasquali C, Curcio CB, Gentile P, Cervelli G. PRL platelet rich lipotransfer: Our experience and current state of art in the combined use of fat and PRP. *Biomed Res Int* 2013;**434191**.

17. Arner P, Arner O, Ostman J. The effect of local anesthetic agents on lipolysis by human adipose tissue. *Life Sci* 1973;**13**(2):161–9.

18. Girard AC, Festy F, Roche R. New insights into lidocaine and adrenaline effects on human adipose stem cells *Aesth Plast Surg* 2013; **37**:144–52.

19. C. Brandi, D'Aniello C, Grimaldi L, Bosi B, Del I, Lattarulo P, Alessandrini C. Carbon dioxide therapy in the treatment of localized adiposities: Clinical study and histophysiological correlations. *Aesthetic Plast Surg* 2001;**25**:170–4.

20. Knighton DR, Hunt TK, Scheuenstuhl H, Halliday BJ, Werb Z, Banda MJ. Oxygen tension regulates the expression of angiogenesis factor by macrophages. *Science* 1983;**221**:1283–5.

21. Hodson L. Adipose tissue oxygenation: Effect on metabolic function. *Adipocyte* 2014 Jan 1;**3**(1):75–80.

22. Cihantimur B, Herold C. Genital beautification. *Aesthetic Plast Surg* 2013;**37**:1128–33.

23. Gimble J, Guilak F. Adipose-derived adult stem cells: Isolation, characterization, and differentiation potential. *Cytotherapy* 2003;**5**:362–9.

Radiofrequency; fractional CO_2 laser; depigmentation techniques

Pablo Gonzalez Isaza

As demand for cosmetic gynecology procedures increases, patients search for procedures that may be performed on an outpatient basis with minimal discomfort, short downtime, and rapid return to sexual activity. In the text that follows, I will review:

• Fractional CO_2 laser and radiofrequency (RF) treatment for labia majora redundancy and vaginal laxity;
• fractional laser treatment for vulvar hyperpigmentation;
• other (chemical) treatments for vulvar hyperpigmentation.

Fractional laser and RF treatment for vaginal relaxation

Vaginal relaxation is the loss of the optimum structural architecture of the vagina and surrounding musculature and connective tissue layers. This process is generally associated with natural aging and is especially affected by childbirth. During the vaginal relaxation process, the vaginal muscles become relaxed with poor tone, strength, and support, and internal and external diameters can increase dramatically; under these circumstances the vagina is no longer at its optimal physiologically functioning state. Masters and Johnson pioneered studies that concluded that sexual gratification is directly related to the amount of frictional forces generated during intercourse [1]. Vaginal relaxation has a detrimental effect on sexual gratification.

The incidence of this condition is unknown. In an international survey of urogynecologists, 83% of 563 respondents described vaginal laxity as an unreported condition by their patients; the majority considered laxity a self-reported bothersome condition that impacts sexual function and relationships [2]. Dr. Alexandros Bader utilizes the term "vaginal relaxation syndrome" (VRS) and opines that VRS is an anatomical defect of the vaginal walls present in 8 of 10 patients after 1 or more vaginal deliveries (personal communication, "Vaginal Tightening Using Double Wave Diode Laser," submitted for publication). Non-invasive treatments such as pelvic floor exercises and electrostimulation can show an improvement in these patients, but efficacy is limited and patient adherence to treatment may not be optimal.

Both fractional laser and RF energy may be delivered to the vaginal walls by devices with vaginal-shaped cones. Salvatore *et al.* reported an increase of 50% in vaginal tone after one session of a fractional CO_2 laser system (MonaLisa Touch DEKA Laser Systems, Florence, Italy; FemiLift, Alma Lasers, Tel Aviv, Israel) [3].

The use of a fractional CO_2 laser for vaginal tightening relies on the concept that a carefully controlled fractional CO_2 laser can be utilized to heat deeper structures. The therapeutic goal is to stimulate connective tissue activation and reorganization with subsequent tissue revitalization. This process is similar to other procedures approved for the treatment of human skin laxity, in which increased collagen formation appears to contribute to the mechanism of action. Sekiguchi *et al.* reported an experience with 30 post-menopausal women who complained about vaginal relaxation and poor satisfaction during sexual relationships. Non-surgical non-ablative RF energy was applied and tolerated well by the patient, with important changes in vaginal laxity perception and sexual satisfaction during intercourse in the subjects, before and after the treatment protocol [4].

Numerous reports of short-term improvement in both vaginal tone and mild urinary incontinence are being reported at meetings and anecdotally, but all reports are retrospective and have not withstood the test of prospective evaluation and adequate follow-up. Treatment protocols are being developed by industry, and treatment units are available. Reliable, well-powered prospective data awaits collection. It is likely these units will be used and/or misused prior to the collection and publication of reliable, prospective, evidence-based data. The ability of these units to produce tightening of the proximal vagina is exciting. Even if temporary (duration of effect touted by industry is ~18–36 months after 3 treatments spaced 1 month apart), this could produce a welcome additive effect to surgical tightening of the pelvic floor, with the possible addition of maintenance of continence.

Another possible use for both RF and fractional CO_2 laser units may be to aid in temporary tightening and improvement in sexual function for women after childbirth and in women planning future parity.

Millheiser *et al.* claim that women report a decrease in sexual satisfaction following vaginal delivery; they found that after a complete treatment with monopolar non-inavasive RF energy (Viveve Medical Corp., Sunnyvale, CA), 100% of patients reported a statistically significant improvement in vaginal laxity and sexual function that was maintained through 12 months. No serious adverse events were reported [5].

The success of minimally invasive laser procedures on both vaginal tone and mild genuine stress urinary incontinence have been reported following the use of different Er:YAG laser technologies [6,7]. The results indicate an improvement in vaginal laxity and even in the mild and moderate stages of stress urinary incontinence. The main limitation of this type of technology lies in the lack of effectiveness on tissues with a high water component. The high water absorption of the Er:YAG wavelength, 10 times that of carbon dioxide, limits the diffusion of energy deeply into the tissues, resulting in only temporary effects [8]. Controlled studies with longer follow-up are needed to confirm these findings.

RF energy, applied with a broad 15.20 mm "wand" to the labia majora via a protocol consisting of three monthly spaced treatments, produces measurable diminishment of labia majora redundancy lasting ~12–24 months, as reported in a series of patients (N = 30) (Dr. Red Alinsod, personal communication.). Again, controlled prospective study results are yet to be forthcoming (see Figure 15.16).

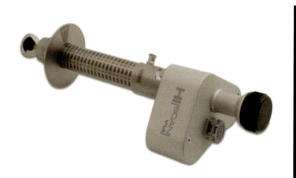 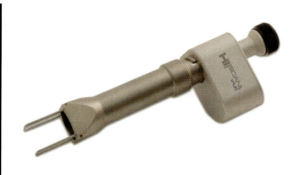

Figure 15.16 Hi Scan 360-degree vaginal probe and vulvar hand piece. Reprinted with permission of Deka M.E.L.A., Florence Italy.

Fractional laser and miscellaneous treatments for vulvar hyperpigmentation

In our practice in South America, and in other practices worldwide, "lightening" therapy for vulvar and perineal hyperpigmentation is a common request among women seeking cosmetic gynecology procedures. Hyperpigmentation of the perianal and vulvar regions can be caused by aging, hormonal changes from pregnancy, infections (syphilis), and medical conditions such as contact dermatitis and tight-fitting underwear, in addition to ethnically related hyperpigmentation (Table 15.1).

The first people to try "intimate skin bleaching" (specifically anal bleaching) were women and men in the adult entertainment industry. With the advent of HD (high-definition) TV, the demand for this treatment among this group has dramatically increased. Mainstream Hollywood film stars adopted this treatment once nudity became more prevalent in movies. However, it was not until the introduction of Brazilian waxing that intimate skin bleaching become more mainstream; once hair is removed women may notice hyperpigmentation.

Table 15.1 Differential diagnosis of vulvar hyperpigmentation.

	Melanocyte Increase	Melanin Increase
Genetic	• Lentigines • Peutz-Jeger Syndrome	• Neurofibromatosis • Nevus De Becker • Efelides
Chemical drug related	• MSH	• Arsenic • Psoralens • Bergamota • Cytostatics
Endocrine		• Addison's disease • Kwashiorkor • Intestinal malabsorption • ACTH excess
Physical	• UVR	• Trauma • Ionizing radiation exposure
Inflammation/ infection		• Post-inflammatory hyperpigmentation • Lichen planus • Lupus erythematosus • Psoriasis • Pitiriasis versicolor

The use of minimal undergarments not only makes the perirectal area more visible, prompting many women to bleach the perianal area, but the actual use of G-string type undergarments causes the perianal and inguinal area to become darker secondary to rubbing of the material (usually nylon) against the skin, causing chronic irritation. Frequent users of G-strings tend to have darker perianal and vulvar areas.

Physiopathology

Pigmentation is caused by the combination of pigments localized in the dermis and epidermis and includes (a) oxygenated hemoglobin of arterioles and capillaries; (b) deoxygenated hemoglobin of venules; (c) deposits of carotenes or unmetabolized bile salts and other exogenous pigment (drug, metals, etc.), and (d) melanin, the main component of racially determined skin coloration.

Skin lightening agents ("cosmoceuticals")

Ingredients such as azelaic acid, lactic acid, retonic acid, salycylic acid, and pyruvic acid gently lighten the skin and reduce the activity of tyrosinase, the enzyme responsible for "darkening" in the lower layers of the skin. Soothing anti-oxidant agents such as vitamin C, bearberry extract, licorice extract, and mulberry extract provide a gentle moisturizing treatment to protect while continuing to lighten the skin.

Products that contain hydroquinone are believed to be linked with negative side effects such as liver damage, thyroid problems, and cancer [9]. Prolonged use of hydroquinone can thicken collagen fibers, resulting in a spotty skin appearance and scarification called ochrindosis. For this reason hydroquinone has been banned in numerous countries across Europe and Asia.

Mercury may also be toxic. Long-term mercury use strips skin of its natural pigment. Prolonged exposure can cause cancer, mercury poisoning, and liver or kidney failure [10].

Physical treatments

Microdermabrasion is a dermatologic procedure utilizing a mechanical medium for exfoliation to gently remove the outermost layer of dead skin cells from the epidermis. Most commonly, microdermabrasion uses two parts: an exfoliating material like crystals or diamond flakes and a machine-based suction to gently lift up the skin during exfoliation. It is a non-invasive procedure and may be

Table 15.2 Agents purposed to have vulvar hypopigmentation effects.

Arginine	Lactic Acid	Azelaic Acid	Mandelic Acid
• Moisturizing properties • Anti-inflammatory effects • Nitric oxide precursor	• Moisturizing properties • Skin lightener • Bactericidal properties • Stimulates cell differentiation	• Skin lightener • Bactericidal • Anti-oxidant	• Exfoliative properties • Stimulates ground matrix components production • Bactericidal • Moisturizing properties

Table 15.3 Cosmoceutical peeling regimens.

Agent	Mechanism of Action	Dose	Side Effects
KOJIC ACID: *Aspergillus phenielium* 5-hydroxymetil-4H pyrane 4-1 derivate	• Direct inhibition of tirosinase enzyme through the union of a Cooper molecule	1 gm BID for 90 days	• Contact dermatitis
LICORICE (GLABRIDINA) (GLYCORRIZAGLOBRA) EXTRACT	• Anti-inflammatory and bleaching properties • Inhibits UVB-induced pigmentation • Disperses melanin • Tirosinase inhibition affecting melanocyte DNA	1 gm QD 4 weeks Poor bleaching properties; should be used in combination therapy	• Not known
ARBUTIN DEOXYARBUTIN VACCINIUM LEAF DERIVATE VITISIDAEA (GLUCONOPIRANOSIDA 3%)	• Tirosinase inhibition • Inhibits melanocyte differentiation • Non-direct toxicity on melanocytes • Bleaching properties • Pigment suppression 63% effectivity	1 gm BID 2 weeks	• Paradoxical hyperpigmentation if concentrations above 3% are used
HYDROQUINONE (HQ Benzene-1-4diol 2%)	• Direct melanogenesis inhibition • Tirosinase inhibition • Toxic effect on melanocyte	1 gm BID 2 4 WEEKS	• Local irritation • Post-inflammatory hyperpigmentation • Oocronosis • Carcinogenesis in animals
NIACINAMIDE NICOTINAMIDE B COMPLEX 3.5% retinyl palmitate	• Hydrosoluble • Inhibits melanin transfer to keratinocyte • Reduces hyperpigmentation • Increases skin elasticity and hydration	1 gm BID 4 weeks	• Not known
AZELAIC ACID	• Tirosinase inhibition • Cytotoxic effect on melanocytes	1 gm BID 12 weeks	• Local irritation
EDELWEISS complex (violet cream)	• Oligonucleotides act blocking gene transcription • Melanogenesis modulator • Bleaching effect in normal and hyperpigmented skin	1 gm BID 8 weeks	• Not known

performed in-office by a trained skin care professional. It may also be performed at home using a variety of products that are designed to mechanically exfoliate the skin. As these treatments do not affect the basal layer of the skin, they have sub-optimal effects on depigmentation.

Laser treatments

Laser devices such as a fractional CO_2 laser have important advantages including a finding of 30% more collagen production than the Er:YAG laser [11], resulting in better cosmetic results.

The term "fractional" refers to the fact that only a fraction of skin is treated by producing columns of heat, leaving surrounding dermal tissue intact. The result is a safer treatment with less downtime.

Laser may be used for vulvar hyperpigmentation in selected cases with well- established protocols to prepare the skin before and after treatment. The most common protocol used is to prepare the skin with low potency topical steroids 2–3 days prior to laser application. Two sessions 2 months apart are sufficient to lighten the skin of the vulva and perianal region with long-term results (personal experience of author). Fractional CO_2 laser acts via an indirect photothermolysis effect generating epidermal exchange, thus increasing vulvar capability to retain water molecules, and is a safe procedure that may be performed on an outpatient basis with a high degree of satisfaction [11].

Miscellaneous vulvar and perineal lightening techniques
Self- applied treatments

The best creams for vaginal bleaching are specifically formulated for sensitive areas. These creams, while slightly more expensive than normal skin lightening creams, have been prepared using ingredients such as vitamin B3, lemon juice, mulberry and bearberry extract, and licorice extract. Commercially available products advertise themselves as specifically formulated for specific conditions; however, no peer-reviewed

proof exists. Medical supervision is helpful to diminish the risk of post-inflammatory hyperpigmentation, which has been seen with the use of these products.

Superficial Peeling

Superficial peeling aims to restore skin color and texture and should be applied by a health care provider (Tables 15.2 and 15.3).

References

1. Masters, WH, Johnson VE. *Human Sexual Response*. Toronto: Bantam Books, 1966.
2. Pauls RN, Fellner AN, Davila GW. Vaginal laxity; a poorly understood quality of life problem. Survey of physician members of the International Urogynecological Association (IUGA). *Int Urogynecol J* 2012;**23**:1435–48.
3. Salvatore S, Nappi RE, Zerbinati N, et al. A 12-week treatment with fractional CO_2 laser for vulvovaginal atrophy: A pilot study. *Climacteric* 2014;**17**:363–9.
4. Sekiguchi Y, Utsugisawa Y, Azikosi Y, et al. Laxity of the vaginal introitus after childbirth: Nonsurgical outpatient procedure for vaginal tissue restoration and improved sexual satisfaction using low-energy radiofrequency thermal therapy. *J Wom Health* 2013;**22**:775–81.
5. Millheiser LS, Pauls RN, Herbst SJ, Chen OT. Radiofrequency treatment of vaginal laxity after vaginal delivery: Non-surgical vaginal tightening. *J Sex Med* 2010;**7**:3088–95.
6. Vizintin Z, Rivera M, Fistonic I, et al. Novel minimally invasive VSP Er:YAG laser treatments in gynecology. *J Laser Health Acad* 2012;**1**:46–58.
7. Lee MS. Treatment of vaginal relaxation syndrome with an Er:YAG laser using 90 and 360 scanning scopes: A pilot study and short term results. *Laser Ther* 2014;**23**: 129–38.
8. Goldberg D. Lasers for facial rejuvenation. *Am J Clin Dermat* 2003;**4**:225–34.
9. Levitt J. The safety of hydroquinone: A dermatologist's response to the 2006 Federal Register. *J Am Acad Dermatol* 2007;**57**:854.
10. Anneta E, Resko D. Cosmoceuticals: Practical applications. *Dermatologic Clinics* 2009;**27**(4):401–16.
11. Hunzeker C. Fractionated CO_2 laser resurfacing: Our experience with more than 2000 treatments. *Aesth Surg Jour* 2009; **29**:317–22.

CHAPTER 16

Surgical risks and untoward outcomes

Otto J. Placik

Northwestern University Feinberg School of Medicine, Chicago, IL, USA

Good judgment comes from experience and a lot of that comes from bad judgment.

Will Rogers

Introduction

Scope

Although cataloging a complete list of risks of vulvo-vaginal procedures is unlikely, I will detail a range of potential complications. Surgical procedures considered include:

A Mons reduction/liposuction/lift
B Labia majora reduction
C Elective clitoral surgery: clitoral hood reduction or clitoral unhooding or clitoropexy
D Labia minora reduction
E Vaginoplasty/perineoplasty or "vaginal rejuvenation"
F Hymenoplasty/hymenorrhaphy
G Labia majora augmentation

Many of the complications will be discussed in the relevant chapters devoted to each topic. Additional procedures, including the G-Shot, O-Shot, and the range of non-surgical aesthetic enhancement procedures such as bleaching or hair removal or ornamentation/pigmentation/piercing/adornment will not be reviewed here but also have a unique set of adverse outcomes. For clarification purposes, the G-Shot is a registered trademark name for the clinical procedure of the Gräfenberg spot (G-spot) augmentation by sub-cutaneous injection of fillers that initially was performed with commercially available collagen but now is accomplished with a variety of other agents. The O-Shot is also another registered trademark, an abbreviation of the Orgasm Shot. In this procedure autologous derived platelet-rich plasma (PRP) is injected around the clitoris and vagina to provide relief to women complaining of stress urinary "incontinence and with sexual dysfunction" by activating the female orgasm system [1]. There is presently no information in peer-reviewed literature regarding the O-Shot.

For transgender women, there are, in addition, a number of surgical procedures intended to reconstruct both the internal and external genital structures. A discussion of these will be reviewed in Chapter 13. Chapter 17 is devoted to revisions and re-operations. Aside from the procedures of labiaplasty and vaginoplasty, there is relatively little data regarding the incidence or frequency of undesirable outcomes among transgender aesthetic procedures, but it can be assumed to be similar in incidence to comparable procedures performed on natal females.

Disclaimer: Beauty is in the eye of the beholder. Unlike traditional functional procedures with a defined objective (e.g., removal of uterus), aesthetic procedures are more difficult to assess in terms of favorable versus undesirable results. The popular media puts increasing focus and attention to the evolving aesthetics of the female pudenda [2]. One of the most critical issues is the subjective nature of beauty and the patient versus the practitioner's ability to attain the desired endpoint. Thus, an outcome that may be judged favorably by the surgeon may be viewed as less than desirable by the patient. The establishment of reasonable expectations in the pre-operative discussion thus becomes paramount in importance.

Within the context of the pre-operative assessment, the aesthetic goals must be reviewed as they pertain to

---

Female Genital Plastic and Cosmetic Surgery, First Edition. Edited by Michael P. Goodman.
© 2016 John Wiley & Sons, Ltd. Published 2016 by John Wiley & Sons, Ltd.

changes being made. The surgical limitations and potential consequences of those changes must be discussed so that the patient has a realistic expectation of the surgeon's intended surgical approach. If the surgeon and patient are not in agreement, this must be resolved prior to surgery. Photographs are often useful to help understand the patient wishes but also to provide objective evidence that is not skewed by unrealistic expectation or fuzzy recollection of the patient's pre-operative state. Patients who are not willing to accept the surgeon's pre-operative aesthetic goals are not good candidates for surgery. Other "red flags" for patient dissatisfaction are discussed below.

As with any aesthetic procedure on paired organs, symmetry is typically expected. Inability to accomplish this may be viewed as a failure. It is well worthwhile to explain pre-operatively that asymmetry is normal. The intended goal of surgery is *less* asymmetry and *not* perfect symmetry. An explanation pre-operatively is exactly that. After surgery, an explanation is viewed as an excuse.

Disclaimer: Sexual function is a highly complex matter not dictated solely by physical appearance or structure. Unfortunately, marketing of these procedures may result in unrealistic expectations of enhancing sexual performance among patients seeking the surgery. At the initial evaluation, it must be explained that alterations in the shape and contour of the external genitalia and a decrease in caliber of the vaginal canal may be successful, yet not resolve sexual dysfunction or relationship conflicts. The examiner should ask about a history of psychosexual insults and the patient's hopes for surgery.

In general, as in any surgical procedure, preventing complications begins with assessing surgical risk via a thorough history and physical to identify goals, expectations, comorbid conditions, and the functional/aesthetic anatomy. Procuring information and patient education are invaluable in achieving successful outcomes. Bleeding diatheses must be excluded in this particularly vascular area. Identifying a history of tobacco use and implementing a strategy for cessation at least 3–4 weeks pre-operatively is advised. A medication history with overview of prescription and over-the-counter medications and herbal supplements should be documented in order to prevent adverse drug reactions or implement restrictions. Nutritional status and special diet must be considered. Screening for body dysmorphic disorder (BDD) can be completed, but recent studies by Goodman

et al.'s group have shown that typical testing BDD instruments may not be valid in the presence of genital functional and aesthetic concerns in women [3,4]. Suffice it to say that women who have previously undergone a variety of body alterations and/or allude to you that they are interested in a narrow and specific result are suspect and should encourage additional evaluation. Bacterial or fungal vulvar conditions should be noted and treated. Sexually transmitted diseases including a history of genital herpes should be elicited and, if present, treated with appropriate prophylactic therapy. Hormone status as well as atrophic conditions may be ameliorated with topical estrogen preparations peri-operatively. A sexual history and function evaluation are advisable and may include a variety of well-established questionnaires such as the Arizona Sexual Experience Questionnaire or the Female Sexual Function Index [5]. Bowel and bladder assessments are critical. Gauging patient compliance with written pre- and post-operative instructions is essential. This includes [1] preparing and educating patients for managing constipation, [2] timing of sexual activity limitations and restrictions, and [3] active involvement in scar intervention with massage and/or dilators, if indicated. Do discuss the patient's support network for recovery.

A general discussion of the risks, alternatives, and benefits with the patient followed by informed consent may include but is not limited to pain (acute and chronic with pain contracts for those already receiving narcotic analgesics), bleeding, infection (appropriate anti-viral, anti-fungal, antibacterial prophylaxis), hematoma, wound breakdown or delayed healing (explaining this is more common in smokers and timing of management/repair), unfavorable scarring, contour irregularity, asymmetry, swelling, altered sensation, pigmentation irregularities, dyspareunia, vulvodynia, potential effects of subsequent pregnancies, need for additional surgery or revisionary procedures, financial responsibilities, and issues related to insurance coverage or elective payment policies. Options for anesthesia are to be offered and weighed.

Whereas the history is commonly acquired with the patient clothed utilizing a variety of intake forms or methods, the physical examination is performed subsequent to the introduction and in the presence of another individual with tradition dictating that at least one is a female. A careful descriptive evaluation of the external and/or internal genitalia (as appropriate) must be carried out and documented. During the physical examination, the physician should note if the findings corroborate complaints as they relate to severity, protrusion, pouching, erythema, redundancy, laxity, and the presence of associated findings such as varicosities, hemorrhoids, cystocele, rectocele, prolapse, and so forth.

Psychometric evaluation may be warranted using validated instruments described in Chapter 18. Laboratory testing is indicated by the history including endocrine evaluation or dictated by anesthesia requirements. Urodynamic studies may be advised if suggested by the history and useful in the surgical planning. Drawing during the consultation is a fabulous method of documenting and is well worthwhile in visual versus verbal recall; computer imaging may be a good fit in this regard. Post-operative instruction sheets and informed consent documents have been presented elsewhere (Chapters 7 and 12). Other "red flags" for an untoward outcome and dissatisfied patients, which I have identified in my practice, include "soft findings" such as:

- *No eye contact*
- *Partner does most of the talking*
- *Passive approach*
- *Office staff reports difficulty*
- *Non-compliant (too late to appointment, failure to pick up prescriptions, disregarding instructions, etc.)*
- *Problems with previous procedures (revisions)*
- *Too busy to listen*
- *Referral to third person likes and dislikes*
- *Adverse response to revision suggestion*
- *Excessive touching during examination*

Surgical technique

A brief comment about the use of various technologies to accomplish the surgery is needed here. Many proponents may tout one surgical method as superior to another in achieving desired results and minimizing complications despite common knowledge that a definitive surgical method is almost never unanimously agreed upon. Outstanding and experienced surgeons, including the contributing authors, use a variety of instruments and technologies with excellent outcomes, and this may include scalpels, scissors, cautery, laser, radiofrequency, and other modalities. Suture techniques and closure methods similarly vary as well with comparable results.

Procedure-specific risks

Each of the respective procedures and the untoward outcomes will be briefly reviewed; redundancy is inevitable, with commentary on:

a How to avoid
b How to deal with them (or not) "in the moment"
c How to deal with them in the long term

A Mons reduction/liposuction/lift

1 *Wound healing complications/scarring*

a *How to avoid*: Operate on nutritionally sound and stable patients. Be aware of patients who are prone to keloid scarring. Get smokers to quit at least 4 weeks prior to surgery. Avoid devascularizing flaps by excessive undermining or tension. Minimize use of electrocautery in deeper fatty tissues and along skin edge. Develop assessment and treatment plans with use of the Pittsburgh Rating Scale as a validated tool [6]. Perform a layered repair incorporating approximation and suspension of the superficial fascia system (SFS) [7]. Plan incisions with attention to anticipated garment wear to conceal scars. Controversy exists with regard to the use of vertical scars; these may be more visible than horizontal reductions or can cause labia majora distortion. These may be placed as a single midline wedge-type excision or as two paramedian incisions extending into each labia majora. I have generally recommended avoiding these but in massive weight loss patients they may be required to reduce excess horizontal width (Figure 16.4). Patients should be informed about the potential for adverse healing and cicatricial alopecia (loss of hair growth within the scar). Studies have shown that while the vascularity of the mons may improve, that of the abdominal flap, particularly in the midline, may be compromised. This may ultimately affect wound healing along the incision. Therefore, minimize wide undermining or liposuction of the abdominal flap. On an anecdotal basis, I have personally found so-called antibacterial sutures (i.e., Vicryl Plus™) to be problematic, with a high incidence of extrusion. I therefore avoid them.

b *How to deal with them (or not) "in the moment"*: Conservative wound care with dressing changes. Two to three times a day wound cleansing with gentle water irrigation or sitz baths is recommended. Intermittent use of cleansers (Cetaphil, Restoraderm, or CeraVe™) is acceptable but should be minimized.

Light application of the associated moisturizing creams with non-adherent dressings such as Telfa™ are suggested. Negative pressure wound therapy may be of use. Consider use of hyperbaric oxygen. Consider injections with triamcinolone.

c *How to deal with them in the long term*: Scar revision at a later date deferred by 4–6 months when scar is mature and stable. Silicone gel and/or sheeting and the use of a high SPF sunblock are beneficial in promoting scar maturation, flattening of the scar, and minimizing prolonged erythema or pigmentation irregularities. Consider injections of hypertrophic scars with triamcinolone beginning with 10 mg/ml. Other agents claiming benefits include allium cepa preparations or copper-containing creams or electromagnetic modalities. Scar massage and the use of the Graston™ Technique may be beneficial. Laser hair removal may be useful in decreasing the occurrence of inclusion cysts along the suture line. Alternatively, cicatricial alopecia and hairless areas along the normal hair-bearing portions of the mons may be camouflaged with a tattoo simulating the appearance of hair follicles.

2 *Asymmetry*

a *How to avoid*: Almost impossible to avoid. Asymmetry should be established as an acceptable outcome within surgical expectations. Explain to the patient that symmetry may not be achievable due to several factors including wound healing as well as other associated anatomic (i.e. musculoskeletal) or physiologic factors. Measuring and marking the patient in the supine and standing positions with the mons on simulated tension are useful. Mark with attention and respect to hairline and midline vulvar cleft as reference points. Be aware of pre-existing scars. Use consistent tension along mons when making incision. Suspend mons symmetrically along rectus fascia. Follow pre-operative markings. With liposuction, pay attention to volumes removed from each portion of mons.

b *How to deal with them (or not) "in the moment"*: Adjust sutures as needed to correct asymmetric pull. Avoid over-resection with liposuction. Consider fat grafting when necessary. Not always treatable.

c *How to deal with them in the long term*: See A1c above. Fat grafting may be long- term solution. Scar revision to alter height or direction of scar. This is best deferred for 6–9 months.

3 *Infection*

a *How to avoid*: Administer prophylactic antibiotics. Perform an adequate prep with attention to sterile technique. When patients report a history or have physical findings of intertrigo or erythema in the suprapubic crease, I will often recommend that topical anti-fungal agents, such as 1% clotrimazole cream, be applied to the area twice a day for 1 week pre-operatively, although success of this is anecdotal. Although povidone-iodine agents are traditionally used for the vulva, there is increasing off-label use of chlorhexidene gluconate solutions with low concentrations of alcohol [8]. Avoid dead space.

b *How to deal with them (or not) "in the moment"*: Drain and obtain wound culture and sensitivity studies with empiric antibiotics while awaiting results. I commonly employ topical Silvadene™ while culture results are pending. Rapidly progressive infections may be suggestive of necrotizing fasciitis or Fournier's gangrene, particularly in high-risk individuals with certain conditions (diabetes, alcoholism, malnutrition, immunocompromised or immunosuppressed); however, these patients are certainly poor candidates for elective vulvovaginal plastic/cosmetic surgery. This will require aggressive treatment with radical debridement with appropriate monitoring and the suggested use of hyperbaric oxygen therapy. Wound care with dressing changes. The use of a 50% dilution of Dakin's solution (also described by Hegger as 0.025% sodium hypochlorite) was both bactericidal and non-toxic to tissues and with favorable effects on wound healing (9,10).

4 *Hematoma/bleeding/bruising*

a *How to avoid*: Exclude history of coagulopathy. Insure cessation of aspirin and NSAIDs for at least 10 days pre-operatively. Be aware of blood pressure during peri-operative period. Accomplish meticulous hemostasis during the procedure. Apply compression dressings where possible across incisions.

b *How to deal with them (or not) "in the moment"*: Use of suture ligation for obvious vessels, electrocautery for pinpoint bleeding. Emergently evacuate an expanding hematoma with possible drain placement or fibrin glue or quilting sutures and compression dressing. Transfusion is unusual unless the patient has a coagulopathy. Aspiration of an established and stable hematoma undergoing liquefaction at 7–10 days may suffice but may be better performed with a liposuction cannula. Smaller hematomas can be managed conservatively with pressure and time.

5 *Seroma* (Figure 16.1).

a *How to avoid*: Be aware of lymphatics and perform subdermal dissection over femoral region to preserve vasculature and drainage system. Quilting sutures may also help.

b *How to deal with them (or not) "in the moment"*: Repeated aspiration is typically sufficient. If recurrent, consider sclerosis with surgical talc or doxycycline/tetracycline and quilting sutures and/or percutaneous drain such as a SeromaCath™.

c *How to deal with them in the long term*: Chronic seroma may require excision of an associated pseudo-cyst and ablation of dead space. Rarely, lymphatic ligation may be required.

6 *Edema*

a *How to avoid*: See 5a above. Swelling is normal and to be expected. Patients should be prepared for this outcome. Some physicians favor the use of intraoperative steroids. Consider use of NSAIDS post-operatively after assuring a period of adequate hemostasis. Cold compresses are generally administered. Instruct patients in minimizing dependency or unnecessary mobilization of the area. Recommend gentle compression garments.

b *How to deal with them (or not) "in the moment"*: Prolonged use of compression wear with cold compresses. Prescribe manual lymphatic drainage by certified therapist.

c *How to deal with them in the long term*: Same as 6b above.

7 *Pain/alteration in skin sensation*

a *How to avoid*: Be informed and educated about anatomic variability of the ilioinguinal innervation to the pubis. Caution with dissection over femoral neurovascular structures [11].

b *How to deal with them (or not) "in the moment"*: I prefer use of long-term absorbable sutures rather than permanent sutures to minimize nerve entrapment or ligation or suture granulomas. Local anesthetics are most common form of management administered intraoperatively. Longer lasting anesthetics such as Exparel™ with or without the use of a nerve block technique are less commonly instituted. Even less frequent is the use of indwelling catheters from a pain pump. Local anesthetics are supplemented with oral medications such as narcotic analgesics and delayed use of NSAIDs or COX-2 inhibitors such as Celebrex. Cold compresses provide some analgesic effects.

c *How to deal with them in the long term*: Excision of neuromas is rarely needed. Remove permanent suture material. Provide referral to pelvic therapist for ultrasound therapy and scar desensitization. Consider referral to pain management specialist.

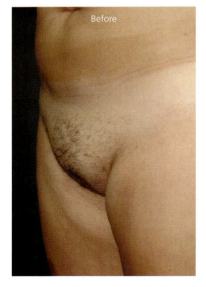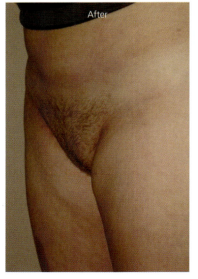

Figure 16.1 Recurrent seroma requiring repeated aspiration and sclerosis. Source: O. Placik. Reproduced with permission.

8 *Contour irregularities*

As is the case with liposuction anywhere else on the body, the most common complaint is insufficient volume reduction and/or lax skin with irregularities (Figure 16.2).

a *How to avoid*: When performing liposuction, the use of smaller cannulas and staying as deep as possible will minimize irregularities. With a pubic lift, attention must be paid to the thickness of the mons versus the abdominal flap. Patients should appreciate that long-term changes may be due to subsequent pregnancy, weight loss or gain, and aging.

b *How to deal with them (or not) "in the moment"*: Beveling the thicker mons flap may diminish the prominence or bulge of the mons and provide a smoother transition from the abdomen to the mons. Alternatively, sharp defatting of the deeper or superficial fatty layers may help to debulk a particularly thick mons pubis.

c *How to deal with them in the long term*: The use of "lipomassage" techniques such as Endermologie™ of the mons may help mitigate the cellulite-type appearance of unevenly performed liposuction. Fat grafting of depressions via lipoinjection techniques may also be beneficial.

9 *Anesthetic/allergies*

a *How to avoid*: A thorough history with review of medication and latex sensitivities and allergies is essential. Avoid use of triggering agents when indicated. Perform desensitization, when necessary, under supervision of an allergist. Management of sleep apnea and comorbid conditions should be addressed with possible pre-operative anesthetic consultations when general anesthesia or IV sedation is administered. Patient's health status should be optimized when undergoing general anesthesia. Perform procedures in facilities commensurate with patient's health status. Adhesives and tape or sutures

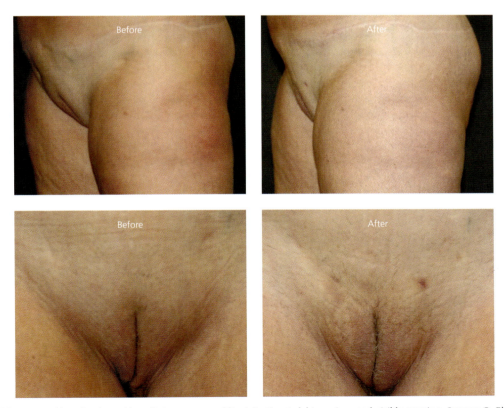

Figure 16.2 Mons pubis reduction with radiofrequency and lipoinjection to labia majora and visible scarring. Source: O. Placik. Reproduced with permission.

should not be used in individuals with a history of sensitivity.

b *How to deal with them (or not) "in the moment"*: Protocols and medications for managing anaphylactic reactions as well as hyperthermia should be in place. Topical allergic reactions should be treated with discontinuation of offending agents with possible topical or systemic therapy. Anaphylaxis requires emergent treatment.

10 *Need for revisionary surgery*

a *How to avoid*: Follow standards of care and exercise good judgment in carrying out all aspects of pre-, intra-, and post-operative care. Be cautious with liposuction and avoiding over- or undercorrection. Anticipate and explain potential for recurrent laxity and hairline displacement with need for hair removal particularly in massive weight loss patients. Complete a layered repair to disperse wound tension.

b *How to deal with them (or not) "in the moment"*: Have an existing written policy in place or as part of the informed consent to discuss the need for revisionary surgery. Need to be handled on a case-by-case basis. Most can be performed under local anesthesia.

c *How to deal with them in the long term*: Most revisions should be deferred for a minimum of 6–9 months to allow sufficient time for scar maturation and contraction.

11 *Financial issues*

a *How to avoid*: A clear-cut financial policy agreement should be provided to patient prior to surgery. Issues of health insurance coverage or non-coverage in the case of elective surgery should be discussed pre-operatively.

b *How to deal with them (or not) "in the moment"*: Have a designated office staff manage financial matters. Physician should focus on treatment. Insurance issues may be more efficiently handled by third parties or outsourced.

12 *Diversion of urine stream*

a *How to avoid*: Measure patient in standing position with simulated upward displacement of mons to assess skin resection and final position but adjust intraoperatively. Stay at least 5 cm above vulvar cleft. Suspend SFS to abdominal wall fascia but to not place excessive cephalad tension. Monitor vulvar distortion while placing SFS anchoring sutures.

b *How to deal with them (or not) "in the moment"*: Adjust suspension sutures if noting marked vulvar distortion. While many patients actually report alteration in the urine stream, it did not appear to be problematic and some noted diminished bladder incontinence in one study [7].

c *How to deal with them in the long term*: Not necessary. Ultimately, if symptomatic elevation and release and advancement of mons could provide some relief but is not described nor recommended.

13 *Suture granulomas*

a *How to avoid*: Use longer lasting absorbable sutures rather than permanent sutures.

b *How to deal with them (or not) "in the moment"*: Exploration and excision is typically sufficient and will resolve the problem.

14 *Dissatisfied patients*

a *How to avoid*: Pre-operative review of good, bad, and average results may help physician to understand patient expectations. Discuss overall body contour and BMI to put regional treatment in context of overall proportions. Ask patient about familiarity with others who have undergone the procedure and review the spectrum of responses and results from surgery.

b *How to deal with them (or not) "in the moment"*: See patients at regular periods during post-operative period. Allow sufficient time for healing to become stable. Review pre-operative discussions and overview of before and after photographs. Perform revision surgery if acceptable goals can be established and realistically accomplished.

c *How to deal with them in the long term*: Second opinions from colleagues may provide re-assurance of acceptable outcome. Consider support groups. Possibly refer patients for cognitive behavioral therapy in instances of BDD.

B Labia majora reduction

Sometimes performed with mons reduction and labia minora reduction, labia majora reduction may be a stand-alone procedure.

1 *Wound healing complications/scarring/color*

a *How to avoid*: See A1a above. If possible, place the final scar so that it lies in the non-hair bearing portions of the labia to diminish risk of keloid and cicatricial alopecia. Layered sutures with attention to repair Colles' fascia will help to distribute wound tension and minimize irregularities. A few interrupted vertical mattress sutures will evert the wound edges in this area where there is a tendency for inversion along the inter-labial sulcus.

b *How to deal with them (or not) "in the moment"*: See A1b above.

c *How to deal with them in the long term*: Much of this is discussed in A1c above. Pertinent changes are added here. For major defects, a variety of flaps (V-Y, gluteal, medial thigh, pudendal, gracilis or rectus abdominis flaps) have been utilized in the reconstruction of extirpative defects following oncologic resection but are not generally capable of delivering aesthetic quality results [12]. However, a wound of this size is highly unlikely and the vast majority can be completed with excision, residual local tissue re-arrangement, and scar revision at a later date. On occasion, medial and inward rotation of the hair-bearing portion of the labia majora may result in alteration in the direction of hair growth that may irritate the labia minora; in this instance, hair removal (shaving, electrolysis or laser) may alleviate the discomfort.

2 *Asymmetry*

a *How to avoid*: See A2a above. Point out anatomic features that contribute to asymmetry. If larger resections are planned, consider the use of "tailor tack" sutures to assess the final result and potential on final appearance prior to completing definitive wound suture. Be aware of leg positioning in the lithotomy position to assure the least degree of asymmetry and the effect on labia distortion.

b *How to deal with them (or not) "in the moment"*: Adjust sutures as needed to correct asymmetric pull. If principles of under-resection are practiced early in one's career, sequential resection of the larger side will result in a satisfactory outcome. These are not always treatable as some features of asymmetry cannot be corrected.

c *How to deal with them in the long term*: Scar revision may be used to alter height or direction of scar. This is best deferred for 6–9 months. Further reduction of the larger side may be contemplated. Augmentation of the smaller side may be more difficult; one may consider the use of fat grafting via lipoinjection. This may require multiple stages. One may try to simulate the appearance and assess the patient's response using injection of saline (short term) or fillers such as Resytlane™ for a longer result.

3 *Infection*

a *How to avoid*: Do not operate on patients who have recently depilated and have folliculitis. Advise patients not to shave the night prior to surgery. Otherwise, follow precautions as discussed in A3a above.

b *How to deal with them (or not) "in the moment"*: Managed identically to measures described above in A3b.

4 *Hematoma/bleeding/bruising*

a *How to avoid*: The area is highly vascular and hematoma may occur. This gives more reason to follow the precautions followed in A4a above.

b *How to deal with them (or not) "in the moment"*: See management described in A4b above (Figure 16.3).

5 *Edema*

a *How to avoid*: Edema will occur and is to be expected but is less than the labia minora. Be aware of lymphatics and perform limited subdermal dissection to preserve the vascularity and drainage system of the flaps. Minimize strangulating effect of sutures and incisions. Place sutures more loosely than other parts of the body to anticipate the marked swelling that occurs. Remaining precautions are similar to those discussed in A6a above.

b *How to deal with them (or not) "in the moment"*: Same as A6b above.

6 *Pain/alteration in skin sensation*

a *How to avoid*: Be informed and educated about the different sensory innervation of the anterior and posterior parts of the labium majus. The anterior third of the labium majus is supplied by the ilioinguinal nerve (L1) and genital branch of the genitofemoral nerve to the pubis, whereas the posterior two-thirds are supplied by the labial branches of the perineal nerve (S3), and the lateral aspect is also innervated by the perineal branch of the posterior cutaneous nerve of the thigh (S2) [13]. Dissection in the depths of the inter-labial sulcus at the level of the meatus is to be avoided.

b *How to deal with them (or not) "in the moment"*: Long-term absorbable sutures are not used here but instead sutures such as Monocryl or Vicryl Rapide™ are employed. Otherwise pain management mirrors A7b above.

c *How to deal with them in the long term*: In the early phases, referral to a pelvic therapist for desensitization while anticipated nerve recovery or dysesthesias

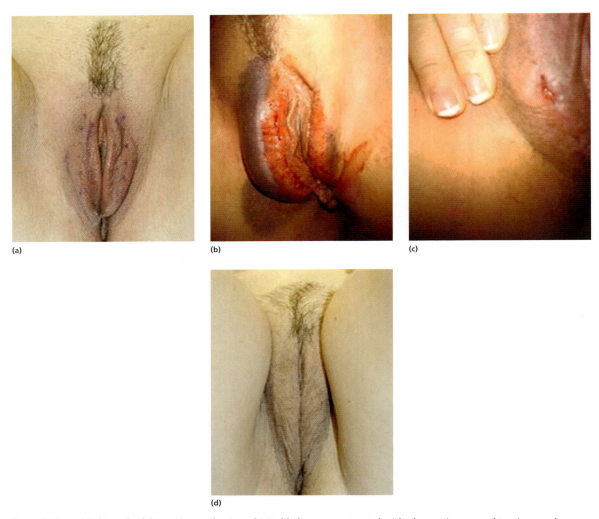

Figure 16.3 (a) Markings for labia majora reduction. (b) Stable hematoma treated with observation wound tension results in (c) slight superficial edge deshiscence treated with wound care. (d) Healed at 3 months without surgical intervention. Source: O. Placik. Reproduced with permission.

resolve may be beneficial. A variety of modalities such as external massage or ultrasound may be employed. Superficial wound dehiscence with any technique may produce an area of tissue attenuation and thinning that causes tenderness and hypersensitivity. Resection and approximation of normal tissues often produces resolution.

7 *Contour irregularities*

These are generally minimal in this area.

a *How to avoid*: Repeatedly assess wound tension during closure, Attention should be paid to equal distribution of skin on either side of the incision to avoid "bunching" that may lead to "dog-ears." Use only interrupted or running continuous inverting sub-cutaneous sutures, incorporating the fascia to provide symmetric wound approximation. It has been suggested to repair any Colles' fascial defects with a small-caliber running suture. Closure may be via sub-cuticular absorbable or interrupted nylon skin sutures removed +1 week later.

b *How to deal with them (or not) "in the moment"*: Meticulous attention to wound closure should minimize the occurrence of contour irregularities. If noted at the time of surgery, remove and replace the sutures until a satisfactory outcome is achieved. As stated above radiofrequency treatment may diminish or eliminate minor irregularities. Some surgeons have used laser resurfacing or radiofrequency treatment but this is not a conventional approach and is likely best for only minor irregularities

  c *How to deal with them in the long term*: The use of scar massage and passage of time (6–9 months) typically results in resolution of most minor irregularities with scar maturation and remodeling. Patients are generally re-assured during this time and discouraged from undergoing scar revision unless performed for marked wound separation. Widened scars can be revised at 6–9 months. Scalloping of the wound edges may be treated with excision and closure or with radiofrequency resurfacing.

 8 *Anesthetic/allergies*
  Identical to A9 above.
 9 *Need for revisionary surgery*
  Identical to A10 above.
 10 *Financial issues*
  Identical to A11 above.
 11 *Suture granulomas*
  Identical to A13 above.
 12 *Dissatisfied patients*
  Identical to A14 above.

C Elective clitoral hood surgery

This can include various procedures such as [1] clitoral hood size reduction, or [2] clitoral unhooding (unroofing of phimotic central hood), or [3] Other hood manipulations not previously described in Chapter 8. Many other terms have been used such as clitoroplasty, clitoral hood removal, clitoral hoodectomy, hoodplasty, and dorsal slit surgery but are not specifically referenced here. The complications will be discussed below as they refer to each of these

 1 *Wound healing complications/scarring*
  a *How to avoid*: Operate on nutritionally sound and stable patients. Be aware of patients who are prone to keloid scarring. Get smokers to quit at least 4 weeks prior to surgery. Avoid devascularizing flaps by excessive undermining or tension. Minimize use of electrocautery in deeper fatty tissues and along skin edge. Ensure your history and physical examination exclude the potential for lichen sclerosus. Physical examination should evaluate the presence of piercings

that may interfere with healing of the incisions. When unhooding is performed for lichen sclerosus, clobetasol is typically prescribed but should be discontinued 2–4 weeks prior to surgery. Be aware of any adhesions, particularly in mobilizing the hood for surgery. Incorporate a layered repair of incisions. With any procedure on the clitoral complex, excessive manipulation of the glans proper may induce injury with scarring that may result in iatrogenic adhesions. In the case of a hood reduction, excessive skin removal may produce retraction and unintended exposure of the clitoris. Controversy exists with incision design for hood reduction; some surgeons prefer divergence of the superior limbs of the incisions versus others who recommend convergence. Converging superior scars may produce greater edema in the circumcised tissues of the hood. Vertical incisions parallel the vascular supply and are commonly employed.

  b *How to deal with them (or not) "in the moment"*: Conservative wound care with dressing changes. Consider use of hyperbaric oxygen. Consider injections of hypertrophic scars with triamcinolone beginning with 10 mg/ml.

  c *How to deal with them in the long term*: Scar revision at a later date deferred by 4–6 months when scar is mature and stable. Silicone gel may be beneficial in promoting scar maturation, flattening of the scar, and minimizing prolonged erythema or pigmentation irregularities. Other agents claiming benefits include allium cepa preparations or copper-containing creams or electromagnetic modalities.

 2 *Asymmetry*
  a *How to avoid*: Almost impossible to avoid. Asymmetry should be established as an expected surgical outcome. Explain to patient that symmetry may not be achievable due to several factors including wound healing as well as other associated anatomic (i.e., musculoskeletal) or physiologic factors. Measuring and marking the patient in the supine and standing positions with the skin on simulated tension are useful. If larger resections for the clitoral hood are planned, consider the use of "tailor tack" sutures to assess the final result and potential on asymmetric hood retraction. Mark with attention and respect to the midline vulvar cleft and inter-labial sulcus as reference points. Be aware of pre-existing scars or piercings or adhesions from lichen sclerosus. Use consistent

tension or retraction along hood when making incision. Follow pre-operative markings and take intra-operative swelling into account with under-resection rather than over-resection.

b *How to deal with them (or not) "in the moment"*: Adjust sutures as needed to correct asymmetric pull. Consider inferiorly based flaps from the labia minora when necessary in the event of over-resection. Similarly, skin grafting from the locally redundant tissues of the contralateral hood or labia minora can be performed but are less reliable than flaps and will require quilting stitches or a stent-type dressing. Not always treatable.

c *How to deal with them in the long term*: See C1c and 2b above. In addition V-Y advancement flaps of the clitoral hood can be considered based on Buck's fascia [14]. Scar revision to alter height or direction of scar. This is best deferred for 6+ months. (See Figures 17.12–17.15 in Chapter 17.)

3 *Infection* (Figure 16.6)

a *How to avoid:* See A3a above.

b *How to deal with them (or not) "in the moment"*: See A3b above.

4 *Hematoma/bleeding/bruising*

a *How to avoid*: See A4a above.

b *How to deal with them (or not) "in the moment"*: See A4b above. Use of suture ligation for obvious vessels, electrocautery or bipolar cautery for pinpoint bleeding. Emergently evacuate expanding hematoma with possible drain placement or fibrin glue.

5 *Edema*

a *How to avoid*: Be aware of lymphatics and perform subdermal dissection to preserve vasculature and drainage system, which is accomplished by staying superficial to Buck's fascia. Avoid horizontal incisions across hood; however, these are occasionally recommended for clitoropexy. Place sutures loosely to anticipate the marked swelling that occurs. Swelling is normal and to be expected. Patients should be prepared for this outcome. Consider use of NSAIDs post-operatively after assuring a period of adequate hemostasis. Cold compresses are generally administered. Instruct patients in minimizing dependency or unnecessary mobilization of the area. Recommend gentle compression garments.

b *How to deal with them (or not) "in the moment"*: Prolonged use of compression wear with cold compresses. Prescribe manual lymphatic drainage by a certified therapist.

6 *Pain/alteration in skin sensation*

a *How to avoid*: Educate patients about expectations and the potential for sensitivity particularly with an unhooding. The incidence of dyspareunia following elective clitoral surgery is not well described but has been reported as a complication. Be informed and educated about anatomic variability of the internal and external pudendal innervation of the vulvar structures [15]. The dorsal nerve of the clitoris pierces through the perineal membrane approximately 2.4–3.0 cm lateral to the urethral meatus and travels on the membrane for 1.8–2.2 cm to the ischiopubic ramus, where it travels along the antero-lateral surface of the clitoral body for 2.0–2.5 cm. Dissection in the depths of the inter-labial sulcus at the level of the meatus is to be avoided. Be cautious when operating lateral to the midline and deep to Buck's fascia. It is not well known that the undersurface of the prepuce has many sensory nerves and direct surgery in this location is generally not advised unless indicated for lysis of adhesions [16]. When performing an unhooding, it may therefore be preferable to create flaps that preserve the undersurface of the prepuce rather than resect it. Over-zealous hood reduction may produce an exposed clitoris with initial hypersensitivity followed eventually by decreased sensitivity secondary to desensitization from chronic stimulation.

b *How to deal with them (or not) "in the moment"*: Transvaginal pudendal nerve blocks are useful for limiting pain in the immediate post-operative period. I prefer avoiding paramedian surgery deep to fascia of the clitoral hood. Deep dissection over the clitoris should be limited. Local anesthetics are the most common form of management administered intraoperatively. Longer lasting anesthetics such as Exparel™ with or without the use of a transvaginal pudendal or other local nerve block technique are less commonly instituted after the fact and are better implemented prophylactically. Local anesthetics are supplemented with oral medications such as narcotic analgesics and delayed use of NSAIDs or COX-2 inhibitors. Cold compresses provide some analgesic effects. Although the topical post-operative use of Dermaplast™ is conventionally recommended by gynecologists, I have found that patients have experienced improved pain relief with conservative use of Neo To Go First Aid Antiseptic/Pain Relieving Spray™.

c *How to deal with them in the long term*: In the early phases, referral to a pelvic therapist for desensitization while anticipated nerve recovery or dysestheisas resolve may be beneficial. A variety of modalities such as external massage or ultrasound may be employed. Chronic pain is an exceptionally difficult problem to manage in this area. Neurorrhaphy, neurolysis, or excision of neuromas of the dorsal nerve of the clitoris is best performed by an individual with experience. In the event that a patient complains of excess sensitivity from an over-zealous resection and clitoral exposure, the residual hood may be advanced using a V-Y flap technique [17]. Consider referral to pain management specialist.

7 *Contour irregularities*

These are generally minimal in this area particularly for unhooding or clitoropexy.

a *How to avoid*: When performing hood reduction, repeated assessment of wound tension and closure should be exercised throughout the procedure. Excessive wound tension may result in skin necrosis, separation, and irregularities. I relieve tension and "tack" wound edges with a few interrupted deep dermal sutures, followed by a sub-cuticular suture with buried knots, followed by a third and reinforcing layer of a few loosely tied simple interrupted sutures. Radiofrequency has been used to "resurface" the wound edges by "feathering" at the conclusion of the procedure (personal communication, Red Alinsod MD).

b *How to deal with them (or not) "in the moment"*: See B7b above.

c *How to deal with them in the long term*: See B7c above.

8 *Anesthetic/allergies*

Identical to A9a above.

9 *Need for revisionary surgery*

Identical to A10 above.

10 *Financial issues*

Identical to A11 above.

11 *Suture granulomas*

Identical to A13 above.

12 *Dissatisfied patients*

Identical to A14 above.

13 *Sexual dysfunction*

a *How to avoid*: Please read initial disclaimer. It is clear that there is a public perception and (many patients will) question if surgery on the clitoral

complex will enhance sexual function. The answer is more difficult, and this must be relayed to the patient prior to undergoing surgery. Sexual dysfunction may be due to an excessively prominent or covered clitoris or the awareness of an "unattractive" clitoris in addition to other factors such as medical endogenous or exogenous endocrine conditions, psychological maturity, as well as the individual's and sexual partner's understanding. However, this needs to be elucidated through a history and physical in consultation with other therapists. Critics have stated that the resection of erogenous and sensate tissue is likely to be responsible for impaired sexual arousal following these procedures [18]. In another study of 407 patients, only 166 patients returned a follow-up questionnaire (41%) [19]. Of these 166 patients, 22.9% [38] reported a positive increase in sexual sensation, whereas 5.4% (9 of 166) described a negative change, but 8 of those 9 rated their satisfaction with the procedure as an 8–10. Sexual function may be assessed with a variety of short validated sexual function surveys such as the Arizona Sexual Experience Questionnaire or the Female Sexual Function Index [5]. "Measuring sexual function after clitoral surgery is as important as anatomical and cosmetic assessment" [20]. However, long-term sexual function is difficult to measure and compromise can occur following clitoral surgery [21]. Lean *et al.* recommend that clitoral surgery be performed by a specialized surgeon with methods that [1] minimize damage to the neurovascular structures, [2] avoid excision of sensitive and erectile tissue, and [3] deliver a desirable aesthetic result within anatomic considerations [20].

b *How to deal with them (or not) "in the moment"*: Patients with diagnosed sexual dysfunction should be counseled prior to surgery with regards to the source of the problem and expectations for correction.

c *How to deal with them in the long term*: Second opinions from colleagues may provide re-assurance of acceptable outcome. Consider support groups. Possibly refer patients for cognitive behavioral therapy in instances of BDD.

D Labia minora reduction

Although exact numbers are not available, this is probably the most common aesthetic vulvovaginal procedure performed by a variety of surgical disciplines; much controversy exists about the broad range of treatment options. The incidence of complications is not clearly known; reports cite risks ranging from a high of 7% to a low of 2.65% [20,22–25]. In one study evaluating combined labiaplasty (labia minora reduction) and/or clitoral hood reduction in 176 individuals, patient self-reported complications were cited as 9.5% (n = 15) and were attributable to comments such as "did not heal right, stitches came out, needed a revision" (n = 6), prolonged healing/pain (n = 5), dyspareunia (n = 3), and excessive bleeding (n = 1) [23]. These were not classified according to surgical technique. Labia minora reduction may be accomplished using many different described approaches such as edge trim (aka sculpted edge, amputation, [curvi]linear resection, etc.), wedge, or fenestration (de-epithelialization) methods. A variety of other techniques (inferior wedge, V-Y advancement, Z-plasty, W-plasty, etc.) exist and essentially are modifications of the above three procedures. Incisions or tissue ablation are carried out using scalpel, scissors, electrocautery, laser, radiofrequency, and other modalities. An ongoing debate about the benefits of the "edge" versus the "wedge" is abundant in the literature and common at every meeting. A recent study of the edge technique reported only one complication of asymmetry in more than 100 patients over a 10-year period [26]. In another series of over 812 modified linear resections of the labia minora and clitoral hood (termed a "composite reduction labiaplasty"), complications included only a "few cases of wound dehiscence requiring surgical correction" [27]. At the heart of this controversy is the goal of preserving the labial edge and minimizing scar. While this may seem rational, it is the color, thickness, and irregularity of the edge that many patients find undesirable. Given the delicate balance between form (aesthetic considerations) and function, this is an ongoing debate with experienced surgeons performing both.

The complications will be discussed below as they refer to each of these.

1 *Wound healing complications/scarring/color/tag/cyst*

  a *How to avoid*: Operate on nutritionally sound and stable patients. Get smokers to quit at least 4 weeks prior to surgery. Do not operate on diabetics not in meticulous control. Be aware of patients who are prone to keloid scarring. True keloids are exceptionally rare in this area of modified epithelium and thick scars are more likely due to hypertrophic scarring from delayed healing. Physical examination should

evaluate the presence of piercings or prior birth trauma (fistulae or tears) that may interfere with healing of the incisions. Look for vascular malformations or varicosities (commonly associated with prominent external hemorrhoids), particularly after childbearing. It is best to avoid varicose areas or refer for venous treatment prior to surgery. Lymphatic malformations are even less common but should be excluded in the physical examination. Although superficial edge dehiscence occurs frequently, this commonly heals uneventfully with wound care. This is also discussed in D7 below. Avoid devascularizing flaps by excessive undermining or tension. Superficial wound dehiscence with any technique may produce tags or an area of tissue attenuation and thinning with potential fistula or sinus tract formation (Figure 16.10; see Chapter 17, Figures 17.5, 17.12–17.14), which cause tenderness and hypersensitivity. If at all possible, avoid bifurcating or trifurcating incision lines ("T-ing incision line"), as the risk of superficial or deep separation at the site of the bi/trifurcation is significant (Figure 16.4). In all cases, evert the wound edges to avoid inclusion cysts or overlapping with superficial dehiscence. In one small study comparing 12 linear edge resections to 7 wedge resections, the authors state the latter had a higher wound dehiscence rate (28.5% vs. 8.3%) but better aesthetic results [28].

There is a longer learning curve for the V-wedge, to acquire the judgment to estimate the angle of the resected tissues. Excessive tension may result in partial (Figures 16.5 and 16.6; Figure 17.7, Chapter 17) or complete wound dehiscence (Figure 17.8, Chapter 17). Early on, it is best to under-resect to minimize this difficult problem. On occasion, one may see color discrepancies (Figure 17.6, Chapter 17) with the superior flap not matching the color of the inferior flap, and this is not always correctable. Modifications are required to treat clitoral hood redundancy. Redundant tissues of the vaginal fourchette may be addressed with a conservative "U-shaped" local resection.

Criticisms of the edge (linear resection) technique include the possibility of over-resection (Figure 16.7; Figure 17.9, Chapter 17), creation of an irregular corrugated edge or truncated appearance, or visible scar along the leading edge. One must take great care, as discussed elsewhere in this chapter, to avoid tight, running, or interlocking sutures; this technique, common to general and undertrained

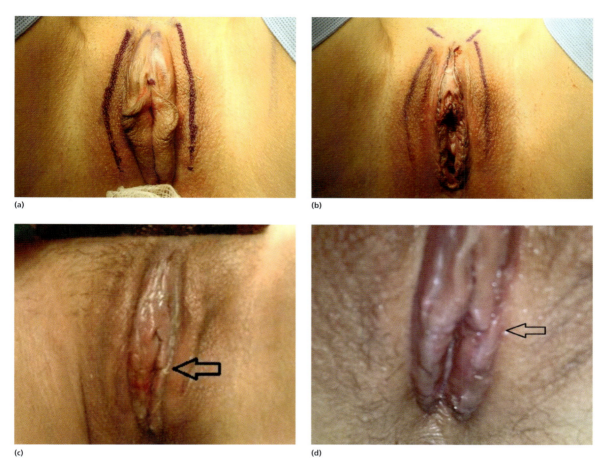

Figure 16.4 (a) Intraoperative view of labiaplasty, RCH, linear resection. (b) View at conclusion of procedure showing intact suture line with trifurcation bilaterally allowing hood/distal frenular fold resection. (c) Post-operative day 10 view with dehiscence at trifurcation of labia minora, clitoral frenulum, and clitoral hood. (d) Cell phone view of patient at 4 weeks showing healing but small gap along leading edge. Patient considering revision. Source: O. Placik. Reproduced with permission.

general gynecological surgeons, produces the results seen in Figures 17.17 and 17.18, Chapter 17. With the edge resection, wound tension is less of a concern unless the labia are especially thick. In this case, a gently beveled incision may be performed along the medial and lateral edges to create a "debulking" effect and the creation of a tapered (as opposed to a blunted) leading edge to the reduced labia. It is generally advised that edge resections be limited to tissue distal to Hart's line (visible sebaceous glands sometimes referred to as Fordyce spots located along the medial aspect of the labia minora). Proximal to this is an area of mucosal epithelium of the vagina essential defined as the vestibule that may produce

unfavorable healing when directly approximated to the stratified squamous epithelium of the lateral surface of the labia minora. This can produce a dry or tethered sensation with intercourse. If wound healing complications ensue, there is a potential for vulvar vestibulitis or pain syndromes as well as diversion of the urinary stream when marked scarring occurs.

With fenestration methods, wound separation may result in a fistula or delayed healing due to inverted wound edges and painful scarring. I recommend avoiding full thickness resection in the "window" and prefer de-epithelialization of the area. When de-epithelialization is completed, limited (2 mm) undermining at the periphery of the fenestration allows a layered repair with wound edge eversion. Specific methods and sutures are discussed in Chapter 8. Estrogen receptors are known to be pre-

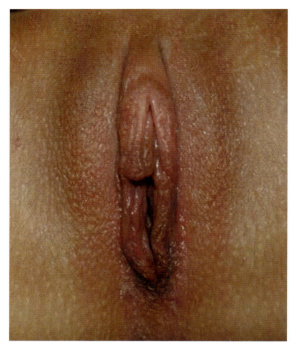

Figure 16.5 Patient with right-sided wedge dehiscence. Source: C. Hamori. Reproduced with permission

sent in the labia minora and have been identified in resected specimens [29]. To assist in healing postoperatively, topical estrogen creams may be useful to assist in post-operative healing, although this is generally reserved for hormonally deficient patients or those reporting symptoms compatible with atrophy [30]. In hormonally diminished patients prescribe this peri-operatively for a minimum of 3–4 weeks prior and 4–6 weeks afterward.

b *How to deal with them (or not) "in the moment"*: See B1b above. Off-label use of topical estrogen cream has been suggested for those with hormone deficiency or atrophy.

c *How to deal with them in the long term*: See B1c above. Consider injections of hypertrophic scars with triamcinolone beginning with 10 mg/ml. Skin tags or cysts, may occur with any approach, and can be excised at +4 months.

2 *Asymmetry*

a *How to avoid*: See B2a above. Traction or tension can easily distort markings. Measure and mark with attention and respect to the midline vulvar cleft and inter-labial sulcus as reference points. Be aware of preexisting scars or piercings or scars from birth trauma/repair. Use consistent tension or retraction along hood when making the incision. Follow pre-operative markings and take intraoperative swelling into account with under-resection rather than over-resection.

b *How to deal with them (or not) "in the moment"*: See B2b above. Consider superiorly based flaps or V-Y from

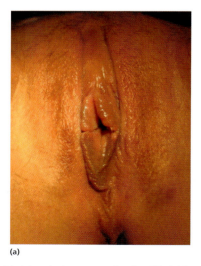
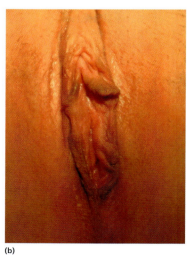

(a)   (b)

Figure 16.6 Patient with (a) early (post-operative day 10) dehiscence following wedge resection, and (b) late results, 2 months post-operatively following conservative wound care. Source: M. Goodman. Reproduced with permission.

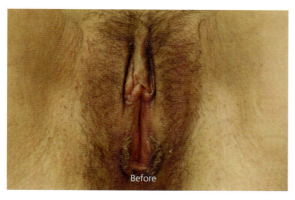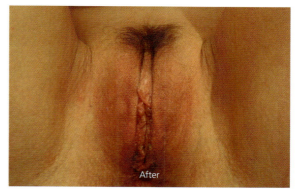

Figure 16.7 Over-resection of left labia minora with subsequent correction. Source: O. Placik. Reproduced with permission.

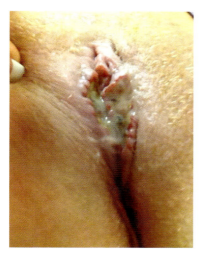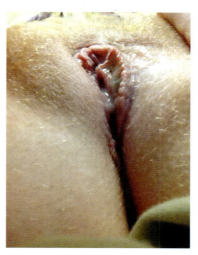

Figure 16.8 Two views of infected and dehisced linear edge resection labiaplasty occurring in the first week post-operatively. Patient sought consultation following surgery elsewhere. Source: M. Goodman. Reproduced with permission.

the clitoral hood when necessary in the event of over-resection. Similarly skin grafting from the locally redundant tissues of the hood or contralateral labia minora can be performed but is less reliable than flaps and will require quilting stitches or a stent-type dressing. Some features of asymmetry cannot be corrected.

c *How to deal with them in the long term*: The reconstructive use of V-Y advancement flaps of the clitoral hood, based on the vascular supply of Buck's fascia, transposed to the labia minora deficit can be considered [14]. Scar revision may be used to alter height or direction of scar. This is best deferred for 6–9 months.

3 *Infection* (Figure 16.8)

a *How to avoid*: Administer prophylactic antibiotic/ anti-viral/anti-fungal agents as indicated. Administer prophylaxis (400 mg acyclovir or 1,000 mg valcyclovir) 10 days before and after surgery) for patients with a history of herpes genitalis. Perform an adequate prep with attention to sterile technique. Avoid dead space during incision closure.

b *How to deal with them (or not) "in the moment"*: See A3b above.

4 *Hematoma/bleeding/bruising* (Figure 16.9)

a *How to avoid*: The occurrence rates of hematoma have been reported to vary from 4–7%. This seems particularly high given verbal communications with experienced practitioners but does warrant attention [31–33]. See A4a above. Observation of the patient for a minimum of 15 minutes following conclusion of the procedure as well as cessation of the vasoconstrictor

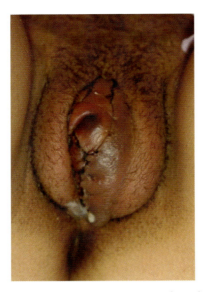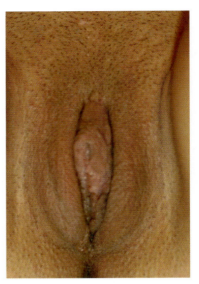

Figure 16.9 Post-operative hematoma treated conservatively, with spontaneous resolution and 3-month appearance. Source: O. Placik. Reproduced with permission.

effects of epinephrine or other agents may be considered. Instruction in stool softeners and bowel laxatives as well as activity limitations to minimize increased venous congestion from straining.

b *How to deal with them (or not) "in the moment"*: See A4b above.

5 *Edema* (Figure 16.11 and Figure 17.4, Chapter 17)

a *How to avoid*: See B5a above. Felicio reports that combined labial and clitoral hood procedures have an increased tendency for edema; therefore surgery may be staged but is typically performed at the same time for convenience purposes [25].

b *How to deal with them (or not) "in the moment"*: See A5b above.

c *How to deal with them in the long term*: Same as A5b above.

6 *Pain/alteration in skin sensation*

a *How to avoid*: Educate patients about expectations and the potential for hypersensitivity. While some patients experience an initial loss of sensitivity, hypersensitivity is not uncommon between day 4 and lasting up to 3 weeks. Concerns have been raised with permanent loss of sensation and/or dyspareunia. While sensory nerve endings are undoubtedly resected, this author's personal experience and the literature notes little effect on sensation using two-point discrimination and no significant

effect on sexual function [18]. Dissection in the depths of the inter-labial sulcus at the level of the meatus is to be avoided. Be cautious when operating lateral to the midline and deep to Buck's fascia. Be aware of Hart's line and perform the majority of your resections distal to this, as this anatomic landmark technically distinguishes the labia minora from the vestibule. Pain syndromes in this area may result in vestibulodynia. When performing an unhooding it may therefore be preferable to create flaps that preserve the undersurface of the prepuce rather than resect it.

b *How to deal with them (or not) "in the moment"*: Transvaginal pudendal nerve blocks are useful for limiting pain in the immediate post-operative period or if the local infiltration does not provide sufficient analgesia. Please read A7b above. Cold compresses provide some analgesic effects. Although the topical post-operative use of Dermaplast™ is conventionally recommended by gynecologists, I have found that patients have experienced improved pain relief with conservative use of Neo To Go First Aid Antiseptic/ Pain Relieving Spray™.

c *How to deal with them in the long term*: See B6c above. Chronic pain is an exceptionally difficult problem to manage in this area. Diagnosis is essential and this is likely known by the surgeon performing the initial

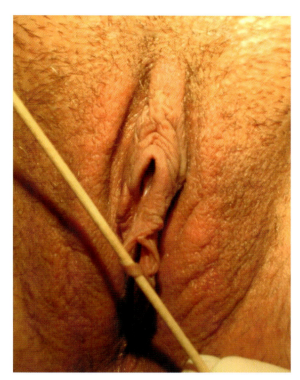

Figure 16.10 Fistula following wedge resection, secondary to rejection subcutaneous 4-0 Vicryl suture. Source: M. Goodman. Reproduced with permission.

procedure. Neurorrhaphy, neurolysis, or excision of neuromas of the dorsal nerve of the clitoris is best performed by an individual with experience. Consider referral to pain management specialist.

7   *Contour irregularities*

a *How to avoid*:   When performing labia minora reduction, repeated assessment of wound tension and closure should be exercised throughout the procedure, especially with the wedge techniques. Excessive wound tension may result in skin necrosis, separation, and irregularities. Running locking sutures provide excellent hemostasis in the perineum and are commonly utilized by many practitioners in this anatomic region; however, they have a greater tendency for wound edge irregularities that may occur with wound edge strangulation that is aggravated by tissue swelling in the post-operative period, and for this reason should be avoided. See wound closure technique in B and D5a and A6a

above. Radiofrequency has been used to "resurface" the wound edges at the conclusion of the procedure (personal communication, Red Alinsod MD).

b *How to deal with them (or not) "in the moment"*:   See B7b above.

c *How to deal with them in the long term*:   See B7c above.

8   *Anesthetic/allergies*
Identical to A9 above.

9   *Need for revisionary surgery*
See A10 above and Chapter 17.

10 *Financial issues*
Identical to A11 above.

11 *Suture granulomas*
Identical to A13 above.

12 *Dissatisfied patients*
Identical to A14 above.

13 *Sexual dysfunction*
Please read C13 as well as comment below.

a *How to avoid*:   Sexual dysfunction may be due prolapse of excessively long labia into the vaginal cavity with intercourse or to ulceration or the perception of an unacceptable appearance in addition to other factors, such as medical endogenous or exogenous endocrine conditions, psychological maturity, as well as the individual's and sexual partner's understanding. While sexual function may improve with labiaplasty, the procedure should not be touted as such, as noted here and elsewhere in this text.

E Vaginoplasty/perineoplasty ("vaginal rejunvenation")

The techniques available for performing perineoplasty/ vaginoplasty or "vaginal rejuvenation," as it is referred to in the lay press, vary from one practitioner to another. The specific approaches are addressed in Chapter 9. A clear appreciation of the sexual function goals to be achieved is essential. Patients must understand the consequences of the smaller diameter introitus and vaginal canal and the implication for increasing sexual friction and contact but not necessarily sexual intimacy. Although inadequate reduction in size is a common complaint, excessive reduction is also possible and may produce vaginismus. The approach will commonly dictate the nature of the complications. In the vast majority of cases, this is typically accomplished using a modification of a colporrhaphy approach along the

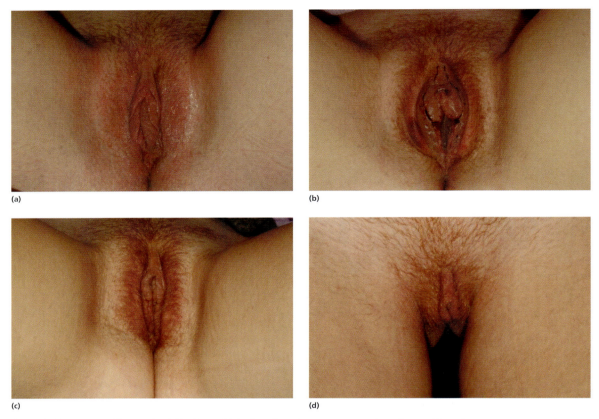

(a)   (b)

(c)   (d)

Figure 16.11 (a) Pre-op linear/edge labiaplasty. (b) Profound persistent post-operative edema without hematoma or wound dehiscence lasting nearly 3 weeks and treated conservatively. (c) and (d) Post-operative result shows relatively large clitoral hood but satisfactory healing. Source: O. Placik. Reproduced with permission.

posterior vaginal wall plus a plastic reconstruction of the introitus (perineoplasty) with significant elevation and bulking of the perineal body. There are unique considerations for each of the other approaches. Therefore, anterior or lateral incisions on the vaginal vault will have a different set of complications specific to the anatomic structures encroached such as the urethra or bladder or suspensory ligaments. The complications and considerations discussed here will relate solely to the posterior vagina/pelvic floor.

Incisions or tissue ablation are carried out using scalpel, scissors, electrocautery, laser, radiofrequency, and other modalities. The incidence of complications is not clearly known and in one study evaluating combined vaginoplasty (defined in this study as work on the proximal vagina) and perineoplasty (lower one-third to one-half of the distal vagina) in 47 individuals,

patient self-reported complications were cited as 16.6% (n = 8) and were attributable to prolonged healing/pain (n = 1), dyspareunia (n = 2), excessive bleeding (n = 2), sensations of being too tight (n = 2), and infection (n = 1) [23].

1 *Wound healing complications/scarring/fistula*

   a *How to avoid*: Operate on nutritionally sound and stable patients. Get smokers to quit at least 4 weeks prior to surgery. Patients with risk factors that increase the potential for increased abdominal pressure and stress on the repair should be addressed preoperatively and include obesity, chronic obstructive pulmonary disease (coughing), chronic constipation, and occupations requiring straining and bearing down. True keloids are exceptionally rare in this area of modified epithelium and thick scars are more likely due to hypertrophic scarring from delayed healing.

History should include inquiries regarding urinary continence, flatus/fecal incontinence and fecal retention, and hemorrhoids in addition to birth trauma, tears and repairs, and prior surgery. Urodynamic studies may be justified. Physical examination should evaluate the presence of prior birth trauma (fistulae or tears) that may interfere with healing of the incisions as well as rectocele or cystocele. The integrity of the levator ani muscles and posterior wall may be assessed by asking the patient to bear down or perform Kegel exercises, as well as with the assistance of a perineometer. A bidigital examination is performed to gain an appreciation for the thickness of the rectovaginal septum especially just proximal to the hymenal ring. Avoid devascularizing flaps by excessive undermining or tension. Superficial wound dehiscence with any technique may produce an area of tissue attenuation and thinning that causes tenderness and hypersensitivity. Layered repairs will help to diminish tension along the wound edge.

The reader is again referred to Chapter 9 on marking and estimating the final vaginal size and suture selection. It is generally preferable to perform limited undermining of the vaginal lining in a progressive fashion as the muscle is exposed and repaired. Be extremely cautious when dissecting just proximal to the hymenal ring where the rectovaginal septum may be particularly thin. The lining is then resected in a conservative fashion to diminish wound tension once the muscle approximation is finished. Slight redundancy is acceptable. This will optimize the vascularity of the wound edge and limit dead space where a hematoma or abscess may develop. Similarly, it is always better to err on the side of undercorrection versus over-correction when completing the mid-vaginal resection and muscle repair. Excellent visualization with an assortment of retraction devices such as the Lone Star™ retractors and drapes with "rectal condoms" and/or vigilant and repeated examination of the rectum while performing both elevation of the vaginal flaps and the ensuing muscle repair will minimize the potential for inadvertent injury or suture of the rectal mucosa. In the event of a rectal injury, avoid excessive use of electrocautery. Interpositional implants, particularly alloplastic materials, are generally not advisable at the time of primary repair and have become a hotbed of controversy and litigation. Layered repairs should incorporate approximation of the bulbospongiosus (crown suture) and the transverse perineal muscles followed by a separate layer for wound edge eversion. The final layer should ensure that the wound edges are everted into the vaginal cavity. Inversion is more likely to cause wound dehiscence and separation. This is especially important at the level of the vaginal fourchette and sufficient laxity should be permitted for a tension-free repair with the legs abducted. Wound breakdown in this area is common and prone to hypersensitivity particularly with sexual activity; the use a few interrupted vertical mattress sutures of 5-0 Monocryl™ in this area takes tension off of the mucosal closure.

Scarring/hemorrhoids/fissures are not uncommon in this region. The posterior extent of the repair commonly encroaches on the perianal tissues, and it is especially important to elicit a history and to conduct a physical examination of hemorrhoids or fissures. These may complicate the procedure and quite often produce additional pain that may exceed the perineoplasty due to a thrombosed hemorrhoid or fissure exacerbation. Make surgical resections taking previous incisions into consideration and incorporating them into the surgical plan. Parallel scars in the perineum may lead to an intervening area of poorly vascularized tissue.

Topical vaginal estrogenization for 1–3 months preoperatively has been shown to increase the vaginal vascularization in peri-/post-menopausal women and may be considered in this group of patients. Incorporation of a layered repair of incisions (i.e., levators first layer; rectovaginal fascia second layer; mucosa/epithelium third layer along with elimination of "dead space") is crucial.

Last, the need for refraining from sexual penetration in the post-operative period should be discussed and is generally advised for a minimum of 6–8 weeks. Resuming activity prior to this may result in wound disruption and discomfort.

b *How to deal with them (or not) "in the moment"*: (Figure 16.12) Conservative wound care with dressing changes. Two to three times a day wound cleansing with gentle water irrigation or sitz baths is recommended.

In the event of a violation of the rectal mucosa, thoroughly irrigate the wound and perform an imbricated and layered repair of the rectal mucosa making sure the edges are everted into the rectum.

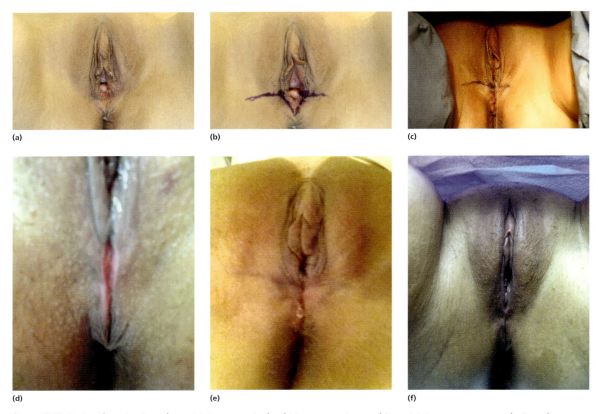

Figure 16.12 Vaginoplasty/perineoplasty. (a) Pre-operatively. (b) Intraoperative markings. (c) Appearance at conclusion of procedure showing intact perineum. (d) Post-operative day 1. (e) Patient's cell phone photograph showing superficial wound edge breakdown on day 12. (f) Appearance of healed wound at 6 weeks treated conservatively with dressing changes. Source: O. Placik. Reproduced with permission.

Alternatively, consider intraoperative consultation with a colorectal surgeon. Follow with a layered repair of muscle. Ensure that the patient will remain on stool softeners for 2–3 weeks. In the post-operative periods, this is very important because narcotic analgesics tend to be constipating. An enterotomy will typically heal uneventfully but, if a fistula develops, referral to a specialist is compulsory. Consider use of hyperbaric oxygen. Topical estrogen cream has been suggested for those with hormone deficiency or atrophy. Patient's enthusiasm for testing the results of surgery has commonly ended in early resumption of sexual activities with wound dehiscence. In most instances, this is treated conservatively.

c *How to deal with them in the long term*: See B1c above.

2 *Asymmetry is less of a concern here than with surgery on the other paired structures.*

a *How to avoid*: Almost impossible to avoid. Asymmetry is normal. Explain to patient that symmetry may not be achievable due to several factors including wound healing as well as other associated anatomic (i.e., musculoskeletal) or physiologic factors. Follow pre-operative markings especially at the vaginal fourchette where the labia minora approximate each other.

b *How to deal with them (or not) "in the moment"*: Adjust sutures as needed to correct asymmetric pull. Not always treatable as some features of asymmetry cannot be corrected.

c *How to deal with them in the long term*: See E1c and 2b above.

3 *Infection*

   a *How to avoid*: See A3a above.

   b *How to deal with them (or not) "in the moment"*: See A3b above.

   c *How to deal with them in the long term*: See E3a and b above for acute infections. In most instances, chronic infections are rare and should be excluded and treated pre-operatively.

4 *Hematoma/bleeding/bruising*

   a *How to avoid*: Exclude history of coagulopathy. Ensure cessation of aspirin and NSAIDs for at least 10 days pre-operatively. Be aware of blood pressure during peri-operative period. Accomplish meticulous hemostasis during the procedure especially in patients with hemorrhoids, as there are numerous dilated varicosities that may require ligation intraoperatively. This author has found placement of a resorbable stay suture 1 cm proximal to the apex of the resection left long (6–7 cm) extremely useful for retraction and placement of additional figure-of-eight hemostatic sutures in the rare event of bleeding at the conclusion of the procedure or in the early post-operative period. Observation of the patient for a minimum of 15 minutes following conclusion of the procedure as well as cessation of the vasoconstrictor effects of epinephrine or other agents may be considered. Instruction in stool softeners and bowel laxatives as well as activity limitations to minimize increased venous congestion from straining and the Valsalva effects are recommended. While bleeding is the primary concern, clotting and subsequent deep venous thrombosis also needs to be addressed when patients undergo general anesthetic. In this event, compression stockings and sequential compression devices are used. Chemoprophylaxis is utilized only if its pre-operative risk assessment warrants it. At the conclusion of the procedure vaginal packing may be utilized if temporary compression is desired.

   b *How to deal with them (or not) "in the moment"*: See A4b above. In persistent oozing a saline-soaked vaginal pack may be used overnight for tamponade but will require a Foley catheter, and hospitalization for observation may be considered with a voiding trial prior to discharge.

5 *Edema*

   a *How to avoid*: See B5a above.

   b *How to deal with them (or not) "in the moment"*: Prevention is best as described above. Prescribe

manual lymphatic drainage by certified therapist in severe cases. Gentle ambulation may assist in lymphatic circulation. Pelvic tilt or elevation can help when the patient is supine.

6 *Pain/alteration in skin sensation/dyspareunia/spasm*

   a *How to avoid*: Educate patients about expectations and the potential for dyspareunia and need for vaginal dilation exercises and prevention of spasm. Tight musculofascial plication will commonly result in spasm that will be painful and aggravated by defecation. A pre-operative bowel prep and post-operative use of stool softeners for 2–3 weeks may be considered. The possibility of vaginal dilation exercises and the need for patient participation should be discussed pre-operatively. Some authors claim that posterior colporrhaphy (performed for various reasons and not necessary for elective enhancement of sexual function) may have an incidence of dyspareunia ranging from 21% to 27% [34]. If presently "partnered," ask patients to describe their partner's erect penis size using an approximation with their thumb and forefinger. The size of the postsurgical introitus and degree of tightening may differ for patients whose partners are on the larger or smaller sides of the size spectrum.

   The surgeon should be informed and educated about the innervation. Whereas the lower vagina and perineal skin is supplied by the posterior labial branches of the pudendal nerve (S2, S3, and S4), the upper vagina is innervated by the splanchnic nerves (S2, S3, and occasionally S4) [13,35]. In addition to local infiltration, modified epidural catheters with pain pumps using agents such as 0.25% bupivacaine or pudendal nerve blocks with off-label use of Exparel™ can provide longer term pain control.

   b *How to deal with them (or not) "in the moment"*: Transvaginal pudendal nerve blocks are useful for limiting pain in the immediate post-operative period or if the local infiltration does not provide sufficient analgesia. See A7b above.

   c *How to deal with them in the long term*: In the early phases, referral to a pelvic floor physical therapist will be beneficial. A variety of modalities such as external massage or ultrasound applied internally or externally may be employed. Dilation with cone-shaped dilators, progressing ~3 mm every 2–3 weeks, along with finger massage application of estrogen and possibly testosterone-containing ointment or gel will be helpful. Refractory cases (not specifically related to vaginoplasty) have responded to botulinum toxin; the author has used this with good results in two patients [36]. Superficial wound dehiscence with any technique may produce an area of tissue attenuation and thinning that causes tenderness and hypersensitivity and may recurrently tear with resumption of coitus. Resection and approximation of normal tissues often produces resolution (Figure 16.13). In rare instances, this has been associated with a recurrent subclinical herpes infection (detected only by biopsy) and concurrent treatment with anti-viral therapy is also considered prior and subsequent to surgery.

7 *Urinary retention*

Retention is rarely encountered with solely posterior wall dissection but is not uncommon with anterior and upper vaginal dissection.

a *How to avoid*: Inquire about history of urinary retention. Treat and manage pain as discussed above in E6. Achieve meticulous hemostasis. Be aware of this and anticipate post-operatively. Ask patient to void prior to discharge. The editor has found the administration of 1 mg lorazepam ~4 hours post-operatively and at bedtime day of surgery to be helpful in reducing retention, especially in anxious patients (personal communication).

b *How to deal with them (or not) "in the moment"*: Straight catheter with assessment of retained volume. Be on the lookout for other causes of mechanical blockage such as a hematoma.

c *How to deal with them in the long term*: Ongoing urine retention requires evaluation with urodynamic and diagnostic imaging or radiologic studies.

8 *Contour irregularities*

These are generally not a concern with regards to the vagina and relate primarily to the perineum and are dealt with in E2 above.

9 *Anesthetic/allergies*

Identical to A9 above.

10 *Need for revisionary surgery*

Identical to A10 above.

11 *Financial issues*

Identical to A11 above.

12 *Suture granulomas*

Identical to A13 above.

13 *Dissatisfied patients*

a *How to avoid*: Pre-operative discussions relating to expectations are more important here than in nearly any other female genital procedure. Unlike other elective procedures, patients are seeking improved sexual function and are less likely to be concerned with appearance. Appearance concerns relate primarily to the appearance of prolapsed hymenal fragments or visibility of the introitus. Review of photographs of sample before and after photographs may help the physician understand patient expectations as well as giving the patient an understanding of anticipated outcomes. Inform patients about limitations and risks of excessive reduction.

b *How to deal with them (or not) "in the moment"*: See patients at regular periods during post-operative period. Allow sufficient time for healing to become stable. Review pre-operative discussions. Dissatisfaction will typically fall into one of two categories: too tight or too loose. To avoid the former, it is best to avoid aggressive plication. In the instance it is too tight, vaginal dilators and stretching exercises will, in most instances, result in progressive relaxation and accommodation. Liberal use of lubricants may help to ease the sensations of tightness, and pelvic floor physical therapists may be extremely helpful. Perform revision surgery with myofascial release if acceptable goals or resection of permanent suture or materials were used. This can be extremely complex surgery and referral to a specialist should be considered. Surgery should be performed only if realistic goals can be established and accomplished. Prior to addressing concerns of too loose a repair, discuss the complications of further reduction with potential for sensations of undesirable tightness or traction or vaginismus especially with sexual activity. Traditional methods for promoting vaginal tone such as Kegel exercises and pelvic floor exercises under the supervision of a pelvic floor physical therapist should first be attempted for 6–9 months prior to surgical intervention.

c *How to deal with them in the long term*: See A14c above.

14 *Sexual dysfunction*

Please read C13 as well as comment below.

a *How to avoid*: Please read initial disclaimer. It is clear that there is a public perception (and many patients believe) that a tighter, smaller vagina will improve sexual function. The answer is more difficult and this must be relayed to the patient prior to undergoing surgery. Sexual dysfunction may be due

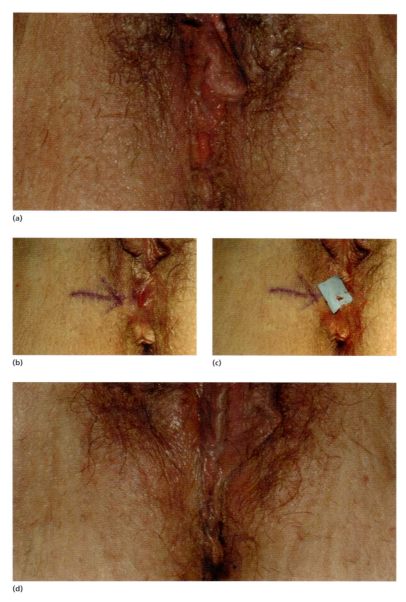

Figure 16.13 (a) Perineoplasty patient with marked dyspareunia attributable to neuroma. (b) Pre-operatively, arrow shows location of neuroma. (c) Neuroma excised. (d) Post-operative result with successful resolution of pain. Source: O. Placik. Reproduced with permission.

a combination of real or perceived impressions of a large vagina, Not infrequently, women interpret excessive natural autogenous lubrication as being attributable to a loose vagina. This must be distinguished from a physically large vagina conservatively measured as snugly admitting two fingers (highly variable). Issues of self-image and confidence directly relate to sexual function. Therefore, some patients may interpret certain aspects of vaginal appearance and relate these to feelings of a large vagina. A patent introitus or visible hymenal fragments are common complaints of women presenting for surgery. An appreciation for age-related changes as they relate to orgasm, satisfaction, and discomfort is important [37]. In one such study, where patients underwent combined vaginoplasty and perineoplasty, 38.7% of patients rated their sexual function as "good to great" pre-operatively, whereas this increased to 86.6% post-operatively [23].

b *How to deal with them (or not) "in the moment"*: See C13b above. Treatment of psychosexual issues, body image, and the rationale for a vaginal tightening procedure are addressed elsewhere.

c *How to deal with them in the long term*: See C13c above. Second opinions from colleagues may provide re-assurance of acceptable outcome. Consultation with sex therapists for management of dysfunction may provide an additional option. Referral to support groups may be beneficial. Possibly refer patients for cognitive behavioral therapy in instances of BDD or sexual therapist in instances of dysfunction.

F Hymenoplasty/hymenorrhaphy

The difficulties in discussing untoward outcomes of hymenoplasty stem from the fact that it is a procedure shrouded in mystery. There are few published reports on this procedure in peer-reviewed literature and the reports describe techniques that have not been verified in multicenter trials. These entail a broad range of procedures that are inadequately described or documented due to the tremendous controversy with the procedure. Therefore much of this is based on personal knowledge and experience. It appears that each practitioner develops a technique with which she/he becomes comfortable. This is further complicated by the desired goals of each patient, which vary and may be culturally defined. Whereas some simply request bleeding upon vaginal penetration, others may request a visually intact hymen that should approach a visualized ideal; that is, a fully intact membrane with a central small aperture. Clearly the latter is difficult to achieve.

It must be explained to the patient that this is not a tightening procedure, as this is a common misunderstanding. Furthermore, because this is essentially a procedure performed for cultural reasons, the specific traditions of the relevant culture should be appreciated in order to satisfy the patient's intended results. In most instances, bleeding with sexual penetration is the purpose. With this in mind, a simple adhesion is usually adequate and this is relatively straightforward. However, due to the avascular and thin tissues involved, the repairs are prone to breakdown. Careful inspection post-operatively, usually at 3–4 weeks, is necessary to assure the adhesion is intact. Too early or too aggressive inspection may cause wound separation and failure of the repair (Figure 16.14). On occasion, if the repair is performed 3 weeks prior to consummation, and even if the adhesion dehisces, there may be sufficient granulation tissue present to produce bleeding with sexual penetration. Some cultures dictate that a third party performs an examination to confirm the intact hymen. In these rare circumstances, a more thorough repair should be undertaken several weeks to months to allow for satisfactory healing and time for revisionary procedures.

l *Wound healing complications/scarring*

a *How to avoid*: As with most other procedures, operate on nutritionally sound and stable patients. Get smokers to quit at least 4 weeks prior to surgery.

Interestingly this is one of the few areas where scarring is highly desirable in order to achieve a surgical adhesion that accomplishes the intended goal; however, evolution has created a tissue that is intended to break down as a normal process. Because this area is prone to wound separation, this is likely the most common complication of surgery, although exact numbers are not known. For this reason, one must perform multiple points of surgical adhesion with the anticipation that a portion of the repairs will fail. One should attempt to accomplish a tension-free repair. This is one of the few areas where minimal if any epinephrine or electrocautery is used in order to avoid tissue necrosis or diminished vascularity. Surgery may be bloodier for this reason. It is imperative to approximate raw tissues with sutures that do not strangulate tissue. Patients are instructed to avoid examining the wound for a minimum of 3 weeks and to simply perform hygiene with gentle non-penetrating perineal irrigation. Depending on the goals of surgery, timing is important. While 4-0 chromic suture is commonly utilized, this author find that is more likely to promote inflammation and dehiscence and now favors 5-0 Monocryl™. Other causes for failure include mechanical disruption and tampon use or douching. Most practitioners advocate strict activity limitation for at least 3 weeks post-operatively. In rare

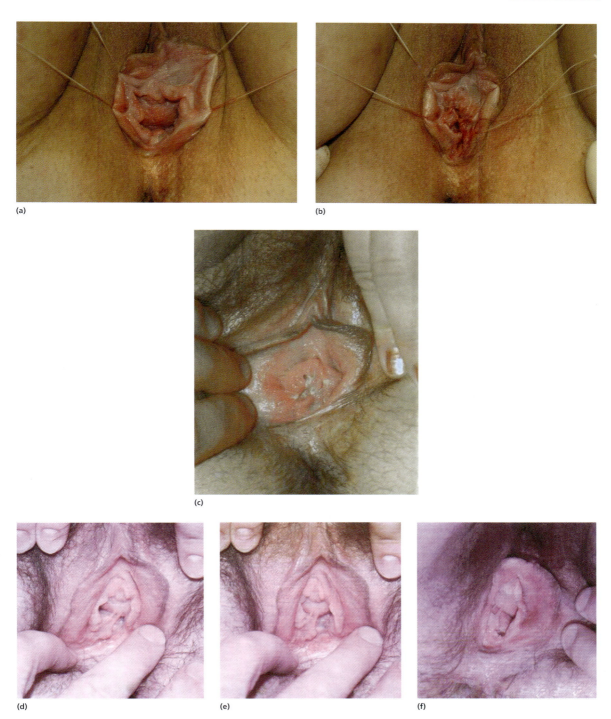

Figure 16.14 Intraoperative views of hymenoplasty patient at (a) beginning and (b) conclusion of the procedure with multiple (3) adhesions accomplished. (c) Early post-operative views provided by patient showing aggressive examination with apparent intact repair. (d)–(f) Late views provided by patient showing dehiscence of nearly all repairs. Source: O. Placik. Reproduced with permission.

instances an overly aggressive repair may produce scarring that will not tear with penetration.

b *How to deal with them (or not) "in the moment"*: If wound separation occurs shortly before anticipated coitus, sufficient granulation tissue may be present to cause the desired bleeding with penetration. Alternatively, a simple suture of 4-0 chromic may be placed across the hymenal ring to act as a mechanical barrier and reproduce bleeding with coitus. This is generally only effective in the week or 2 prior to intercourse as the suture will dissolve. The patient may need to be counseled that the suture could be potentially detectable. If sufficient time permits or a visually intact hymen is desired, it is best to wait at least 3 months before repeat anticipated repair. Unfortunately, prior to 3 months, the tissues are immobile and edematous and not generally amenable to repair. As stated earlier, in the rare event that the repair results in an especially prominent or strong scar that is resistant to penetration, surgical release may be required.

2 *Asymmetry*

Not an issue but patient's perceived ideals of the appearance may not be realistic.

a *How to avoid*: Impossible to avoid. While the idealized image of an intact hymen is a membrane with a central aperture, this is nearly impossible to achieve. An intact hymen may present with a variety of appearances. Explain to the patient that the idealized concept is not likely achievable. It is better not to operate than to leave the patient with the impression that this is obtainable.

3 *Infection*

a *How to avoid*: Extremely uncommon; however, the incidence is not known.

b *How to deal with them (or not) "in the moment"*: See A3b above.

c *How to deal with them in the long term*: See E3a and b above.

4 *Hematoma/bleeding/bruising*

a *How to avoid*: These are limited due to the diminished vascularity in this area and the absence of a dead space. See E4a above.

b *How to deal with them (or not) "in the moment"*: Typically observation and pressure are sufficient to control bleeding. Be cautious about excessive use of cautery because this may cause necrosis. Silver nitrate or battery-powered cautery may be sufficient.

5 *Edema*

a *How to avoid:* See A6 above.

b *How to deal with them (or not) "in the moment":* See E5b above.

6 *Pain/alteration in skin sensation*

a *How to avoid*: Pain is usually minimal to moderate and the procedure is typically well tolerated. Intraoperatively, one alteration in protocol is the use of local anesthetics *without* epinephrine. Standard analgesics are prescribed post-operatively.

b *How to deal with them (or not) "in the moment"*: See E6b above.

c *How to deal with them in the long term*: See E6c above.

7 *Anesthetic/allergies*

Identical to A9 above.

8 *Need for revisionary surgery*

Identical to A10 above.

a *How to avoid*: This may be difficult to avoid due to the inherent nature for wound breakdown (see F1a above). One should anticipate a revision rate higher than other procedures and plan for it as discussed earlier with timing scheduled according to cultural dictates and anticipated consummation. Prepare patients for the potential of a revision.

b *How to deal with them (or not) "in the moment"*: Have an existing written policy in place or as part of the informed consent to discuss the need for revisionary surgery. Circumstances and treatment need to be handled on a case-by-case basis. Most can be performed under local anesthesia.

c *How to deal with them in the long term*: Most revisions should be deferred for a minimum of 3–5 months to allow sufficient time for scar maturation.

9 *Financial issues*

Identical to A11 above.

10 *Dissatisfied patients*

a *How to avoid*: Establish a clear idea of the patient's goals, which may be influenced by her specific cultural standards. Furthermore, dissatisfaction may result from patient's believing a hymenoplasty will tighten the vaginal canal. Explaining the differences of a hymenoplasty, perineoplasty, and vaginoplasty are well worth the time to help patients comprehend anticipated outcomes. Pre-operative discussions reviewing the variable appearance of an intact hymen may allow patients to accept a reasonable facsimile.

b *How to deal with them (or not) "in the moment"*: The success of the procedure is most commonly measured by the ability to bleed at the time of coitus and secondarily to the appearance of an intact hymen. This is unique because patient satisfaction is determined by a single short-lived event, whereas most procedures are intended to provide long-lasting results. Unfortunately, there is no way to deal with them in the moment because if it fails, the opportunity is lost. In some cultures, the consequence of an unsuccessful operation can be serious and can lead to dissolution of the marital contract, social isolation, financial ruin, and public humiliation of the woman and her family and/or the potential for physical harm. This is best prevented by completing a successful surgical adhesion and confirming this remains intact post-operatively. While numerous social agencies are making attempts at education and changing the public's opinion and perceptions, efforts are ongoing.

c *How to deal with them in the long term*: If patients are dissatisfied because an idealized hymenal appearance has not been accomplished, the surgeon must determine if this is a realistic possibility and communicate this to the patient. Surgical revision is an option at this point. See F1b above regarding timing.

G Labia majora augmentation

When patients report dissatisfaction with redundant or loose skin of the labia majora, options include both augmentation to restore lost volume or cutaneous resection; most surgeons prefer the more predictable and longstanding outcomes afforded by labia majora cutaneous reduction discussed in section B above. Because labia majora "involution" or atrophy or laxity is infrequently managed with augmentation but more commonly treated by reduction, this subject is addressed in a more abbreviated fashion and the reader is referred to the section above for a more generalized discussion of surgical complications. Augmentation, when performed, is typically accomplished with autologous fat injections or with commercially available fillers composed of hyaluronic acid or injectable poly-L-lactic acid (i.e. Sculptra).

1 *Wound healing complications/scarring/necrosis/cysts/ nodules/granulomas*
   a *How to avoid*: See A1a above for a general discussion of complications. Wound healing is less of a concern here because incisions are minimal and most augmentations are achieved using injections. Be aware of patients who are prone to keloid scarring. Getting smokers to quit at least 4 weeks prior to surgery is especially true for fat grafting. Adipose tissue injections commonly result in partial fat resorption and attempts at over-correction to compensate for this effect may produce cysts or fibrosis [38]. On occasion, infection occurs (discussed below and shown in Figure 16.15). Fat graft harvesting and preparation techniques as well as stem cell or platelet-rich plasma supplementation is controversial. No standard approach has been established, with strong advocates existing for every method. There are a few general principles to which most proponents adhere. To enhance graft take, excessive grafting is not advised; it is often better to graft in multiple sessions to achieve larger volume corrections. Anecdotally, practitioners may limit injections to no more than 10–15 cc per side. If greater volume is necessary, it has been advised that the patient return for staged treatments. Grafts are best placed in the superficial sub-cutaneous plane immediately beneath the dermis where the blood supply is greatest. Multiple passes with a small cannula using a threading technique are advised for optimal "seeding" of the grafts. Proponents argue about the size as well as the use of a sharp or blunt-ended cannula. Debate rages about whether these factors produce an increase in survival. In any event, a depot technique is to be avoided for this will certainly result in necrosis. The deeper tissues of the labia majora, contained by Colles' fascia, are inherently less vascular and more prone to fat necrosis. In rare instances, excessive fat grafting has been reported to produce pronounced visibility of the labia majora in tight clothing and may be associated with increased perspiration [39]. Similar considerations with the use of injectable fillers include homogenous dispersion. Some fillers such as poly-L-lactic acid have been associated with granuloma formation. A more dilute preparation with 10 cc versus the recommended 5 cc as well as aggressive massage following injections is reported to decrease this risk. Alternatively, the use of 4–5 cc of hyaluronic acid (Restylane™) diluted 2:1 (for a final volume of 12–15 cc) or 1.5–3 cc of calcium hydroxyapatite (Radiesse™) prepared with a similar dilution have been used to diminish the formation of "bumps" and accomplish greater volumes [40].

b *How to deal with them (or not) "in the moment"*: In the event of palpable or visible or pronounced cyst

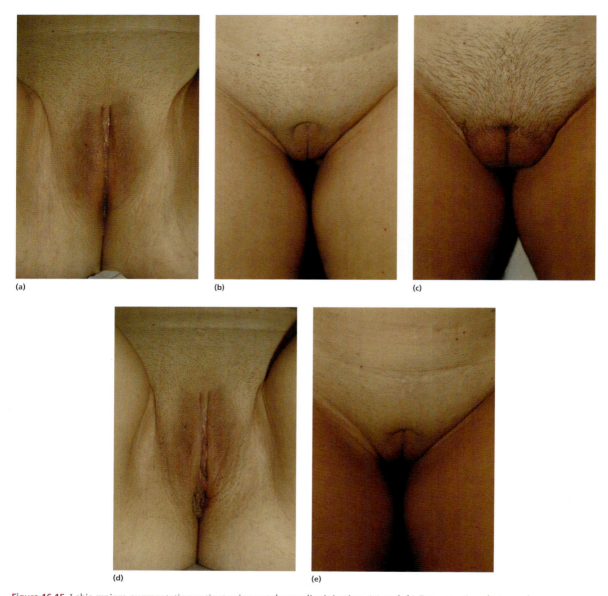

Figure 16.15 Labia majora augmentation patient using autologous lipoinjection. (a) and (b) Pre-operative photographs. (c) Infection with photo taken immediately prior to drainage procedure. (d) and (e) Post-operative view 4 months later. Patient is contemplating additional lipoinjection. Source: O. Placik. Reproduced with permission.

formation following fat injection, aspiration (on a single or on multiple attempts) may produce a satisfactory outcome. Fibrotic nodules may be treated with steroid injections performed once a month for up to 3–4 sessions beginning with triam-cinolone 10 mg/ml and progressing up to 40 mg/ml.

Overly aggressive injections may result in atrophy. Similar treatment has been advised for granulomas following poly-L-lactic acid [41].

c *How to deal with them in the long term*: Rarely chronic cysts or painful nodules may require excision. The majority of these cysts or masses will resolve spontaneously by 6 months. Repeated lipoinjection procedures may be necessary to achieve the desired volume augmentation. At this point in time, most practitioners utilize non-permanent fillers that require ongoing injections in order to maintain volume. The frequency will depend on the product used and the individual's response.

2 *Asymmetry*

a *How to avoid*: See A2a above. Point out anatomical features that contribute to asymmetry including the size and shape of the labia majora as well as the depth of the inter-labial sulcus. Although computer imaging software has been used to estimate volume restoration for the face or breast, I am not aware of its use for achieving augmentation of the genitalia or accomplishing greater symmetry. Certainly this is an available option. Be aware of leg positioning in the lithotomy position to assure the least degree of asymmetry and the effect on labia distortion.

b *How to deal with them (or not) "in the moment"*: If recognized by the physician immediately, additional volume can be added to the smaller side with additional fat or filler. Rarely if ever is the larger side made smaller. If this is desired, liposuction can remove fat. If hyaluronic fillers have been utilized, injection of hyaluronidase (after appropriate skin testing) may accomplish enzymatic digestion. However, this is not a precise process and one must be prepared to lose all of the filler volume. Poly-L-lactic acid and calcium hydroxyapatite cannot be immediately reversed and will require time for dissolution of the volume. In most instances of asymmetry following augmentation most patients will report dissatisfaction with the smaller side. Shape discrepancies are not exclusively due to volume discrepancies and some features of asymmetry cannot be corrected by volume correction alone.

c *How to deal with them in the long term*: Chronic asymmetry treatment is essentially the same as immediate treatment. Timing is less of an issue than with other surgical procedures. Whereas one should likely wait 3 months for additional fat grafting in the event of undercorrection, the use of fillers such as hyaluronic acid can be injected at any time, poly-L-lactic acid at 6–12 week intervals and calcium hydroxyapaptite every 3 months. Fat grafting may require multiple stages. One may try to simulate the appearance and assess the patient's response using injection of saline (short term) or fillers such as Resytlane™ for a longer

result. The long-term effects of tissue expansion (internal or external) are well known for reconstructive purposes elsewhere in the body, such as the breast; however, the use of labia majora expansion following labiaplasty surgery is not standardized.

3 *Infection*

a *How to avoid*: See A3b above. On an anecdotal basis, using similar principles of fat grafting to the buttock, some practitioners will add antibiotics to the fat at a dose of 1 gram of cefazolin (or 300 mg of clindamycin in penicillin/cephalosporin allergic patients) per 500–1,000 cc of fat.

b *How to deal with them (or not) "in the moment"*: Management is similar to that discussed in A3b above.

4 *Hematoma/bleeding/bruising*

a *How to avoid*: The area is highly vascular and hematoma may occur but is highly unlikely. However, it is advisable to follow precautions reviewed in A4a above.

b *How to deal with them (or not) "in the moment"*: See A4b above.

5 *Edema*

a *How to avoid*: Due to the vascularity of the area and the capacity of the space contained by Colles' fascia, swelling will occur and is to expected but is remarkably less than the labia minora. Patients should be prepared for this inevitability. Some physicians favor the use of intraoperative steroids. Otherwise see measures discussed in A6a above.

b *How to deal with them (or not) "in the moment"*: See A6b above.

6 *Pain/alteration in skin sensation*

a *How to avoid*: See B6a above. Topical anesthetics such as BTL cream (benzocaine 20%, lidocaine 6%, and tetracaine 4%), Anecream™, LMX5™, or EMLA™ may ease the discomfort of injections. Be aware of application over an expansive area and the potential for toxicity or adverse reactions. In additional to local infiltration, fillers typically contain local anesthetics and may be further diluted with additional local anesthetic as described in G1a above.

b *How to deal with them (or not) "in the moment"*: See A7b above.

c *How to deal with them in the long term*: See A7c above. Resection of tender nodules may produce a resolution to this problem.

7 *Contour irregularities*

These are generally minimal in this area and the reader is referred to G2 above.

8 *Anesthetic/allergies*
See A9 above.
9 *Need for revisionary surgery/treatment*
See A10 above.
10 *Financial issues*
See A11 above.
11 *Dissatisfied patients*
See A14 above.

Summary

A thorough understanding of the patient and anatomy with careful peri-operative care and surgical execution will minimize risks and the potential for untoward outcomes. However, even in ideal circumstances, complications will occur. Options for surgical management are discussed in Chapter 17.

References

1. http://www.oshot.info/.
2. Placik OJ, Arkins JP. Plastic surgery trends parallel Playboy magazine: The pudenda preoccupation. *Aesthet Surg J* 2014;**34**:1083–90.
3. Goodman M, Fashler S, Miklos JR, Moore RD, Brotto LA. The sexual, psychological, and body image health of women undergoing elective vulvovaginal plastic/cosmetic procedures: A pilot study. *Am J Cosmet Surg* 2011;**28**:219–26.
4. Goodman M, Placik OJ, Dalton T, Matlock D, Simopoulos A, Hardwick-Smith S. Two year outcomes of the Vaginal Aesthetic Surgery Evaluation (VASE-2) of body image, genital perception and sexual satisfaction in women undergoing female genital plastic/cosmetic surgery. In press.
5. Goodman MP. Female cosmetic genital surgery. *Obstet Gynecol* 2009;**113**:154–9.
6. Ching S, Thoma A, McCabe RE, Antony MM. Measuring outcome in aesthetic surgery: A comprehensive review of literature. *Plast Reconstr Surg* 2003;**111**:469–80.
7. Bloom JM, Van Kouwenberg E, Davenport M, Koltz PF, Shaw RB, & Gusenoff JA. Aesthetic and functional satisfaction after monsplasty in the massive weight loss population. *Aesthet Surg J* 2012;**32**:877–85.
8. Solutions for surgical preparation of the vagina. Committee Opinion No. 571. American College of Obstetricians and Gynecologists. *Obstet Gynecol* 2013;**122**:718–20.
9. Heggers JP, Sazy JA, Stenberg BD, Strock LL, McCauley RL, Herndon DN, Robson M. C. Bactericidal and wound-healing properties of sodium hypochlorite solutions: The 1991 Lindberg Award. *J Burn Care Res* 1991;**12**:420–4.
10. Altunoluk B, Resim S, Efe E, Eren M, Benlioglu C, Kankilic N, Baykan H. Fournier's gangrene: Conventional dressings versus dressings with Dakin's solution. International Scholarly Research Notices, 2012.
11. Rab M, Dellon AL. Anatomic variability of the ilioinguinal and genitofemoral nerve: Implications for the treatment of groin pain. *Plast Reconstr Surg* 2001;**108**:1618–23.
12. Salgarello M, Farallo E, Barone-Adesi L, Cervelli D, Scambia G, Salerno G, Margariti P. A. Flap algorithm in vulvar reconstruction after radical, extensive vulvectomy. *Ann Plast Surg* 2005;**54**:184–90.
13. https://www.inkling.com/read/grays-anatomy-standring-40th/chapter-77/lower-genital-tract.
14. Alter GJ. Labia minora reconstruction using clitoral hood flaps, wedge excisions, and YV advancement flaps. *Plast Reconstr Surg* 2011;**127**:2356–63.
15. Yavagal S, de Farias TF, Medina CA, Takacs P. Normal vulvovaginal, perineal, and pelvic anatomy with reconstructive considerations. *Semin Plast Surg* 2011;**25**:121.
16. Cold CJ, McGrath KA. Anatomy and histology of the penile and clitoral prepuce in primates. In: *Male and Female Circumcision*, pp. 19–29. New York: Springer, 1999.
17. Hamori CA. Postoperative clitoral hood deformity after labiaplasty. *Aesthet Surg J* 2013;**33**:1030–6.
18. Ginger VA, Cold CJ, Yang CC. Structure and innervation of the labia minora: More than minor skin folds. *Female Pelvic Med Reconstr Surg* 2011;**17**:180–3.
19. Alter GJ. Aesthetic labia minora and clitoral hood reduction using extended central wedge resection. *Plast Reconstr Surg* 2008;**122**:1780–9.
20. Lean WL, Hutson JM, Deshpande AV, Grover S. Clitoroplasty: past, present and future. *Pediatr Surgery Int* 2007;**23**:289–93.
21. Minto CL, Liao LM, Woodhouse CR, Ransley PG, Creighton SM. The effect of clitoral surgery on sexual outcome in individuals who have intersex conditions with ambiguous genitalia: A cross-sectional study. *Lancet* 2003;**361**:1252–7.
22. Pourcelot AG, Fernandez H, Legendre G. Quelle technique chirurgicale utiliser en cas d'hypertrophie des petites lèvres?. *Gynécol Obstét Fertil* 2013;**41**:218–21.
23. Goodman MP, Placik OJ, Benson III RH, Miklos JR, Moore RD, Jason RA, Matlock D, Stern BH, Stanton RA, Kolb SE, Gonzalez F. A large multicenter outcome study of female genital plastic surgery. *J Sex Med* 2010;**7**:1565–77.
24. Rouzier R, Louis-Sylvestre C, Paniel BJ, Haddad B. Hypertrophy of labia minora: Experience with 163 reductions. *Am J Obstetr Gynecol* 2000;**182**:35–40.
25. Felicio YA. Labial surgery. *Aesthet Surg J* 2007;**27**:322–8.
26. Chang P, Salisbury MA, Narsete T, Buckspan R, Derrick D, Ersek RA. Vaginal labiaplasty: Defense of the simple "clip and snip" and a new classification system. *Aesthet Plast Surg* 2013;**37**:887–91.
27. Gress S. Composite reduction labiaplasty. *Aesthet Plast Surg* 2013;**37**:674–83.

28. Marchitelli CE, Sluga MC, Perrotta M, Testa R. Initial experience in a vulvovaginal aesthetic surgery unit within a general gynecology department. *J Low Genit Tract Dis* 2010;**14**: 295–300.

29. Martin-Alguacil N, Pfaff DW, Kow LM, Schober JM. Oestrogen receptors and their relation to neural receptive tissue of the labia minora. *BJU Int* 2008;**101**:1401–6.

30. Prorocic M, Vasiljevic M, Tasic L, Dzatić O, Brankovic S. The management of fusion of the labia minora pudendi in adult women using a radiosurgical knife. *Clin Exp Obstet Gynecol* 2012;**40**:170–3.

31. Munhoz AM, Filassi JR, Ricci MD, Aldrighi C, Correia LD, Aldrighi JM, Ferreira MC. Aesthetic labia minora reduction with inferior wedge resection and superior pedicle flap reconstruction. *Plast Reconstr Surg* 2006;**118**:1237–47.

32. Heusse JL, Cousin-Verhoest S, Aillet S, Watier E. Mise au point sur les techniques de nymphoplastie de réduction [Refinements in the labia minora reduction procedures]. *Ann Chir Plast Esthét* 2009;**54**:126–34.

33. Maas SM, Hage JJ. Functional and aesthetic labia minora reduction. *Plast Reconstr Surg* 2000;**105**:1453–6.

34. Ostrzenski A. Vaginal rugation rejuvenation (restoration): A new surgical technique for an acquired sensation of wide/smooth vagina. *Gynecol Obstet Invest* 2011;**73**:48–52.

35. Patten J. *Neurological Differential Diagnosis*. New York: Springer, 1982.

36. Ferreira JR, Souza RP. Botulinum toxin for vaginismus treatment. *Pharmacol* 2012; **89**:256–9.

37. Aslan E, Beji NK, Gungor I, Kadioglu A, Dikencik BK. Prevalence and risk factors for low sexual function in women: A study of 1,009 women in an outpatient clinic of a university hospital in Istanbul. *J Sex Med* 2008;**5**: 2044–52.

38. Triana L, Robledo AM. Refreshing labioplasty techniques for plastic surgeons. *Aesthet Plast Surg* 2012;**36**:1078–86.

39. Alinsod R. Awake in-office Barbie labiaplasty, awake in-office labia majora plasty, awake in-office vaginoplasty, awake in-office labial revision. Presented at the Congress on Aesthetic Vaginal Surgery, November 2011, Tucson.

40. Jesitus J. Injectables, RF energy aid female genital rejuvenation. April 1, 2012. Available at: http://cosmeticsurgery times.modernmedicine.com/cosmetic-surgery-times/ news/modernmedicine/modern-medicine-feature-articles/ injectables-rf-energy-ai?id=&sk=&date=&pageID=2 (accessed November 1, 2014).

41. Bauer U. Injectable poly-L-lactic acid (PLLA): Practical approaches to optimize outcomes. *Internet J Plast Surg* 2009;**7**(1).

CHAPTER 17
Revisions and re-operations

Michael P. Goodman

Caring for Women Wellness Center, Davis, CA, USA

The only reason why some people become lost in thought is that it's unfamiliar territory.

Paul Fix

Occasionally, your patient will consider her result sub-optimal. Occasionally, you will consider the result sub-optimal. These occurrences may or may not coincide. On one hand, it is not rare for a surgeon to view post-operative results and, either secondary to faulty technique, poor post-operative patient compliance, or adverse healing conditions, say to himself or herself, *"could be better."* The patient may be satisfied, as her expectations have been met with the debulking and non-visualization of previously protruding labia minora. On the other hand, you may consider the results excellent, only to have your patient tell you, "you know, that little edge bothers me" or "the right side is a little bigger than the left" or "see that flap there?"

It is not unusual for a patient to view her labia much more intensively post-operatively than she did prior to surgery and to be dissatisfied with slight or modest asymmetries, skin tags, discolorations, "protrusions," or "dog-ears." It is not rare for your patient who pre-operatively swore that her posterior commissure or clitoral hood needed no work, either because "it did not bother her" or to avoid extra costs associated with a more complex procedure, to after surgery acutely note the appearance of these entities, which now appear more prominent to her than prior to her surgery.

This author considers revisions and re-operations separated points along the same axis. There are times when an extensive "revision" might be considered a true "re-operation." This will be covered shortly.

A "revision" is a situation where both the surgeon and the patient are generally satisfied with the outcome, save for small area(s) of "dog-ear(s)," modest dissymmetry, area(s) of pigmentation, area(s) of mild scarring secondary to healing by secondary intention, small separation of the leading edge of a V-wedge-type repair, a small fistula, and so forth.

The usual reason that a patient wishes a revision is a minor/modest irregularity that either aesthetically or functionally "bothers" her.

Factors influencing patients' decisions for *revisions*

1 "Dog-ears"; small polypoid-appearing projections along the suture line; minor irregularities of, or at the end of, the suture line.
2 Symmetry—(area of) one labum larger than the other.
3 Area(s) of darker pigmentation.
4 Trim of edges produced by minor separation at leading edge of apex of V-wedge repair.
5 Minor trim of edge of frenular fold, left long to avoid operating in close proximity to the clitoral glans.
6 Removal of portion of delayed absorbable suture that failed to absorb.
7 Repair of minor fistulous tract(s) produced by extrusion of suture material. (Major repairs involving reconstruction should be considered re-operations.)

Female Genital Plastic and Cosmetic Surgery, First Edition. Edited by Michael P. Goodman.

A "re-operation" or "re-do" is a situation where, more or less, a second labiaplasty or hood reduction or posterior commisurectomy or more major surgical procedure is performed secondary to one or more of several factors that have made the outcome of the original procedure unacceptable for the patient. In this text, I will mostly concentrate on revisions, as, in my and other aesthetic vulvovaginal surgeons' experience, the request and actual performance of a revision of some sort will occur approximately once every 20–25 cases, the majority of which are minor revisions to aid in symmetry. Most all revisions are accomplished by the original surgeon, while most often the patient turns to another surgeon to accomplish a "re-do."

Factors influencing patients' decisions for *re-operations*

1 *Grossly inadequate* tissue removal the first time.
2 *Excessive* labial tissue removal with mucosa to interlabial fold suturing, with or without excessive, ptotic clitoral hood folds.
3 Patients' decisions to secondarily remove tissue (e.g., hood, posterior commissure, labia majora) they had elected to defer during first procedure.
4 Major breakdown of the original procedure (e.g., major separation of V-wedge; major dehiscence of curvilinear incision).
5 Gross dissymmetry.
6 Disfigurement or major "grooving" secondary to injudicious use of large caliber, running (±interlocked) strangulating suture closure of the labiaplasty incision.

Revisions

A revision should not be entertained in most cases until a minimum of 3–4 months (and in many cases 6 months) from the original procedure. There are two reasons for this. First, it takes 3 months or more until the tissue has healed sufficiently that the results at this time are likely to be what the patient will experience ongoing. Prior to this time, "softening" and other tissue changes continue to occur in this "work in progress." The second reason is that the process of re-vascularization takes time, and it will be a minimum of 3–6 months until the area you have previously worked on may

have re-vascularized sufficiently for the surgeon to expect a normal healing process in the area.

Circumstances
1 *Surgical and post-operative factors*:   Several surgical situations increase the potential that a revision may be requested. Significant edema, secondary to excessive use of cautery, post-operative bleeding into the incision, injudicious activities by the patient, or other unknown factors can lead to dissymmetry. Tearing out of suture(s) may lead to gaps and healing by secondary intention, or "divots" in the suture line. Failure to bevel the ends of incision lines can lead to abrupt transitions and dog-ears. Failure to curve incision lines upward in V-wedge also may lead to "dog-ear" formation in the lateral portion of the suture line.
2 *Patient factors*: The importance of judicious post-operative self-care has been emphasized elsewhere in this text. Injudicious activities lead to excessive edema and wound separation, leading to desire for revision or re-operation.
3 *Physician factors*: Two factors come into play here. First is a failure in the patient-physician interaction and outcome negotiation. The physician must listen carefully to the aesthetic goals of his/her patient, while also assessing the anatomic realities so as to skillfully counsel the patient regarding the propriety of her desires as they relate to her specific anatomy in order to agree on a reasonable goal or compromise. This also involves expectations: the surgeon must carefully prepare the patient for an "approximate" rather than a specific result; when discussed results are not forthcoming, a revision is frequently on the horizon. While the physician must listen carefully to his/her patient's goals, so must he/she share garnered expertise to counsel the patient as to the best operative procedure, as appropriate. For example, if a patient has a very prominent clitoral hood, but only wishes a labiaplasty and no revision of hood size, the surgeon must counsel the patient and document in the medical record that, after surgery, her hood will appear quite prominent and that he or she would advise some mitigation of this size at the initial surgery.

Patient presentation
Frequently the patient requesting a revision will contact her surgeon one or several times during the recovery period noting dissymmetry, excess swelling,

separation, and so forth, concerned that "it is not even." Most certainly she will mention this at her 4- to 6-week post-op exam. The author advises document-ing this on the medical record, while at the same time kindly but firmly notifying the patient that the inci-sion is a "work in progress" and will go through additional changes "softening" and "re-arranging itself" before she can assess the "final" result at or after 3–4 months. Take note of the area she may be dissatisfied with and reassure her that if it is still a problem for her *after 3 months*, you will be happy to effect a small revision to better meet her aesthetic goals, and document this discussion.

Your negotiation with the patient and decision whether and when to proceed

In the end, you wish your patient to be satisfied. While some anxious and/or dysmorphic patients will slip your notice and make up a portion of patients wishing revision, more often it is a specific area that the patient finds unsatisfying that she wishes removed/revised. It is imperative that you and your patient reach a clear agreement as to exactly what she wishes revised, and to document this both in writing and photographically (see revision form below). Be clear that revisions will not be ongoing, certainly if you elect to not charge a fee (the "standard" for the majority of minor revisions). Most experienced surgeons will perform one minor revision free of charge but may charge for any further "revisions."

How to effect revisions: procedure, equipment, setup, anesthesia, surgical venue

Most revisions require only a local sterile prep and minimal draping; usually a sterile towel and fenestrated drape will suffice. Equipment may be limited to forceps, needle holder, Metzenbaum scissors, and some sort of cutting tool (fine scissors, RF, laser, scalpel, electrosurgical needle) and minor cautery equipment. This is where a contact laser fiber or radiofrequency needle comes in handy; both are superior for revisions secondary to their exquisite "scrolling" capacity. However, a fine-tipped electrocautery device, fine plastic surgery scissors (Keye, etc.), or scalpel + Bovie will suffice. Procedures lend themselves to an office setting, utilizing local anesthesia (see Chapter 14.)

Situation-specific operative techniques

1 *"Droopy" labia majora repair ("festoons")*:   Repair procedure involves a "tear-drop" incision inside the festooned "droopy" areas at the base of the repaired labum majus. Layered closure with or without a "tailor tack" as per labiaplasty majora technique described in Chapter 8 is utilized (Figure 17.1).

2 *Broadened vertical repair scar mid labum majus*: Secondary to placement, weight gain, or genetics a labum majus repair suture line may be visible and broaden. This is a "revision" only the brave would attempt, as the odds of recurrence are great. A re-repair may be contemplated, attempting to place the scar in the inter-labial fold, but as a secondary repair this is unlikely to be successful unless a significant enough amount of labum majus remains to enable incision re-location. My advice here is to make certain you have advised the patient and documented that the labia majora suture lines may be visible and will not be hair-bearing (usually not a problem).

3 *"Dog-ears"; "hypertrophied" irregularity of suture line; pigmented areas; mild dissymmetry*: These repairs suggest themselves. In so many of these minor situations, one patient is perfectly satisfied with the results, while another asks for a revision. The rules are: always wait until 3+ months post-op to consider a revision; make sure the patient understands that the revision may make other areas appear more prominent to her; you only revise when there is an obvious dissymmetry; and there may be a charge for any further revisions

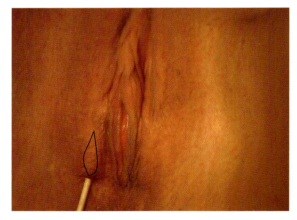

Figure 17.1 Patient 2 years post LP minora + majora. Did not like "droop" bottom right labum majorum. Suggested repair outlined. Source: M. Goodman. Reproduced with permission.

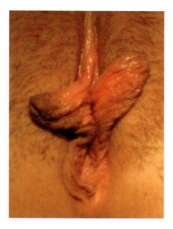
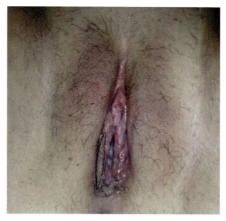

Figure 17.2 Pre- and post-op curvilinear resection. The patient decided against revision. Source: M. Goodman. Reproduced with permission.

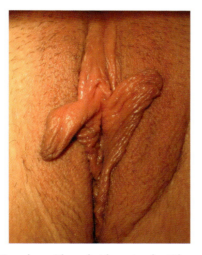
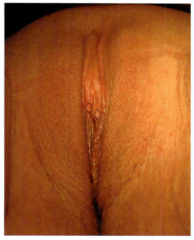

Figure 17.3 Post-op V-wedge, with modest hypertrophy ("dog-ears") at anastamosis site. Potential revision with small diamond-shaped incision lines closed vertically or left to heal by secondary intention (a smooth surface usually re-forms). Source: M. Goodman. Reproduced with permission.

after the first. A simple elliptical excision or shave will usually suffice. For a "shave," sutures are not required. Small excisions may be approximated with an interrupted or sub-cuticular suture line. Examples of possible minor revisions are seen in Figures 17.2 through 17.6.

4 *Separation of V-wedge*: V-wedge incisions may separate. The majority of times, if this occurs, the separation is minor and not of consequence to the patient, or if it is, may be revised with minor simple excision of the separated edge with "contouring" of the labial line.

If the separation is complete, three options present themselves. The labia may be re-wedged and re-approximated if enough labum remains top and bottom to accomplish the re-anastamosis. In this case, the surgeon must make the incision beyond the fibrosed separation area into viable tissue, take care to not put the new V-wedge line under excessive tension, and instruct the patient unreservedly regarding the absolute necessity for lower extremity rest for the first 10 days post-op and a conservative recovery protocol thereafter. A second technique,

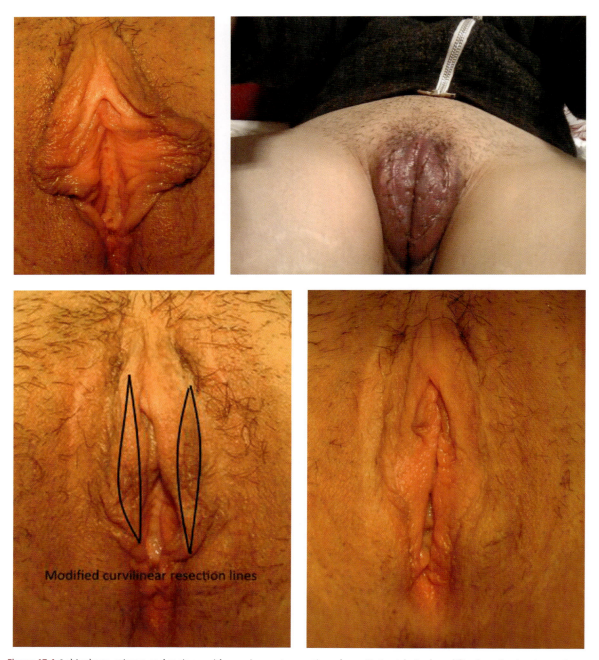

Figure 17.4 Labiaplasty, minora and majora, with massive post-operative edema. Patient desired modification of redundant minora. Final result bottom right panel. Source: M. Goodman. Reproduced with permission.

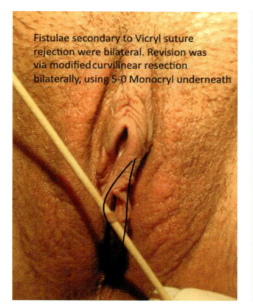
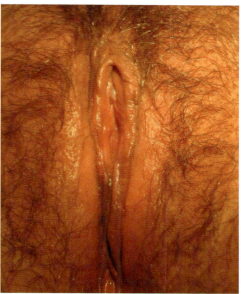

Figure 17.5 Fistulae revised by simple curvilinear excision. Source: M. Goodman. Reproduced with permission.

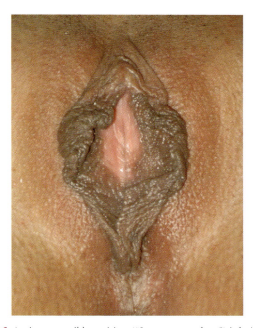
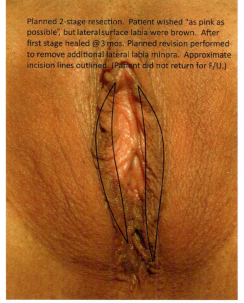

Figure 17.6 At times, possible revision ("2-stage procedure") is built into the pre-operative planning. In this case, the patient desired to be "as pink as possible," but since her brown coloration extended almost to the inter-labial fold laterally, if the patient desired, a second narrow curvilinear resection was planned 3+ months after the first, should she desire. At this time an additional narrow band of labia may be excised without risk of over-excision and exophy of vaginal mucosa. Source: M. Goodman. Reproduced with permission.

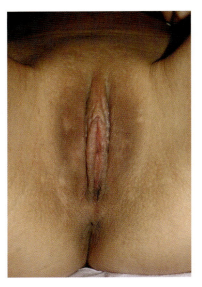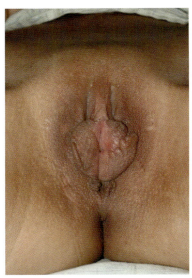

Figure 17.7 Left-sided partial dehiscence following conservative V-wedge labiaplasty, revised/re-operated via a curvilinear incision. Source: O. Placik. Reproduced with permission.

pending availability of tissue, is to bring down, and occasionally up, a "flap" of labum, re-anastamosing it in the "gaped" area. Care must be taken to avoid undue stress/stretch, and to incise deeply enough to assure viability. A third option, the most conservative and carrying the highest success rate, is to convert the separated labial edges into a linear resection, "shaving" off edges superiorly and inferiorly so as to "smoothen" the labia (Figure 17.7). This may only be done if enough tissue remains to effect a cosmetic result and not leave a gaping introitus. Figure 17.8 shows a separated V-wedge incision.

5 *Over-vigorous removal of labia via linear resection*: This is a tough one, as aesthetic fixes are often difficult to achieve. Only the most skilled genital plastic surgeons should undertake the types of flap repairs mandated by over-vigorous removal, if indeed any repair at all can be effected. Oftentimes, the best thing you can do for the patient that sees you is therapy with combined estrogen and testosterone to the introitus to produce ideal epithelization and referral to a good sexual medicine therapist/practitioner to work on sexual and self-image issues. When over-vigorous labial removal is effected, ofttimes the original surgeon has not revised the clitoral hood, and in those patients with "generous" hood epithelium, the hood may be brought down as a flap and over-sewn to a de-epitheliazed portion of the area where the labum

had been totally removed (Figure 17.9). This would be considered at the far end of "revisions," where they morph into "re-operations."

6 *Poor introital healing of perineoplasty*: Occasionally, secondary to either early dehiscence, infection, hematoma, or intercourse/pleasure object insertion prior to full healing, a portion of the introital/perineal incision line may break down. If revision is requested, the same temporal rules must be followed, and this author would wait a minimum of 4–6 months prior to any revision/re-operation. Here also, the line between revision and re-operation is blurry. More often than not, if the major purpose of the initial surgery, vaginal tightening, has been accomplished, and if the cosmesis has not been significantly compromised, revision might be discouraged.

However, if the aesthetic appearance of the introitus is unappealing to the patient, a "mini-perineoplasty," superficially removing separated epithelium and re-anastomosing may be accomplished. In this instance, the patient should be informed about the risk of wound breakdown, as well as the importance of religiously following the surgeon's post-operative activity restrictions.

7 *Perineoplasty over-tightening*: Although this is not a surgical revision, over-tightening somewhere along the perineoplasty incision in the distal one-third to

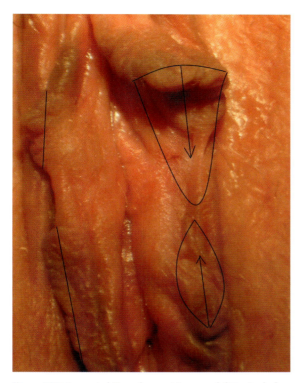

Figure 17.8 Separated V-wedge revision possibilities include shaving edges, seen on right labum, or flaps, depicted on the left labum. In this case, the flaps are brought into approximation and may re-anastamosed to each other at a later time. Alternatively, the labum may be "re-wedged" (not shown), resulting in a smaller labum. Both methods risk re-breakdown. Source: M. Goodman. Reproduced with permission.

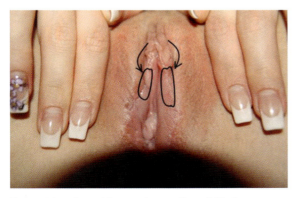

Figure 17.9 Patient with over-vigorous linear labiaplasty. Proposed flap attachment areas are drawn. Source: M. Goodman. Reproduced with permission.

one-half of the vagina is not a rare outcome, occurring ~10–15% of the time according to surgeons polled by the author (this eventuality is more common when V-Wedge LP is performed concomitantly with PP/VP). Most times this is a minor over-correction requiring a short (2–4 weeks) session with progressively larger vaginal dilators, beginning at ~ 2.5–3 cm; at times it is a more major over-correction necessitating 1–2 or more months of progressive dilation, starting with smaller diameter dilators. For peri- or post-menopausal patients, best results are obtained after pre-treating the patient with 2–3 weeks of nightly vaginal estradiol applications, continuing q.o.h.s. when dilations begin and fully through the dilating process.

The most difficult over-tightening to deal with is over-vigorous plication of the levator musculature in the mid-vagina or at the junction of mid- and distal vagina. These "banjo string" over-corrections are best dealt with by making a vaginal incision over the area where the suture may be palpated, carefully dissecting down to the "banjo string" and separating the suture. An alternative is to wait until complete suture absorption (8–10 weeks) and begin careful progressive dilatations. In this case, it may be several months before your patient may resume coitus.

This eventuality must be discussed in pre-operative counseling, and the surgeon should be clear about the time necessary for dilation when beginning the process.

8 *Perineoplasty undertightening*: With the vagaries of healing fibrosis, penile size, and different patient propensities to properly perform post-operative pelvic floor exercises, occasionally patients return requesting "re-tightening."

Requests for additional surgery must be considered on a case-by-case basis. If levator muscle tone is only modest (≤2.5/5, or 10-second perineometer force of ≤10 mm mercury), the author would recommend a minimum of 3–6 months pelvic floor physical therapy with a pelvic floor therapist, or directed work with an APEX™ or In-Tone™-type exercise/biofeedback device. If the patient remains dissatisfied, or for patients whose tone is good but overall tightening sub-optimal, a surgical revision may be deemed appropriate. Revision may consist essentially of re-doing the surgery, albeit not as extensively, as presumably any posterior compartment weakness is already repaired.

SURGICAL REVISION FORM

Patient Name: _____   Date: _____

Procedure: (Minor / Major)_____
_____

When to Schedule: _____

Time Needed: _____

Set-up: (Full / Partial) _____
Sutures: _____

Assistant(s): One / Two ? Sterile: Glove / Gown ? _____

Pre-Med: Yes / No ? _____

Fee?: $_____

Notes: _____

_____

Figure 17.10 Scheduling form for revision.

Consenting for and scheduling revision

Figure 17.10 is the scheduling form the author utilizes in his office. This form may be modified for individual needs.

Additionally, a consent form should be developed for revisions. This form should state that the revision is patient-generated, state specifically and in her own language what the patient wishes performed and why, state the known risks of the revision, and include a disclaimer that with the requested revision the patient waives rights to seek legal redress for undesired outcome from the *initial* procedure. There should be language stating that the surgeon does not agree to perform additional revisions, and that if additional revision is sought by the patient, that the surgeon reserves the right to charge for additional work (see Figure 17.11).

Should you charge?

Most experienced genital plastic/cosmetic surgeons do not charge for minor revisions, as noted above. This is not necessarily the case for "re-dos," as noted below. However, the surgeon would do well to be clear with his/her patient that he/she will revise only once, so the patient should be clear as to her desires. Of course, if the revision is unsuccessful, the surgeon has the option of another revision to "get it right."

Re-operations (aka "re-do")

Reasons for re-operations

One has only to peruse the Internet, or the E! channel, to realize that all cosmetic procedures do not end successfully. An unfortunate but popular term has been applied to poor-outcome cosmetic work: "*botched.*" Female genital procedures are no exception. There are times, either secondary to ineptitude, lack of procedural knowledge, necessary training, or skills on the part of the surgeon, excess caution or timidity on the part of the surgeon, over-aggressive surgery on the part of the surgeon, inability to communicate her aesthetic desires on the part of the patient, injudicious recovery activities on the part of the patient, poor healing, suture rejection, unrealistic expectations or just plain bad luck (e.g., suture rejection), that the patient is significantly dissatisfied and surgery beyond a simple revision is entertained.

There is a blurry line at times between "revision" and "re-operation," and one surgeon's revision might be another surgeon's re-operation. There is, however, a distinction, although very likely it is one of degree. For the purposes of this text, a "revision" is a relatively minor procedure to modify a less than satisfactory outcome from the point of view of the patient and is usually performed by

Consent for Revision

I have come to Dr. _____ requesting revision of *(enter area to be revised*

*here)*_____

_____

For the following reason: *(Enter reason for seeking revision here)* _____

_____

_____

_____ I understand Dr._____will do his/her best to perform this revision to my specifications, but exact results cannot be guaranteed. I understand that symmetry cannot be guaranteed.

_____ I understand that there may be risks associated with this revision, and that they include: infection, abnormal bleeding, separation of suture lines, results not in keeping with my expectations, and other rarer events.

_____ I agree to adhere to the recovery protocol discussed by Dr. _____ and the written instructions I have received.

_____ I understand that only one revision will be performed free of charge, or for a greatly reduced fee. I understand that Dr. _____ may refuse further revision(s), or that there will be a charge for any further work performed.

_____ I understand and agree to hold harmless Dr. _____ for any surgical results produced by my initial surgery.

_____ _____ _____
(Patient)   (Date)   (Physician)

Figure 17.11 Consent form for revision.

the original operating surgeon. A re-operation, aka a "re-do," is essentially re-performing a labiaplasty procedure, by any of the methods discussed in Chapter 8, in order to change the outcome provided by an earlier labiaplasty to one better tolerated by the patient. "Re-dos" are frequently performed by a clinician other than the original surgeon.

How patients present
Patients may express their dissatisfaction at any time during or after their recovery period, but very often they voice their concern early during recovery. It is incumbent on the surgeon to be available to evaluate, support, and reassure while at the same time not be "forced" into any premature revision or re-operation, as the majority of the time the situation will resolve itself. The patient should be offered technical and emotional support, while at the same time be advised of potential alternatives, both from the original surgeon or by a specialized surgeon to whom the patient is referred by the primary aesthetic surgeon.

Of course, any complication noted during the postoperative recovery must be diagnosed and treated expeditiously and appropriately. Sepsis must be appropriately treated; a wound dehiscence may be re-approximated with decent probability of success within the first 36–48 hours, but re-approximation after this time is doomed to failure; it is best wait until full healing has taken place (≥3 months) prior to any intended re-operation.

Should you do it or refer to another?

The patient should always be encouraged to re-visit her initial surgeon for a discussion of whether additional surgery, either revision or re-operation, is mandated. It is incumbent upon the initial surgeon to honestly evaluate the situation and his/her own surgical skills and reach an honest and informed decision whether he/she is prepared to offer an alternate procedure to the patient

that has a decent chance of holding together and satisfying the patient's concerns. If this is unlikely, it is incumbent on the primary surgeon to be of assistance to the patient in a referral to a surgeon with skills and experience to offer the patient a reasonable chance of aesthetic and functional success.

When to initially see the patient for a re-operation; when to have her return to her original surgeon

When a genital plastic procedure "goes wrong" cosmetically, your patient will usually voice her displeasure early on. As noted elsewhere in this text, while it is important to advise and reassure your

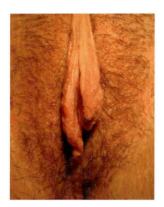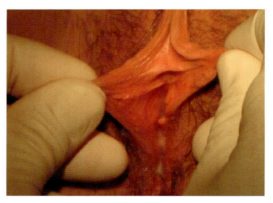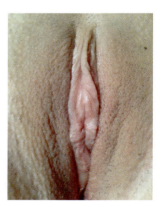

Figure 17.12 The first two photos show labia after an initial V-wedge labiaplasty and revision of a left-sided wound separation. The patient was dissatisfied with the amount of hood and upper labial skin remaining. Re-operation (photo taken by patient at 3 months post-op) consisted of a bilateral curvilinear resection. Source: M. Goodman. Reproduced with permission.

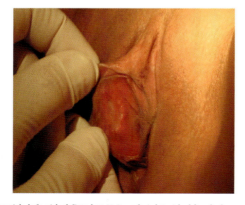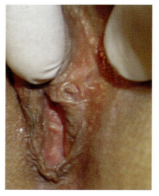

Figure 17.13 Patient with left-sided fistulae X 2 and right-sided healed mucosal surface large ulceration secondary to subcutaneous 4-0 Vicryl rejection and extrusion. Curvilinear revision would be unsatisfactory, as the fistulous tracts are at the level of the vulvar vestibule. The only revision techniques possible would be re-wedge, superior-inferior flap technique, or possibly de-epithelialization technique, depending on the experience of the surgeon. Source: M. Goodman. Reproduced with permission.

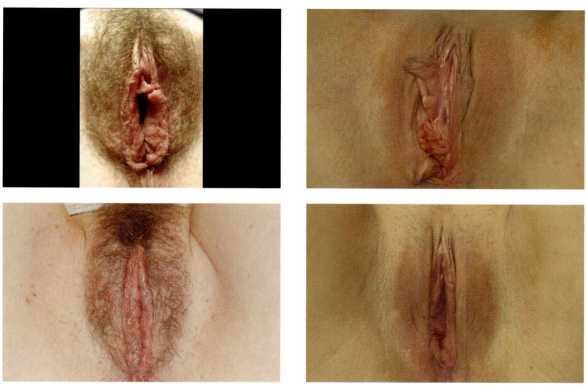

Figure 17.14 Previous linear resection labiaplasty leaving clitoral hood flaps and redundant polypoid-appearing labia. Re-operation performed via curvilinear resection with separate flap resection. Source: J. Miklos and R. Moore. Reproduced with permission.

Figure 17.15 Major revision/re-operation of previous V-wedge labiaplasty with right-sided separation. Re-operation performed via curvilinear resection with attempt to equalize sides. Source: J. Miklos and R. Moore. Reproduced with permission.

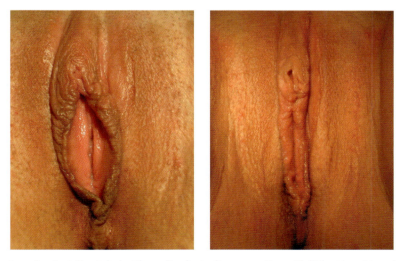

Figure 17.16 Re-operation of patient dissatisfied with results of prior linear resection with little attempt to reduce clitoral hood size, problematic for the patient. Re-operation was another curvilinear resection and reduction clitoral hood, trimming size to patient's specifications. Source: M. Goodman. Reproduced with permission.

patient early on and throughout her recovery, neither a revision nor re-operation should be undertaken early, specifically within the first 3 months after your procedure. A lot of hand-holding is involved, continually re-assuring her that tissue softens, flattens, and changes shape, and for this reason, plus the fact that the re-vascularization necessary to better assure the success of a revision or re-operation is not ideal until at least 3

months, it is best to wait a while before contemplating, much less performing revisionary work.

Ideally, the original surgeon should perform either revision or re-operation if he or she feels qualified, but the patient's best interests, and more often her desires and/or animosity toward her original surgeon may mandate referral to another surgeon. When this is the case, it is to the surgeon's benefit to refer the patient rather than have the patient, on her own, find another surgeon who may not kindly acquit her initial surgeon.

Re-operation techniques

There are no techniques specific for re-operation. The same advisories apply for a re-do as for an initial operation: evaluate the patient's anatomy and her

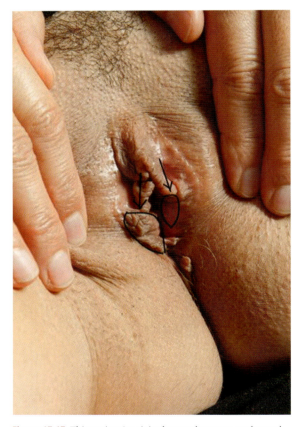

Figure 17.17 This patient's original procedure was performed by a general OB/GYN without specific training in genital plastics. The majority of the left labum majorum was excised to the vulvar vestibule, and both sides were repaired with running intermittently interlocked 3-0 Vicryl resulting in tissue strangulation. How to approach this difficult revision/re-operation? The author suggests excising the irregular polypoid mass representing the strangulated lower labum and denuding the contralateral vestibule below the existing left upper labial remnant, plus producing bilateral flaps and anchoring them below. This emphasizes the murky line between "revision" and "re-operation"! Source: M. Goodman. Reproduced with permission.

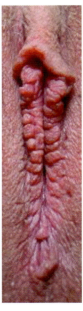

Figure 17.18 Tissue "grooving" secondary to large caliber strangulating surface closure. The only viable revision here, other than linear resection, which would leave no labia and a denuded introitus, would be to "airbrush" the prominent "peaks" of tissue, planing them down gently with an RF needle or touch laser fiber, letting them heal by secondary intention, as developed by Red Alinsod, MD, of Laguna Beach, California. The recovery, aided by analgesics and topical anesthetic gels, may be brutal, but the results are usually excellent, according to Dr. Alinsod. Lots of "hand-holding" here. Source: M. Goodman. Reproduced with permission.

post-operative ideal desires, and design a procedure most likely to meet these goals.

Informed consent; pricing

Informed consent procedures for re-operations may be exactly the same as that used for an initial surgery, as indeed most often this will be the initial time that *you* have operated on this patient. Specific disclaimers regarding outcome that may be compromised secondary to factors beyond your control stemming from the patient's initial surgery may be specifically noted on the consent.

Most surgeons price re-operations and major revisions of work done by another surgeon at or above (usually ~25–50% higher) than the same procedure on a "first-time" patient if the procedure is significantly more challenging secondary to sequelae from the initial procedure. Perusing Figures 17.12 through 17.18

below, one can see that some of these "re-dos" are especially challenging.

Summary

An aesthetic genital plastic/cosmetic surgeon must not only have a plan for successful surgery but must also be savvy regarding how to work with his or her dissatisfied or not fully satisfied patient. *Every* experienced surgeon will be faced with requests for revisions and occasionally re-operation of his/her or another surgeon's work. With time, the surgeon's ability to screen for body dysmorphia and to choose the "right operation on the right patient for the right reasons" will minimize the necessity for revisions or re-operations, but even well-experienced surgeons with >500–1,000 procedures "under their belts" will periodically have the occasion to revise.

CHAPTER 18

Psychosexual issues

Michael P. Goodman

Caring for Women Wellness Center, Davis, CA, USA

It takes a great [wo]man to be a good listener.

Arthur Helps

The decision to undergo genital plastic surgery has a strong psychological and sociocultural basis. There is a robust literature alluding to the importance that appearance, perception of appearance, and actual and perceived function play in a woman's sexual comfort in all realms of sexuality including desire, arousal, and orgasmic function [1–3]. Satisfaction with the visual appearance of the genitalia and self-consciousness about one's genitalia distinctly affect a sexual encounter; greater dissatisfaction with genital appearance is associated with higher genital self-consciousness, which in turn is associated with lower self-esteem and lower motivation to avoid risky sexual behavior [4]. Findings from these studies underscore the detrimental impact of negative genital perceptions on women's sexual well-being. Schick *et al.*, in a study of 217 women, concluded that "interventions that enhance satisfaction with the natural appearance of their genitalia could facilitate the development of a healthy sexual self-concept and provide long-term benefits in terms of sexual safety and satisfaction" [4].

At the same time, it is imperative that these women understand that *they are not abnormal*; that women's genitalia normally come in an array of shapes and sizes, even if they may be changed or affected by age, childbirth, or genetics. Of course, as in other forms of cosmetic surgical alterations, the fact of "normality" may not dissuade the patient in her quest for a size or functional alteration more in keeping with her aesthetic

and/or functional desires [5]. Both in the West and in Islamic cultures, cultural and media influences for a "clean slit" are very strong [6]. This is no different in a discussion of genital reconstruction than it is in a discussion of any other body "re-arrangements" such as breast augmentation or reduction, facial and nasal reconstruction, abdominoplasty, body "shaping" and "sculpting," and so forth. There is, however, a marked difference in degree of concern and effect on self-image when a woman's own genitals are involved.

Vaginal caliber and tone appear to play a role in sexual sensation, stimulation, and orgasmic response [7–9]. Vaginal "relaxation" has detrimental effects on sexual gratification secondary to reduction of frictional forces with resultant diminishment of sexual pleasure [7,10,11]. Ozel *et al.* [12] found that women with prolapse and vaginal relaxation were more likely to report absence of libido, diminished arousal, and more difficulty achieving orgasm. Additionally, it has been shown that vaginal tone affects vaginal sensation and the ability to reach orgasm [13].

It is incumbent upon the FGPS surgeon to be trained and savvy in sexual medicine or, if not, to have the ability to administer and audit the proper sexual function or psychological testing instruments so as to uncover those patients with a sexual function or body dysmorphic disorder (BDD), including eating disorders [14]. These patients should be referred to the proper practitioner to adjudicate their dysfunction prior to or concomitant with proposed cosmetic surgery. Although there is unanimous evidence in the literature [15–17] of improvement in sexual function with elective cosmetic and functional genital plastic surgery in normal women seeking revision (as opposed to patients seeking much more complicated reconstructive procedures for ambiguous genitalia or intersex operations [18], procedures that are unrelated to the elective cosmetic/plastic procedures herein reviewed), these procedures should not be touted as means to directly correct sexual dissatisfaction [19]. Genital plastic surgeons must be acutely aware of some patients' unrealistic expectations that surgery will have a positive impact on a failing relationship. A deep-seated sexual/psychosexual issue including sexual abuse and association of their genitalia with disgust or contamination may encourage some women to seek a surgical solution. Not surprisingly, these women may be disgruntled if the surgery fails to have the desired impact on their sexuality or their relationship. In circumstances such as this, referral to a psychosexual counselor would be more appropriate than surgery, or at the least should precede surgical modification. Surgeons must also be aware of motivational factors. While it is not unusual for the partners of women with robust-sized labia to comment, occasionally derogatorily [20], this should not be the major motivation for a surgical re-adjustment. Given the psychosocial and clinical impact of surgery, extreme caution must be exercised by surgeons performing FGPS [21].

Several testing instruments may be utilized by the genital aesthetic surgeon to uncover patients with primarily a sexual dysfunction (Figures 18.1 and 18.2), but great care must be taken in interpretation. David Veale and co-workers in the UK have validated a questionnaire specifically designed to screen for BDD in women seeking cosmetic, body-altering procedures [22], and his Cosmetic Procedures Screening questionnaire for women seeking labiaplasty (COPS-L) is an excellent tool for a referral psychologist to utilize for patients you are uneasy about performing surgery upon.

For aesthetic clinicians, the Arizona Sexual Experiences Scale (ASEX) or the Female Sexual Function Index, short form (FSFI-6) are two easy-to-administer short-form screening instruments that practitioners may use to, along with interview and intuition, perform an intake screen for sexual dysfunction. Patients who score 19 or higher on the ASEX, or 18 or lower on the FSFI-6, should receive in-depth evaluation prior to a surgical

procedure. However, as Goodman et al. have shown, both in a small pilot study [23] and in a larger, better powered, and time expanded study presently in preparation for submission for publication and discussed in detail below, although a large percentage of women seeking and receiving genital plastic and cosmetic surgical services test positive for body dissatisfaction and exhibit both sexual dissatisfaction and poor genital self-image prior to their surgery, these apparent "dysfunctions" disappear after completion of surgery [23].

Goodman et al. studied the pre-operative sexual function of their patients undergoing a variety of FGPS procedures (Table 18.1) and found pre-operative sexual function in all groups to parallel but be listed as less satisfactory than that of a population of similar-aged women, especially in the group seeking and receiving vaginal tightening procedures [24–29]. It may be difficult to separate a patient with sexual *dys*function from one with perceived sub-optimal sexual function, seeking enhancement. The FGPS surgeon *must* have the comfort, time, and inclination to intimately discuss sexuality and sexual matters with his/her patient, while admitting that this discussion may not be totally comfortable for either party. If the physician does not have the time and/or inclination, proper care and avoidance of failure and medical-legal entanglements mandates pre-operative referral for evaluation.

Goodman and Brotto's group [23] completed a small pilot study in 2011, the first *prospective* study ever of genital plastics, which found that women seeking cosmetic and functional genital modification scored similarly pre-operatively in terms of psychological and sexual function, but that a full 50+% of genital plastic patients qualified at intake as having "moderate" BDD, as quantified by a standard testing instrument, the BDD-YBOCS (Yale Brown Obsessive Compulsive Scale, modified for BDD). Six months post-operatively, a modest improvement in sexual functioning was noted in the study group, while evidence for BDD had *fallen to 7%, lower than the control group*, suggesting a great personal effect of perceived "abnormalities" in this area. This study was criticized for its small sample size and short follow-up period. A more expansive follow-up study, with larger numbers (120 patients undergoing a variety of genital plastic and cosmetic procedures) and a full 2-year follow-up has been performed and has been submitted for publication With 73% follow-up at 6 months, the initial disruptions seen in sexual function, body image, and

Arizona Sexual Experiences Scale (ASEX)
Administered under license from The University of Arizona

Antidepressants can cause sexual side effects in some people. This simple five-question self-evaluation may help you recognize if you're having a problem. If you are concerned about a sexual dysfunction, especially if you have a score in the "sexual dysfunction" range, you may want to talk to your doctor about treatment options with fewer sexual side effects.

For each item, please indicate your OVERALL level during the PAST WEEK, including TODAY.

	1	2	3	4	5	6
How strong is your sex drive?	extremely strong	very strong	somewhat strong	somewhat weak	very weak	no sex drive
How easily are you sexually aroused (turned on)?	extremely easily	very easily	somewhat easily	somewhat difficult	very difficult	never aroused
[FOR WOMEN] How easily does your vagina become moist or wet during sex?	extremely easily	very easily	somewhat easily	somewhat difficult	very difficult	never
[FOR MEN] Can you easily get and keep and erection?	extremely easily	very easily	somewhat easily	somewhat difficult	very difficult	never
How easily can you reach an orgasm?	extremely easily	very easily	somewhat easily	somewhat difficult	very difficult	never reach orgasm
Are your orgasms satisfying?	extremely satisfying	very satisfying	somewhat satisfying	somewhat unsatisfying	very unsatisfying	can't reach orgasm

Total score for the 5 questions:_____

As a general guide to understanding your score, this is how the numbers were interpreted when they were used in clinical studies: a person was considered to have sexual dysfunction if they had either **a total score of 19 or higher; a score of 5 or higher on one question; or a score of 4 or higher on 3 questions**.

Important: This ASEX self-evaluation is provided for your information and to help you understand the types of sexual side effects some people may experience. It was developed and validated by researchers at the **University of Arizona for use in clinical trials** conducted by trained investigators and should not be used to diagnose any conditions. You may wish to use the questions and your answers as a basis for discussion with your doctor.

McGahuey CA, Gelenberg AJ, Laukes CA, et al. The Arizona Sexual Experience Scale (ASEX): Reliability and validity. *J Sex Marital Ther.* 2000;26:25-40.

WXL016-0511   06/11

Figure 18.1 Arizona Sexual Experiences Scale. Source: Goodman *et al.* 2009 [16]. Reproduced with permission from Taylor & Francis.

FSFI – 6 QUESTIONAIRE

(Over the past 4 weeks)

1. How would you rate your level (degree) of sexual desire or interest?		VERY HIGH 5	HIGH 4	MODERATE 3	LOW 2	VERY LOW OR NONE AT ALL 1
2. How would you rate your level of sexual arousal ("turn on") during sexual activity or intercourse?	NO SEXUAL ACTIVITY 0	VERY HIGH 5	HIGH 4	MODERATE 3	LOW 2	VERY LOW OR NONE AT ALL 1
3. How often did you become lubricated ("wet") during sexual activity or intercourse?	NO SEXUAL ACTIVITY 0	VERY HIGH 5	HIGH 4	MODERATE 3	A FEW TIMES 2	ALMOST NEVER OR NEVER 1
4. When you had sexual stimulation or intercourse, how often did you reach orgasm?	NO SEXUAL ACTIVITY 0	VERY HIGH 5	HIGH 4	MODERATE 3	A FEW TIMES 2	ALMOST NEVER OR NEVER 1
5. How satisfied have you been/ with your overall sexual life?		VERY SATISFIED 5	MODERATELY SATISFIED 4	EQUALLY SATISFIED AND DISSATISFIED 3	MODERATELY DISSATISFIED 2	VERY DISSATISFIED 1
6. How often did you experience discomfort or pain during vaginal penetration?	DID NOT ATTEMPT INTERCOURSE 0	ALMOST NEVER OR NEVER 5	A FEW TIMES 4	SOMETIMES 3	MOST TIMES 2	ALMOST ALWAYS OR ALWAYS 1

Figure 18.2 Female Sexual Function Index, short form (FSFI-6).

Table 18.1 FGPS patients' estimation of their preoperative sexual function.

Post-Operative Sexual Function	LP and/or RCH (n = 174) N (%)	VP and/or PP (n = 46) N (%)	LP with VP and/or PP, with or without RCH (n = 31) N (%)
"Poor"	36 (20.7)	13 (28.3)	7 (22.6)
"Fair"	44 (25.3)	25 (54.3)	12 (38.7)
Poor/Fair	80 (46.0)	38 (82.6)	19 (61.3)
"Good"	68 (39.1)	7 (15.2)	8 (25.8)
"Great"	26 (15.0)	1 (2.2)	4 (12.9)
Good/Great	94 (54.1)	8 (17.4)	12 (38.7)

Source: Goodman *et al.* 2009 [16]. Reproduced with permission from Wiley.

genital self-image had disappeared; at 1 year (67% follow-up) genital plastic patients had "better" scores than controls; and at 2 years (48% follow-up) scores on sexual function, body dysmorphia, and genital self-image scales were virtually the same as the control group.

Results from this prospective, community-based study with a control group confirmed the findings of Goodman and Brotto's pilot study: while women undergoing genital plastic surgeries had a significantly increased body dysmorphic score (BDD-YBOCS), a significantly lower genital self-image (FGSIS), and a significantly lower Index of Sexual Satisfaction (ISS) before surgery, all of these parameters reverted to "normal" (i.e., same as control group) by 6 months post-op and stayed in the normal range through 1 and 2 years post-operatively.

David Veale and co-workers have also published results looking at psychosexual outcome after labiaplasty [20]. In a prospective, case-comparison study of 49 patients with follow-up of 11–42 months, improvement was noted in 91.3% at long-term follow-up on the Genital Appearance Satisfaction scale [30] (appearance), and smaller improvements were noted in sexual functioning, findings concordant with Goodman *et al.*'s studies [31].

Cindy Meston, PhD, and her group at the University of Texas at Austin have studied genital self-image and sexual well-being and its influence on sexual function and distress. (personal communication; unpublished data from Dr. Meston). They also wished to learn what type of genital appearance is considered visually appealing to men and women and whether genitalia modified by cosmetic surgery were judged as more attractive compared to unmodified genitalia. In their study, 900 men and women completed online questionnaires to assess genital self-image, sexual satisfaction, functioning, and distress. The Female Genital Self-Image Scale [32], the Relational Concern and Personal Concern subscales of the Sexual Satisfaction Scale—Women, [33] and the FSFI [34], all validated testing instruments, were utilized. Men rated unaltered and altered genitalia as more attractive than women; older participants rated unaltered and altered genitalia as more attractive than younger participants; and men and women of all ages found altered genitalia more attractive than unaltered genitalia. They found that genital self-image was positively correlated with functioning variables including arousal, lubrication, orgasm, satisfaction, and pain and negatively correlated with

sexual distress and concluded that women with positive genital self-image experience higher levels of sexual functioning and lower levels of sexual distress. In their study, female genitalia modified by genital cosmetic surgery were considered more attractive regardless of age and gender.

This chapter is not meant to be a treatise on psychosexual attitudes of women as they relate to their genitalia, nor as a complete guide geared toward therapy of any sexual dysfunction or BDD. Standards of care demand that the genital plastic surgeon go beyond being merely a surgical technician and understand that his or her patient is a living, breathing sexual being, and that the most robust sexual organ she has is between her ears. The normality or abnormality of the patient's psychological and sexual makeup must be taken into consideration as part of pre-and peri-operative workup and intervention for this unique group of women.

References

1. Pujols Y, Meston C, Seal BN. The association between sexual satisfaction and body image in women. *J Sex Med* 2010;**7**:905–16.
2. Ackard DM, Kearney-Cooke A, Peterson CB. Effect of body self-image on women's sexual behaviors. *Int J Eat Disord* 2000;**28**:422–9.
3. Lowenstein L, Gamble T, Samses TV, Van Raalte H, Carberry C, Jakus S, Kambiss S, McAchran S, Pham T, Aschkenazi S, Hoskey K; Fellows Pelvic Research Network. Sexual function is related to body image perception in women with pelvic organ prolapse. *J Sex Med* 2009;**6**:2286–91.
4. Schick VR, Calabrese SK, Rima BN, Zucker AN. Genital appearance dissatisfaction: Implications for women's genital image self-consciousness, sexual esteem, sexual satisfaction, and sexual risk. *Psychol Women Q* 2010;**34**:384–404
5. Goodman MP. Female cosmetic genital surgery. *Obstet Gynecol* 2009;**113**:154–96.
6. McDougall LJ. Towards a clean slit: How medicine and notions of normality are shaping female genital aesthetics. *Culture, Health Sexuality* 2013;**15**:774–87.
7. Pardo J, Sola V, Ricci P, Guiloff E, Freundlich D. Colpoperineoplasty in women with a sensation of a wide vagina. *Acta Obstet et Gynec* 2006;**85**:1125–7.
8. Jannini EA, Rubio-Casillas, Whipple B, Buisson O, Komisaruk BR, Brody S. Female orgasm(s): One, two, several. *J Sex Med* 2012;**9**:956–65.
9. Brody S, Weiss P. Vaginal orgasm is associated with vaginal (not clitoral) sex education, focusing mental attention on vaginal sensations, intercourse duration, and a preference for a longer penis. *J Sex Med* 2010;**7**:2774–81.

10. Shek KL, Dietz HP. The effect of childbirth on hiatal dimensions. *Obstst Gynecol* 2009;**113**:1272–8.

11. Ostrzenski A. An acquired sensation of wide/smooth vagina: A new classification. *Eur J Obstet Gynec Repro Biol* 2011;**15**:897–900.

12. Ozel B, White T, Urwitz-Lane R, Minaglia S. The impact of pelvic organ prolapse on sexual function in women with urinary incontinence. *Int Urogynecol J Pelvic Floor Dysfunct* 2006;**1**:14–7.

13. Kline G. (1982) Case studies of perineometer resistive exercises of orgasmic dysfunction. In: *Circumvaginal Musculature and Sexual Function*, pp. 25–42. Basel, Switzerland: S. Karger, 1982.

14. Veale D, Boocock A, Gournay K, Dryden W, Shah F, Willson R, Walburn J. Body dysmorphic disorder: A survey of fifty cases. *Br J Psych* 1996;**169**:196–201.

15. Abdool Z, Shek C, Dietz HP. The effect of levator evulsion on hiatal dimensions and function. *Am J Obstet Gynecol* 2009;**201**:89.e1–89.e5.

16. Goodman MP, Placik OJ, Benson RH III, Miklos JR, Moore RD, Jason RA, Matlock DL, Simopoulos AF, Stern BH, Stanton RA, Kolb SE, Gonzalez F. A large multicenter outcome study of female genital plastic surgery. *J Sex Med* 2009;**8**:1813–25.

17. Maas SM, Hage JJ. Functional and aesthetic labia minora reduction *Plast Reconstr Surg* 2007;**106**:1453–6.

18. Creighton SM, Minto CL, Steele SJ. Objective cosmetic and anatomical outcomes at adolescence of feminizing surgery for ambiguous genitalia done in childhood. *Lancet* 2001;**358**:124–5.

19. Giraldo F, Gonzalez C, deHaro F. Central wedge nymphectomy with a 90-degree Z-plasty for aesthetic reduction of the labia minora. *Plast Reconstr Surg* 2004;**113**:1820–5.

20. Veale D, Eshkerem E, Ellison N, Costa A, Robinson D, Kavouni A, Cardozo, L. A comparison of risk factors for women seeking labiaplasty compared to those not seeking labiaplasty. *Body Image* 2014;**11**:57–62.

21. Renganathan A, Cartwright R, Cardozo L. Gynecological cosmetic surgery. *Expert Rev Obstet Gynecol* 2009;**4**:101–4.

22. Veale D, Eshkevari E, Ellison N, Cardozo L, Robinson D, Kavouni A. Validation of Genital Appearance Satisfaction scale and COPS-L. *J Psychosomatic Obstet Gynecol* 2013;**34**:46–52.

23. Goodman MP, Fashler S, Miklos JR, Moore RD, Brotto LA. The sexual, psychological, and body image health of women undergong elective vulvovaginal plastic/cosmetic procedures: A pilot study. *Am J Cosmetic Surg* 2011;**28**:1–8.

24. Herbenick D, Reece M. Development and validation of the female genital self-image scale. *J Sex Med* 2010;**7**:1822–30.

25. Avis NE, Zhao X, Johannes C, Orr M, Brockwell S, Greendale G. Correlates of sexual function among multi-ethnic middle-aged women: Results from the study of women's sexual health across the nation (SWAN). *Menopause* 2005;**12**:385–98.

26. Laumann EO, Paik A, Rosen R. Sexual dysfunction in the United States: Prevalence and predictors. *JAMA* 1999;**281**:537–44.

27. Laumann EO, Nickolosi A, Glasser DB, Paik A, Gingell C, Moreira E, Wang T. Sexual problems among women and men aged 40–80 years: Prevalence and correlates identified in the global study of sexual attitudes and behaviors. *Internat J Impotence Res* 2005;**17**:39–57.

28. Hayes RD, Dennerstein L, Bennett CM, Sidat M, Gurrin LC, Fairley CK. Risk factors for female sexual dysfunction in the general population: Exploring factors associated with low sexual function and sexual distress. *J Sex Med* 2008;**5**:1681–3.

29. Hayes RD, Dennerstein L, Bennett CM, Fairley CK. What is the "true" prevalence of female sexual dysfunctions and does the way we assess these conditions have an impact? *J Sex Med* 2008;**5**:777–87.

30. Bramwell R, Morland C. Genital appearance satisfaction in women: The development of a questionnaire and exploration of correlates. *J Reproduct Infant Psychol* 2009;**27**(1):15–27.

31. Goodman MP, Fashler S, Miklos JR, Moore RD, Brotto LA. The sexual, psychological, and body image health of women undergoing elective vulvovaginal plastic/cosmetic procedures: A pilot study. *Am J Cosmetic Surg* 2011;**28**:1–8.

32. Herbenick D, Reece M. Development and validation of the female genital self-image scale. *J Sex Med* 2010;**7**:1822–30.

33. Meston C, Trapnell P. Development and validation of a five-factor sexual satisfaction and distress scale for women: The Sexual Satisfaction Scale for Women (SSS-W). *J Sex Med* 2005:266–81.

34. Rosen R, Brown C, Helmar J, Leiblum S, Meston C, Shabsigh R, Ferguson D, D'Agostino R Jr. The Female Sexual Function Index (FSFI): A multidimensional self-reporting instrument for the assessment of female sexual function. *J Sex Marital Ther* 2000:191–208.

CHAPTER 19

Outcomes

Michael P. Goodman

Caring for Women Wellness Center, Davis, CA, USA

Stuff without knowledge is never enough to get you there… it just won't get you there…

Greg Brown, in his song

Two Little Feet,
paraphrasing naturalist John Muir.

In determining outcomes of a given medical treatment or procedure, several considerations must be evaluated. Certainly, the "risk/benefit" bar is higher for an "elective" compared with an "indicated" procedure. Outcome parameters are simple: Is the patient satisfied… or not? Have her needs been met? Did she or did she not experience an enhancement of her sexual function? Were complications minimal and short-lived or major and disfiguring? Was the time, effort, and financial expenditure worthwhile? Are outcomes reproducible over time and from practitioner to practitioner? And, in outcomes reported in evidence-based literature, is the follow-up period sufficient to make a determination and is the study observational or prospective?

Several moderately to well-powered outcome studies investigate LP, with or without RCH, although all but one are retrospective. Five originate from a single surgeon or group [1–5]; one is multicentered [6]. All outcome studies of vulvar procedures (LP, RCH) in the peer-reviewed medical literature appear to show positive outcome statistics, although parameters are relatively primitive (Table 19.1). All papers leveling criticism at LP as a surgical procedure quote anecdotal information only; all peer-reviewed studies available quote patient satisfaction rates in the 90–95+range [1–6], although all are retrospective.

Three retrospective studies evaluate vaginal procedures [6–8] and all report apparently favorable outcomes

(Tables 19.2 and 19.3). Each study utilizes slightly different outcome parameters. They are similar but may be utilized for qualitative comparison only.

Goodman *et al.* [6] and Pardo *et al.* [7] utilized non-validated questionnaires and noted an 89% and 90% rate of improvement in sexual satisfaction, respectively (Table 19.2). Moore *et al.* [8] utilized the Pelvic Organ Prolapse/Urinary Incontinence Sexual Questionnaire (PISQ-12), a validated and frequently utilized instrument to evaluate several parameters of sexual function in patients with pelvic floor issues (Table 19.3). Compared pre-operatively and post-operatively, the overall sexual function statistically improved except in three categories in which there was no change (desire; pain; partner premature ejaculation). Overall sexual satisfaction improved, as well as subcategories of increased sexual excitement during intercourse as well as an overall increase in intensity of orgasms. No increase in dyspareunia was noted post-operatively.

The single published prospective study (previously discussed in Chapter 18) involving genital plastics has a small sample size, and reviews psychological sexual and body image parameters only [9]. A follow-up of this study, as mentioned in Chapter 18, submitted for publication shows virtually the same findings as the pilot study, noting apparent complete resolution of what appeared to be body image, genital self-image, and

---

Female Genital Plastic and Cosmetic Surgery, First Edition. Edited by Michael P. Goodman.
© 2016 John Wiley & Sons, Ltd. Published 2016 by John Wiley & Sons, Ltd.

Table 19.1 Outcomes, labiaplasty; clitoral hood reduction.

Outcome Parameter Author	MD's Estimate of Good Anatomic Results	Satisfied	Not Satisfied	Satisfied Aesthetically	Satisfied Functionally	"Effect on my sexual satisfaction"	"Effect on partner's satisfaction"	Would Undergo Procedure Again	Complications
Rouzier et al. (1) 163 pts.	93% "good-excellent"	96%	4%	89%	93%			96%	"No surgically-related complications"
Munhoz et al. (3) 21 pts.	85% "good-excellent"	95.2%	4.8%						5/21 (23.8%) "Wound healing problems"
Pardo et al. (2) 55 pts		+ +++ 9% 91%							"No major complications"
Alter (4) 166 pts.		95% (average satisfaction score 9.2/10)	5%	"Improved self-esteem" 93%		"Improvement" 71%		98%	4% "Significant complication"
Goodman et al. (5) 211 pts	96.6% "good-excellent"	96.2%	3.8%			+ to +++ no effect 64% 35.3%	+ to +++ no effect 35.7% 64.3%		(patient: 8.5%, all minor; mostly poor or prolonged healing, pain) (MD: 7.3%, all minor; mostly poor healing/ dyspareunia)

Table 19.2 Outcome studies, perineoplasty/vaginoplasty.

Outcome Parameter / Author	Overall Satisfaction			Patient's Satisfaction with Regard to Width		Physician's Estimate of Results		"Enhancement of my sexual satisfaction"				"Enhancement of partner's sexual satisfaction"		Complications According to MD	Complications According to Patient
Pardo et al. (6) 53 patients	++ 74%	+ 21%	O 5%	Satisfied 96%	Not 4%			Much improved 66%	Sufficiently improved 24%	Poorly improved 6%	Worse 4%			3.8%, "all minor"	
Goodman et al. (5) 81 patients	"Yes" 89%	"No" 11%				++ to +++ 92.6%	+− 7.4%	+++ enhancement 54.8%	+ to ++ enhancement 34.2%	No enhancement 9.6%	Negative enhancement 1.4%	+ to +++ enhancement 82.2%	0 to − enhancement 17.8%	19.7%, "mostly minor, no long-term sequelae"	17.3%, none major

Table 19.3 Compare PISQ-12 between pre-op and post-op in vaginal rejuvenation (N = 60).

PISQ-12	Pre-operative Mean (SD)	Post-operative Mean (SD)	p-value
1. How frequently do you feel sexual desire?	2.6 (1.0)	2.6 (0.9)	0.795
2. Do you climax when having sexual intercourse with your partner?	1.7 (1.4)	2.2 (1.4)	0.012
3. Do you feel sexually excited when having sexual activity with your partner?	2.8 (1.0)	3.2 (1.0)	0.004
4. How satisfied are you with the varieties of sexual activities in your current sex life?	2.3 (1.1)	2.93 (1.1)	0.001
5. Do you feel pain during intercourse?	2.6 (1.2)	3.0 (1.3)	0.055
6. Are you incontinent of urine with sexual activity?	2.9 (1.3)	3.9 (0.5)	<.001
7. Does fear of incontinence restrict your sexual activity?	2.8 (1.3)	3.9 (0.5)	<.001
8. Do you avoid sexual intercourse because of bulging of the vagina?	3.2 (1.1)	3.8 (0.6)	<.001
9. When you have sex with your partner, do you have negative emotional reactions such as fear, disgust, shame, or guilt?	2.4 (1.4)	3.6 (1.0)	<.001
10. Does your partner have a problem with erections that affects your sexual activity?	3.1 (1.1)	3.5 (1.1)	0.010
11. Does your partner have a problem with premature ejaculation that affects your sexual activity?	3.3 (1.1)	3.6 (1.1)	0.085
12. Compared to orgasms that you have had in the past, how intense are the orgasms you have had in the past 6 months?	1.1 (1.0)	2.3 (0.7)	<001
Total	30.3 (6.6) Range 11–46	38.2 (5.2) Range 26–46	<.001

Source: Moore *et al.* 2014 [7]. Reproduced with permission of Taylor & Francis.

sexual satisfaction disparities pre-procedure, to a level experienced by the "control" group at all post-operative points in time. Both of these studies look at pre- and post-operative body image, genital self-image, and sexual function in a heterogeneous group of community women undergoing aesthetic and functional vulvovaginal aesthetic surgery at different locations throughout the United States, paired against an age, educationally, and societally matched group of controls (Goodman *et al.*, submitted for publication, discussed Chapter 18).

Only one study in the literature evaluates LP outcome comparing different surgical techniques. Goodman *et al.* in their 2010 study [6] compared LP outcome by surgical technique and found little difference in overall satisfaction and perception of complications between patients receiving a linear versus a V-wedge procedure, although the V-wedge group did notice a statistically significant improvement in "enhancement of sexual function" (*p* = 0.0215) (Table 19.4).

HP outcome has been little studied. In the only reported case series, 50% of a series of 20 patients were followed after consummation of marriage, and all reported a "satisfactory" outcome, whatever that means [10]. The very nature of, and the secrecy surrounding, cultural hymenoplasty makes it virtually impossible to ascertain outcome parameters via post-operative patient follow-up. In the author's personal experience, most HP recipients do not return for long-term evaluation. The fact that those few that do contact their clinician report success with bleeding at consummation of marriage is statistically irrelevant.

Complication rates from all well-powered LP reports in the literature prior to 2010 have been <5% (all minor), but "complications" were not well-defined, and in some studies it was not clear whether the complications were from the surgeon's or patient's viewpoint [1–4, 11]. Goodman *et al.*'s 2010 study [6] looked at "complications" from both the patient's and surgeon's perspective, asking both whether they considered there

Table 19.4 Outcome by labiaplasty surgical technique.

Method of Labiaplasty	Linear Excision (N = 83) N (%)	Modified V-Wedge (N = 70) N (%)	p Value (LE vs V-W)
Overall patient	80 (96.4)	67 (95.7)	p = 0.83
Satisfaction	3 (3.6)	3 (4.3)	
"Yes"			
"No"			
Patient perception of	76 (91.6)	65 (92.9)	p = 0.77
complication	7 (8.4)	5 (7.1)	
"None"			
"Yes"			
Enhancement of sexual function	(N=80)	(N=67)	p = 0.02
"Negative effect"	2 (2.5)	2 (3.0)	
"No effect"	34 (42.8)	18 (26.9)	
"Mild-moderate	25 (30.8)	18 (26.9)	
enhancement"	20 (24.8)	29 (43.2)	
"Significant enhancement"			

was a "complication from their procedure," asking about subjective evaluations including "prolonged healing," "excessive post-operative bleeding," "poor healing," "feeling…too tight," "separation of repair," "hypersensitivity," and so forth (Tables 19.1 and 19.2). Patient's and surgeon's evaluations listed these occurrences respectively as 8.5%/7.3% for LP/RCH, and 17.3%/19.7% for procedures involving perineal and intra-vaginal work. However, in spite of these apparently relatively high numbers of listed complications, the overall "success" rate for each group, when evaluated by both patients and their surgeons, was 97.2%/96.6% for LP/RCH, 83.0%/91.5% for VP/PP, and 91.2%/97.0% for combined procedures, suggesting that the "complications" listed were minor and/or short-lived, not affecting the perceived effectiveness of the surgery. In any case, no reports list major, ongoing complications from these surgeries, other that the fact that, in a small percentage of patients, they did not accomplish their desired goals. *One must remember, however, that these studies included only accomplished vulvovaginal cosmetic/plastic surgeons, and that complications and complication rates from novice surgeons may be significantly higher, with satisfaction rates lower.*

One has only to peruse online sites, to be involved as a medical-legal expert, or to be in the business of evaluating women who have undergone a genital plastic procedure with a cosmetically or functionally poor outcome to realize that, in the "real world," these statistics may not be entirely valid. The fact is that procedures performed by individuals without formal training in performing plastic and sexual function procedures on women, or without a decent level of experience, fare differently and experience poorer outcomes than those reported in the literature by experienced, competent surgeons.

With all reported studies *from experienced surgeons*, encompassing 6 months to 4 years follow-up, these women and their partners appear to be satisfied both cosmetically and functionally. There appears to be a positive impact on sexual health and an apparently favorable risk:benefit analysis.

Again, comments from patients are revealing: "I was very, very self-conscious about the way I looked. Now I feel free. I just feel normal. Now, I have nothing to hide." And, "I just felt that I keep myself in shape everywhere else…[the surgery] has given me more intense sexual enjoyment" [12]. However, one has only to check the Internet, or look at medical-legal case records, to discover that not all patients are satisfied with results. In this, as in many surgical disciplines, novice surgeons often do not fare as well.

The "statistics" aside, outcome in general is affected by many factors that have been or will be discussed in detail elsewhere in this text. These factors may be categorized as follows.

Pre-operative factors include [1] surgeon's training and experience; [2] patient's general and physical health including smoking status, hormonal milieu, immunological status, average blood sugar, medications, and so forth; [3] patient's general knowledge including preparation by office staff and physician, expectations, and her stress and anxiety level; [4] arrangements made by the patient prior to surgery in regards to her level of activities and recovery; and [5] psychological and psychosexual status. This last pre-operative factor should not be ignored. The genital plastic/cosmetic surgeon would do well to screen carefully body dysmorphia, history of sexual abuse, sexual dysfunction, and stress/anxiety disorder, as these factors, individually or in concert, can affect outcome. Patients with these issues should be referred to the appropriate therapeutic practitioner for evaluation and most likely psychotherapeutic intervention in place of or prior to surgical intervention.

Peri-operative factors include [1] asepsis; [2] the surgeon's skill and attention to detail; choice of technique specifically for her anatomy, tools, and suture materials; and adequacy of anesthesia; and [3] cooperation of patient if performed under local anesthesia.

Post-operative factors include [1] adequacy of post-operative instructions, preferably both in oral and written form, with careful evaluation of the patient's understanding of what is expected of her; [2] patient's clarity and understanding of and her ability to follow through on what is expected of her; adequate icing, minimal tissue "handling," cleanliness; [3] availability of the surgeon for queries and potential complication evaluation; patient's general medical health and hormonal status; and [4] the patient's ability to understand the significant tissue and visual changes (almost day-to-day in the first few weeks!) inherent in the 6-month-long healing process and to be able to minimize the anxiety and stress that may accompany recovery from this surgery in some individuals. Some patients, unfortunately, are their own worst enemies and, while disclaiming that they "are not touching it" will send in photos where they are pulling on the suture line so they can show their surgeon "an opening that they have 'discovered' (*produced!*)."

The most common post-operative event precipitating adverse outcome is excessive or inopportune, often inadvertent, physical activity or tissue handling that results in excessive edema and/or premature suture breakage or release from tissue, resulting in wound separation and prolonged healing. Experienced surgeons notice a real difference in swelling and outcome relating to the care their patient gives her own vulva post-operatively. Remind your patients, both verbally and in writing: "Don't pull on it!" "Don't look at it all the time"! "Baby it!" "Don't go back to 'usual and customary' activities one day before instructed to do so," and…"Sex must wait until you are cleared by your surgeon!" Remind your patient that you have done a careful job, she is paying you a lot of $$s for her surgery, and that she, through a careful recovery, is a partner with you and is in control of her own destiny…That said, every plastic/cosmetic surgeon will still have a small cadre of patients who appear to be on *send* rather than *receive*.

References

1. Rouzier R, Louis-Sylvestre C, Paniel BJ, Hadded B. Hypertrophy of the labia minora: Experience with 163 reductions. *Am J Obstet Gynecol* 2000;**182**:35–40.
2. Pardo J, Sola P, Ricci P, Guilloff E. Laser labiaplasty of the labia minora. *Int J Gynec Obst* 2005;**93**:38–43.
3. Munhoz AM, Filassi JR, Ricci MD, Aldrighi C, Correira LD, Aldrighi JM, Ferreira MC. Aesthetic labia minora reduction with inferior wedge resection and superior pedicle flap reconstruction. *Plast Reconstr Surg* 2006;**118**:1237–47.
4. Alter GJ. Aesthetic labia minora and clitoral hood reduction using extended central wedge resection. *Plast Reconstr Surg* 2008;**122**:1780–9.
5. Hamori C. Aesthetic outcomes of labiaplasty. *Aesthet Surg J* 2011;**31**:987.
6. Goodman MP, Placik OJ, Benson RH III, Miklos JR, Moore RD, Jason RA, Matlock DL, Simopoulos AF, Stern BH, Stanton RA, Kolb SE, Gonzalez F. A large multicenter outcome study of female genital plastic surgery. *J Sex Med* 2010;**7**:1565–77.
7. Pardo J, Sola V, Ricci P, Guiloff E, Freundlich D. Colpoperineoplasty in women with a sensation of a wide vagina. *Acta Obstet et Gynec* 2006;**85**:1125–7.
8. Moore RD, Miklos JR, Chinthakanan D. Evaluation of sexual function outcomes in women undergoing vaginal rejuvenation/vaginolaplasty procedures for symptoms of vaginal laxity/decreased vaginal sensation utilizing validated sexual function questionnaire (PISQ-12). *Surg Tech Int* 2014;**24**:253–60.
9. Goodman MP, Fashler S, Miklos JR, Moore RD, Brotto LA. The sexual, psychological, and body image health of women undergoing elective vulvovaginal plastic/cosmetic procedures: A pilot study. *Am J Cosmetic Surg* 2011;**28**:1–8.
10. O'Connor M. Reconstructing the hymen: Mutilation or restoration? *J Law Med* 2008;**1**:161–75.
11. Lista F, Misty B, Singh Y, Ahmed J. The safety of aesthetic labiaplasty: A plastic surgery experience. *Aesthet Surg J* 2015;**35**:689–695.
12. The most private of makeovers. *New York Times*, November 28, 2004. Available at: http://www.ibiblio.org/pub/electronic publications/stayfree/public/nyt_vaginal_surgery.html.

CHAPTER 20

Pearls for Practice

Michael P. Goodman

Caring for Women Wellness Center, Davis, CA, USA

Knowledge is knowing a tomato is a fruit. Wisdom is not putting it into a fruit salad.

Miles Kingston

Whom to Operate On

- Educated, informed patients, who understand their alternatives.
- Patients who have a specific, isolated complaint, cosmetic and/or functional.
- Patients who are considering surgery *for themselves*, not only to "please" their sexual partner, although that desire may reasonably be part of the equation.
- Patients with reasonable expectations.
- Patients for whom this is not a "spur of the moment" decision.
- Patients who are reasonable *elective* surgical candidates.

Whom Not to Operate On

- Women who expect that plastic/cosmetic surgery will correct a sexual *dysfunction*.
- Patients who choose to not include or inform their sexual partner.
- Smokers, poorly controlled diabetics, uncontrolled hypertensives, post-menopausal women not on HRT.
- Patients with "body dysmorphic disorder," or eating disorder, unless they have a specific isolated anatomic situation and have received clearance from their therapist.
- Patients who may have unreasonable expectations.

- Patients who come in with a photograph and want to "look exactly like *that*."
- Patients with an untreated anxiety disorder, or who appear to be significantly challenged by anxiety-related issues.
- Patients who make you or your staff feel uneasy... *Use your "gut."*

How to Get into Trouble

- Operating on patients you shouldn't be operating on!
- Treating everyone the same: same operation on everyone, making their anatomy fit your technique, rather than the opposite.
- Taking too much off in LP and RCH procedures.
- Over-tightening in the mid-pelvic floor in VJR procedures.
- Operating too close to the clitoral complex.
- Not employing meticulous plastic technique; meticulous hemostasis.
- Guaranteeing a specific result (unreasonable expectations).
- Doing revisions too early. (Wait until at least 3–6 months after surgery to consider revision.)
- Being unavailable for questions and complications.
- Inadequate "informed consent."
- Inadequate patient preparation.

Female Genital Plastic and Cosmetic Surgery, First Edition. Edited by Michael P. Goodman.

How to Stay out of Trouble

- Do not operate on everyone who comes in.
- Be clear, and *document*, that neither you, nor any plastic/cosmetic surgeon, can guarantee a specific outcome.
- Invite your patient to be a part of the decision on specific surgical technique and how much she wants off, or how tight she wants to be, and *document*.
- When a patient asks you to "take it all off," counsel appropriately, and be careful to not remove too much. You always can take a little off later; you cannot add back on!
- Have clear and complete written pre- and post-op instructions and informed consent documents.
- Be facile in different techniques.
- Have a cache of "before and after" photos showing possibilities for differing anatomy and different surgical procedures. Have a file of post-op day 3-4-5 photos as well as photos with "less than ideal" results to share with your patient.
- Dialog clearly with your patient re: reasonable expectations.
- Participate in ongoing advanced study via course, workshop, proctorship, and so forth.
- Be patient; be meticulous.
- Be available for your patient post-operatively.
- Stay informed via seminars, meetings, literature, networking.

What Skills Must the Genital Plastic/Cosmetic Surgeon Possess?

- Caring for, and understanding, women.
- A thorough understanding of the anatomy; what to, and what *not* to do.
- The ability to *listen* to a woman and *her* desires.
- Patience, empathy, and kindness; be worthy of your patient's trust.
- Precision; meticulous surgical technique.
- Knowledge of, and facility in, alternative surgical techniques.
- Availability for follow-up and reassurance.

Patient Protection

1 The patient has the right to know:
  - That her surgeon has the proper level of training and experience to perform her procedure.

- The expected outcome, alternative surgical techniques available, recovery experience and expectations, as well as expected complications and rates of occurrence.
- The wide range of anatomic normality and that she falls within this range. *(Given this, the patient still may reasonably wish to alter her appearance.)*
- A clear explanation of the costs including surgeon's fees and operatory and anesthesia charges as well as potential financial responsibilities for revision procedures.

2 Patients should be screened for sexual dysfunction or body dysmorphic disorder.

Patient and Physician Protection

- Take time with your patient and LISTEN to her. What does she wish to accomplish?
- Is her goal reasonable and one that you, via FGPS, can assist her in reaching?
- Is she depressed? Does she have a sexual dysfunction? A body dysmorphic disorder? Will your surgery help her, *even if it does not turn out exactly as she envisioned?* Some women just become preoccupied with the next "defect" to be fixed.

Physician Protection

- Are you conversant with more than one technique for the procedure? Are you clear on how to listen to the patient's desires and to counsel her so that she can decide which suits her best? Are you familiar with the tools, sutures, anatomy, pitfalls, and immediate and long-term post-operative care?
- *Patients have different anatomies.* One procedure does not fit all. Can you deal with "strange anatomy"?
- Have you performed a sufficient number of similar cases so that, if queried in court, you can support your procedure, your decisions, and your care? What is your training? Proctoring? Are you credentialed *specifically* in *cosmetic labiaplasty* (not just *partial vulvectomy*) at your institution? If you are a novice, have you attended a course of sufficient character to prove in a court of law that you are prepared and trained for the surgery you performed?
- Learn when to say "No." Beware of patients who have unreasonable expectations, who want it "just

so," who bring in a picture and say they "want it just like that." Spend extra time on the patient who already has had several body enhancement procedures. Beware the patient who has a history of negative sexual experiences or feels that surgery will cure a sexual dysfunction.

- Give appropriate informed consent! (See Chapter 7).
- Document…Document…Document.

The mantra of all genital plastic/cosmetic surgeons? "Integrity and honesty in all dealings. Care and attention to detail in surgery."

CHAPTER 21

Standards of care

Michael P. Goodman

Caring for Women Wellness Center, Davis, CA, USA

Only the mediocre are always at their best.

Joan Giraudoux

Standards of care (SOC) are the rules by which the consumer, in this case our patients, may be protected and guaranteed a minimal level of professional competence. Medical SOC are most often delineated by professional societies or organizations. In their absence, they may be forthcoming from hospitals via privileging guidelines, and even by legislation. Over time, "community standards" develop relating to the "usual custom and practice" of members of that community. One would hope that these are high standards, but unfortunately this is not always the case. Often, "standards of care" is a legal rather than a medical definition, a hard fact that physicians only viscerally understand after the papers for a professional liability action have been filed.

Why are standards of care needed?

The territory in which genital plastic and cosmetic procedures are performed is akin to the old "Wild, Wild West," namely, wide open and unregulated. Across the United States, across the world, and within the local community, there presently exists no comprehensive "standard" or cohesive training program for this distinct surgical discipline, part gynecology, part plastic and reconstructive surgery.

Training in women's genital plastic/cosmetic procedures, from labiaplasty (minora or majora) to hood

reduction to hymenoplasty to vaginoplasty for reasons of vaginal tightening and improved sexual pleasure, are *not mandated* in gynecologic residency training programs in the United States and most foreign countries. In fact, *plastic technique* in regards to precise tissue handling, use of fine suture material, plastic closure techniques and procedure design oriented toward aesthetic outcome are not part of traditional gynecologic training. Plastic surgeons certainly are instructed in plastic technique, and receive training in vulvar anatomy, but not all programs teach vulvar surgical techniques, and very few contemplate intra-vaginal anatomy and procedures.

An informed SOC is imperative for patient protection, as there is certainly a difference between good outcome and poor outcome. It is intuitive that surgeons with training specific to genital plastic/cosmetic procedures will on average fare considerably better than surgeons untrained for the specific procedures discussed in this text. A pillar of the Hippocratic Oath is *primum non nocere*. It is within that oath that this chapter is rooted.

An approved OB/GYN residency program teaches its resident staff vulvar/vaginal/pelvic anatomy and extirpative procedures involving the vulva and vagina, most commonly for reasons of malignancy or pre-malignancy. It teaches vaginal wall surgery for reasons of symptoms from a variety of pelvic floor weaknesses. It does not teach plastic labial or clitoral hood procedures or technique. It most often does not take into account the

Female Genital Plastic and Cosmetic Surgery, First Edition. Edited by Michael P. Goodman.
© 2016 John Wiley & Sons, Ltd. Published 2016 by John Wiley & Sons, Ltd.

potential effect of vaginal laxity on sexual activities and sexual satisfaction, and this eventuality rarely plays a part in pre-surgical planning. Pelvic floor procedures planned specifically for reasons of tightening to improve cosmesis, friction, and sexual pleasure are not a traditional part of either OB/GYN or plastic surgery programs.

Many plastic surgery programs incorporate labial and hood aesthetic/reconstructive procedures. Many do not. Very few teach vaginal and pelvic anatomy and the ins and outs of a vaginal floor repair. The "ideal" education is depicted in Table 21.1; the present-day reality in Table 21.2.

Precedent exists in both the gynecologic and plastic surgery communities. If we reasonably ask the questions (and certainly develop or imply SOC guidelines) regarding who is most qualified to perform a radical vulvectomy, general OB/GYN or gynecologic oncologist; who is most qualified to perform a laparoscopic pelvic floor repair, general gynecologist or urogynecologist; who should perform a difficult breast reduction or augmentation, general or plastic surgeon, then we certainly must ask the same question in regards to genital plastic/cosmetic procedures. Should there be training and qualification standards for individuals who claim to be able to perform a cosmetic labiaplasty, a clitoral hood reduction, a hymenoplasty,

or a perineoplasty/vaginoplasty to tighten the vaginal barrel specifically for sexual-related reasons? One certainly can ask the proverbial but legitimate question: *If your family member was having an "XYZ procedure," whom would you want…"* More succinctly, what is, and what will be, the SOC to which the profession must adhere, if any?

Medical versus legal standards of care

Medically, for genital plastic/aesthetic procedures, the SOC *theoretically* demands:

1 Proper ("adequate") *training* in *patient selection.*
2 Proper *training* in *basic techniques* and individual *technique selection.*
3 Proper *training* in basic *plastic* technique.
4 Proper *training* in female *sexuality and body image issues* (so as to be able to know when to refer to a skilled therapist).
5 Proper *training* in giving *informed consent.*

Legally however, this is not necessarily the case. *There is no true MEDICAL definition for SOC*, although the term is firmly established in law [1] and legally defined as "the caution that a reasonable person in similar circumstances

Table 21.1 Ideal training for genital plastic/cosmetic procedures.

Taught in Residency Practitioner	Female Genital Anatomy and Diagnostics and Technique	True Plastic Technique	Labiaplasty, Clitoral Hood Reduction–Specific Technique	Perineoplasty, Vaginoplasty Technique Specific for Tightening and Sexual Pleasure	Women's Sexual and Body Image Issues
OB/GYN	++	++	++	++	++
Plastic surgeon	++	++	++	++	++

Table 21.2 The reality re: genital plastic/cosmetic training.

Taught in Residency Practitioner	Female Genital Anatomy and Diagnostics and Technique	True Plastic Technique	Labiaplasty, Clitoral Hood Reduction–Specific Technique	Perineoplasty, Vaginoplasty Technique Specific for Tightening and Sexual Pleasure	Women's Sexual and Body Image Issues
OB/GYN	++	O	O	+	±
Plastic surgeon	+	++	+	O	+

would exercise in providing care to a patient" [2]. This term (SOC) represents an essential component in a professional liability action in regards to proof that the defendant physician failed to provide the required SOC [1].

As far back as 1860, the Supreme Court of Illinois (in a case argued by none other than Abraham Lincoln) declared that "when a person assumes the profession of physician and surgeon, he [*sic*] must…be held to employ a reasonable amount of skill and care" [3].

"With no clear medical definition for SOC, it remains unclear how this mainly legal concept…compares in status to consensus statements or clinical guidelines that are secured in evidence-based medicine and produced by a representative organization or authoritative medical body" [4]. "Consensus statements should represent views from a broad-based, non-advocatory, balanced and objective panel of experts providing a collective agreement keeping in mind that variation is possible among individuals" (WIH Consensus Development Program) [4].

Clinical practice guidelines produced by specialty organizations, government agencies, and healthcare organizations can assist practitioners and patient decision making regarding appropriate healthcare decisions. A problem here of course is that biases of "experts" may inordinately shape these guidelines. "Modern and scientific healthcare should be firmly set in evidence-based medicine, defined as…best evidence in making decisions about the care of individual patients" [5]. "The term 'SOC' should be used with caution. Currently, it can be self-awarded by either a group of like-minded individuals or by a specialty society or organization and is a term which may be abused with the intention of providing impact and authenticity to a point of view" [5].

Strauss and Thomas [1] suggest that perhaps the term "SOC" should not be used without sufficient supporting evidence (e.g., randomized clinical or unchallenged meta-analyses). SOC is basically a legal term. Negligence in general is legally defined as straying from "the standard of conduct to which one must conform…[and] is that of a reasonable man under like circumstances" [6]. Legally, four elements must be met for a plaintiff to recover damages in a professional liability action: [1] Duty, [2] breach of duty, [3] harm, and [4] causation [7]. For example, in regards to genital plastic/cosmetic surgery, the surgeon has a *duty*

to know how to perform the procedure; it is a *breach of duty* to operate without the proper training. In the absence of a poor outcome, this lack of proper training may be moot, but if there is *harm*, *causation* must be proven by linking surgery in the absence of proper training directly to the bad outcome (*harm.*) This second element, "breach of duty," implies conduct outside of the SOC [8].

Summing up, SOC medically is "the watchfulness, the attention, and the prudence that a reasonable practitioner in the circumstances would exercise" [9]. The problem is that the "standard" is often a subjective issue upon which reasonable people can differ.

Understanding the medical and legal disparities, what can be done to protect our patient from un-/undertrained individuals? Who should protect our patients? Whose duty is it? If we don't police ourselves, others (the tort system) will do it.

Who should perform specific surgical procedures: "credentialing" for genital plastics

Another means by which the consumers—our patients—may be protected and guaranteed a minimal level of professional competence is via credentialing or privileging. It is an ethical imperative that a healthcare practitioner perform only those procedures or therapies that she or he is trained in and familiar with (see "Freestanding Training Programs," below).

A large number of genital plastic procedures are performed in healthcare facilities by un- or undertrained healthcare providers. As it is also true that SOC is largely a retrospective legal rather than medical concept, how is one to proceed in the new field of female genital plastic/cosmetic surgery to assure consumer safety and physician competence?

"Credentialing" is a mechanism designed for protection both of the healthcare institution and the consumer. *Mosby's Medical Dictionary* [9] defines "credentialing" as "examination and review of the credentials of individuals *meeting a set of educational or occupational criteria* and therefore being licensed in their field. Strict credentialing is required by both hospital and managed care accreditation bodies. The process is conducted peridically because of the responsibility of the organization for any claims of malpractice by its staff."

Differing only slightly is *Segen's Medical Dictionary* [10], which defines credentialing as "The process of reviewing a health professional's *credentials, training, experience, or demonstrated ability,* practice history and medical certification or license to determine if clinical privileges to practice in a particular place are to be granted. A much less frequent use of the term applies to closed panels and medical groups and refers to examination of the credentials of a physician or other health care provider to determine whether that provider should be entitled to clinical privileges at a hospital or managed care organization.

The definitions are clear: *training, experience,* and *demonstrated ability* are prerequisites for credentialing, or the "privilege" of utilizing a hospital or outpatient facility to perform a (surgical) procedure.

It may be difficult to determine specific SOC within a given medical community. Who should determine SOC for genital plastic and aesthetic procedures? No distinct specialty organization speaks for practitioners who perform FGPS, and the self-serving nature of such organizations is often suspect. The procedures overlap the fields of gynecology, plastic surgery, urology, and sexual medicine, and no distinct organization presently speaks in a cohesive manner for genital plastic/cosmetic surgeons. Are standards to differ with community? State? Area of the country? Nation? In the present era of the Internet and Google, patients are educated and informed and are mobile, regularly crossing state lines and national boundaries to find qualified, experienced surgeons. In almost every state, or nearby, are trained surgeons with an increasing level of experience.

This confusion does not exist for credentialing; the lines are clearly drawn. Has the practitioner been *trained* (including self-training with evidence of continuing medical education (CME) and sufficient volume of procedures to satisfy credentialing, aka "grandfathering") in the procedure of cosmetic reductive labiaplasty, or for vaginal rejuvenation (VRJ), perineoplasty (PP), or vaginoplasty (VP) for reasons of vaginal tightening? Can the physician produce evidence of *training* and/or *experience* in these specific procedures either in his or her residency, a stand-alone training course, or via the performance of a minimum number of cases, *proven by a case list*? If he/she can, it is the responsibility of the credentialing institution to affirm, frequently by proctoring either from a staff member already privileged in the procedure specified or via video proctoring, the

applicant's *demonstrated ability* to perform the procedure. Additionally, as credentialing is an ongoing process, as in other surgical privileges, the practitioner must affirm his or her continued experience and demonstrated ability by confirming a minimum number of cases ongoing every 2–3 years, as per the requirements of the institution. This is the present standard for surgical procedures. It is curious that this standard is not upheld in the area of plastic/cosmetic genital surgery, a standard made difficult secondary to the lack of an established board willing to take these procedures under its "umbrella."

Because a general surgeon has privileges to perform a mastectomy would not, at most hospitals and surgery centers, confer automatic breast augmentation or reduction privileges. Neither would an institution automatically grant radical vulvectomy/node dissection privileges to a practitioner who has proven experience with only wide local vulvar excision. Unfortunately, hospitals and surgical centers have not noticed that physicians at their institutions are performing labiaplasties and clitoral hood reductions under the false umbrella of "wide local excision, vulva" or "partial vulvectomy." In some cases, the procedure of "labiaplasty" may be included under this umbrella, but it is not the cosmetic procedure becoming the standard of care that is performed most often today.

Part of the credentialing process in many states is surgical proctoring. "Surgical proctoring is a peer review process governed by institutional bylaws and administered through a credentialing committee to objectively monitor, regulate, or oversee surgical privileging for its medical staff. Its primary purpose is to insure safety and quality of care for patients undergoing surgical procedures at the institution" [11]. The surgical proctor is an independent and unbiased monitor acting only to assess the required skills of the proctored physician. The proctor must be proficient in the skills being evaluated and may either hold privileges for the procedure in the same or another institution. Proctoring may be either immediate, on-site, or in the eventuality of unavailability of a suitable proctor, tele-proctoring, or remote evaluation through direct observation of a procedure is possible given the speed, bandwidth, and security of presently available Internet connections. Tele-proctoring may be the most cost-effective method for institutions unable to identify a local proctor for surgical privileging [12].

Suggested minimal standards

It is only a matter of time until hospitals are named in the burgeoning number of professional liability actions involving FGPS. Plaintiffs' attorneys are realizing that another set of deep pockets exist within their reach, namely the institutions that allowed a healthcare practitioner untrained in genital plastic/cosmetic procedures to perform these procedures.

Credible training in the relatively specialized field of genital plastics is difficult to come by. The procedure of cosmetic labia minoraplasty, reduction of excess clitoral hood epithelium, labia majoraplasty, release of a phimotic clitoral hood, hymenoplasty, and VRJ/PP/VP for enhanced sexual function is not presently a part of OB/GYN residency curriculums. Fortunately, there are a small handful of credible training programs around the United States where a surgeon can attend to learn technique, patient selection, equipment, sexual issues, risks, complications, and so forth. However, for patient and facility protection, more formal training programs, either freestanding or sponsored by specialty organizations, in addition to being taught in residency training programs, are necessary.

Post-graduate ("residency") training

It is the goal of post-graduate specialty training programs to instruct their trainees in order to maintain minimum competence in the procedures they are likely to encounter in their professional lives, and this training shifts over time with changes in practice patterns. Although use of an endoscope for diagnostic and minimal operative procedures was taught in OB/GYN residency programs in the 1970s and 1980s, it was not until the 1990s, a full 10 years after the original minimally invasive laparoscopic surgeons began their "operative gymnastics" (the term academicians gave to laparoscopic management of ectopic pregnancy, laparoscopic ovarian surgery, and laparoscopic hysterectomy in the 1980s), that residency programs began including minimally invasive endoscopic procedures into their instructional armamentarium. Similarly, the reality of female genital plastic/cosmetic surgery and the fact that it is community rather than academic surgeons who are qualified to perform these procedures will force residency training programs to incorporate both training in plastic technique and training in specific procedures into their programs. Each program will of course set its own standards. Box 21.1 broadly suggests minimum standards.

Box 21.1 Suggested minimum standards for residency training.

Minimum standards, residency
- Didactic, anatomical, and experiential hours in patient selection, intra- and post-operative care of vulvar reduction patients (LP; CHR).
- Concept of adaptation of anterior and posterior colporrhaphy and perineoplasty for reasons of cosmesis and enhancement of sexual function.
- Sexuality and body image issues involved in genital plastic/cosmetic surgery.
- Observation and performance of a minimum number of procedures.

OB/GYN residents traditionally receive training in wide excision of vulvar lesions, a procedure that bears no resemblance (other than the fact that it is in the same anatomic area) to the plastic surgery–based aesthetic reductions mandated for cosmetic labiaplasty and redundant clitoral hood epithelium. Additionally, residents are taught site-specific repairs for prolapse and herniations of the pelvic floor and vagina, without understanding the sexual nature of many complaints, and technique for modifying these surgeries specifically for assuring vaginal tightening for increased sexual pleasure and the pelvic floor physical therapy techniques utilized to improve results. The plastic tissue–handling techniques mandatory for successful genital aesthetics are not presently taught in most all OB/GYN residencies. Vulvar plastic procedures are "hit or miss," and vaginal anatomy and procedures are only occasionally taught in plastic surgery residency programs.

Freestanding training programs

In the absence of training in residency programs, if a surgeon wishes to become competent in genital plastic/cosmetic procedures, she or he must either learn on his/her own in a hit or miss experiential fashion or attend one of a small handful of training programs or preceptorships available around the United States and Europe. Several well-experienced "mentors" either teach formal courses of 2–3 days in length or act as preceptors and mentors, specifically and personally explaining the specific surgical procedures, risks, patient selection, sexuality aspects, pre- and post-op care, and other aspects of genital plastics to their students.

Surgical courses and preceptorships are designed to provide surgeons with the requisite knowledge and

Box 21.2 Suggested minimum standards for freestanding training programs.

Minimum standards, training course (for OB/GYNs, plastic surgeons)
- Two-day minimum didactic and experiential training in external (LP, CHR) and internal (tightening) procedures.
- Observation of a minimum of two–three procedures, at least one of which is a vulvar procedure.
- Proctorship for first one or two LP-related cases.

Box 21.3 Suggested "grandfathering" standards.

Minimal standards, "grandfathered"
- Operative report evidence of ≥20 labiaplasty/RCH procedures and ≥10 tightening-related perineoplasty-related colporrhaphy/perineorrhaphy procedures.
- Minimum 25 units category 1 CME related to female genital/plastic procedures within the preceding 5 years.

Box 21.4 Suggested CME requirements.

Minimal standards, CME
- 25 units category 1 genital plastic-related CME q 5 years.
- 20 units CME in genital plastic-related literature or women's sexuality-related literature q 5 years.

skills to perform a surgical procedure prior to being proctored at their local institution, if so required. Preceptorships are a mechanism for acquiring the surgical skills to perform specific genital plastic/cosmetic procedures for surgeons already familiar with basic vulvar and vaginal anatomy and surgical technique. Short training programs and preceptorships must not attempt to substitute for lack of surgical training and familiarity with female vulvar and vaginal anatomy and should be available for previously trained and experienced surgeons, preferably board-certified or board-qualified gynecologists or urogynecologists, plastic surgeons, and, in some instances, cosmetic surgeons who have previously completed a general surgery residency. Box 21.2 suggests minimum standards for freestanding preceptorship training programs.

"Grandfathering"

In the absence of training in residency programs and, until recently, freestanding programs, many individuals have "trained" themselves. Similar to early pioneers in virtually all novel surgical disciplines (see early years of minimally invasive endoscopic surgical techniques), many surgeons, via reading the available literature re: technique, speaking personally with other surgeons already practicing genital plastics, and "trial and error," have become proficient in the performance of female genital plastic/cosmetic procedures and, in many cases, are presently training others. Certainly, in any discussion of SOC, credentialing, and minimal training recommendations, these many individuals must be recognized. For credentialing purposes, this may be accomplished by mandating evidence of a minimum number of cases and CME. Proctoring may be more difficult to mandate, as it may be these same individuals who may be called upon to be the proctors. Box 21.3 suggests "grandfathering" standards.

Continuing medical education

Any discussion of credentialing and privileging is incomplete without a parallel discussion of CME. Again, CME may not necessarily be considered part of SOC, but it certainly falls under the umbrella of ongoing privileging requirements. There presently are organizations (ACOG, AAPS, ASAPS, ASPS, AACS, ISCG, etc.) and individuals available to organize worthwhile CME activities for those surgeons wishing to begin, and for those presently holding privileges in female plastic/cosmetic genital procedures. Box 21.4 suggests CME requirements.

Experience and quality of care

Experience counts. The difference between a quality result and a disastrous result is obvious and is directly parallel with training and experience. Developing expertise takes a combination of exposure and practice along with a modicum of inherent luck, talent, or a combination of these [13].

To quote Barbara Levy, MD, in an editorial in the journal *Obstetrics and Gynecology*, "Our challenges in providing excellent surgical care for women are real. It will be critical for us to acknowledge variances in surgical performance and begin to define standard measures necessary to optimize outcomes for our patients. Quality initiatives—efforts to recognize and attempt(s) to reduce variance in outcomes—will, of necessity, involve assessment of both surgical volume and overall surgical experience. A commitment to professionalism and dedication to teaching and promoting surgical intervention should be based on patient outcomes. Data and science, not marketing and expediency, are required if we are to provide optimal care" [13].

What are the goals of establishing minimal SOC, most likely via a process of privileging and credentialing? For the primary goal of protection of our patients' well-being (the expressed reason for SOC mandates), minimum training and experiential guidelines would be set in the privileging process. These guidelines and the credentialing process specifically will result in greater legal protection for both patient and surgeon. As procedures and qualified practitioners are identified and credentialed within medical communities, a workable horizontal and vertical referral process may be established, and clearer "community standards" will be set and available to all.

Equally, if not of greater import, would be the inclusion of vulvovaginal plastic and aesthetic techniques into both plastic surgery and—*especially*—OB/GYN training programs. It is time for residency directors and others responsible for GYN post-graduate education to recognize both the importance of these skills for their graduates and the rights of their patients to quality, experienced attendance. Taking this concept one step further, academic programs certainly could adopt community practitioners into their training programs and make this mainstream or at least begin teaching these procedures or accept their growing popularity.

Are any of these goals and mandates enforceable? As community standards, enforcement is unlikely, but as standards for individual licensed institutions they are eminently enforceable. A practitioner either is or is not allowed to perform a given procedure within an institutional setting via mandates in place for the protection both of the institution and the patients it serves. It is consumer-friendly as a mechanism for physician selection by patients and medical-legal importance related to SOC issues within the tort system.

Can this process be skirted by practitioners operating outside of the traditional licensed facility system? Of course it can; no system of medical checks and balances is foolproof. Facilities outside of the traditional hospital/surgical center model may not require a specific credentialing or privileging process. However, these facilities and practitioners operating within them must still medical-legally adhere to community standards, and if these are set in a manner discussed above, untrained and/or inexperienced practitioners certainly expose themselves to additional risk.

References

1. Strauss DC, Thomas JM. What does the medical profession mean by "standards of care"? *J Clin Oncology* 2009; **27**:192–3.
2. The Legal Dictionary. Standard of Care. Available at: http://www.legal-dictionary.thefreedictionary.com/s+o+c.
3. Richie v. West, 23 III 329 (1860).
4. National Institutes of Health. NIH Consensus Development Paper. Available at: http://www.consensus.nih.gov/ABOUTCDP.htm.
5. Sackett DL, Rosenberg WM, Gray JA, Haynes RB, Richardson WS. Evidence-based medicine: What it is and what it isn't. *BMJ* 1996;**312**:71–2.
6. *Restatement of Torts, Second*. Section 283.
7. Garthe v. Ruppert, 264 N.Y. 290, 296, 190 N.E. 643.
8. Moffett P, Moore G. The standard of care: Legal history and definitions: The bad and good news. *Western J Emer Med* 2011;**12**:109–12.
9. *Mosby's Medical Dictionary*, 8th ed. St. Louis: Elsevier, 2009.
10. *Segen's Medical Dictionary*, Huntingdon Valley, PA:, Farlex, 2012.
11. Heit M. Surgical proctoring for gynecologic surgery. *Obstet Gynecol* 2014;**123**:349–51.
12. Rosser JC, Gabriel N, Herman BA, Murayama M. Telementoring and teleproctoring. *World J Surg* 2001; **25**:1438–48.
13. Levy B. Experience counts. *Obstet Gynecol* 2012;**119**:493–4.

Index

Page numbers in *italics* refer to illustrations; those in **bold** refer to tables

---

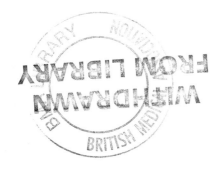